Cardiac Care and COVID-19: Perspectives in Medical Practice

Authored by

Ozgur KARCIOGLU

Prof. FEMAT, Department of Emergency Medicine
University of Health Sciences
Istanbul Education and Research Hospital
Fatih, Istanbul
Turkey

Cardiac Care and COVID-19: Perspectives in Medical Practice

Author: Ozgur KARCIOGLU

ISBN (Online): 978-1-68108-820-4

ISBN (Print): 978-1-68108-821-1

ISBN (Paperback): 978-1-68108-822-8

©2021, Bentham Books imprint.

Published by Bentham Science Publishers – Sharjah, UAE. All Rights Reserved.

need for a court order if at any point you breach any terms of this License Agreement. In no event will any delay or failure by Bentham Science Publishers in enforcing your compliance with this License Agreement constitute a waiver of any of its rights.

3. You acknowledge that you have read this License Agreement, and agree to be bound by its terms and conditions. To the extent that any other terms and conditions presented on any website of Bentham Science Publishers conflict with, or are inconsistent with, the terms and conditions set out in this License Agreement, you acknowledge that the terms and conditions set out in this License Agreement shall prevail.

Bentham Science Publishers Ltd.
Executive Suite Y - 2
PO Box 7917, Saif Zone
Sharjah, U.A.E.
Email: subscriptions@benthamscience.net

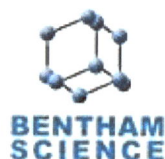

BENTHAM SCIENCE

CONTENTS

PREFACE

The optimal management of patients with cardiac disease warrants a multifaceted approach undertaken in harmony. The recent decades have witnessed major advances in methods for monitoring and interventions aiming to improve outcomes in this outstanding cause of death worldwide. Other than technological improvements, the medical community is aware that this task can only be achieved *via* a mutual collaboration of doctors in the pre-hospital phase, hospital emergency departments, intensive care units, social studies, public health professionals, and bystanders.

For nearly a year, our lives have changed like never before. The current WHO clinical guide documents cite that *'there is no current evidence to recommend any specific anti-COVID-19 treatment for patients with confirmed COVID-19'.*

In order to overcome the pandemic with minimized global losses, the scientific community, healthcare facilities, professional organizations, chambers, and state institutions should work in coordination and unison. Most importantly, only a coordinated approach with all targeted masses reached *via* awareness programmes and campaigns can create a real difference in this pandemic era.

This project, of the book **'Cardiac Care and COVID-19: Perspectives in Medical Practice'** is intended to encompass the advancements regarding diagnoses and treatment modalities for cardiac diseases in general and emergency cardiac conditions to be more specific, with respect to pandemic conditions. Apart from up-to-date descriptions of the problem and delineation of management principles, case examples were also used to highlight complex issues for a concrete understanding of the medical practitioner.

The ultimate objective is to provide a reference source with up-to-date information on the management of cardiac emergencies and resuscitation in the COVID-19 era. We aim to conduct a brief overview of epidemiological features of cardiac emergencies and their sociodemographic factors, measures to be taken for prevention, together with diagnostic and therapeutic procedures to pursue in the pandemic era.

CONSENT FOR PUBLICATION

Not applicable.

CONFLICT OF INTEREST

The author declares no conflict of interest, financial or otherwise.

ACKNOWLEDGEMENTS

Declared none.

Ozgur KARCIOGLU
Prof. FEMAT, Department of Emergency Medicine
University of Health Sciences
Istanbul Education and Research Hospital
Fatih, Istanbul
Turkey

CHAPTER 1

Introduction: Cardiac Disease in the Pandemic Era: Teaching an Old Dog New Tricks?

Abstract: Nowadays, cardiac diseases, both developed *de novo* and acute exacerbations of chronic conditions, remain the most prominent death cause for the middle-aged and elderly, mostly in the developed, industrialized countries.

Since the end of 2019, COVID-19 pandemics have changed our lifestyles fundamentally, and maybe we will never find a way to return to the world of 2019. This catastrophic change had its impact on almost every aspect of our lives, including how we will manage cardiac arrest patients, how to perform perform cardiopulmonary resuscitation (CPR), ACLS, *etc*. A net effect is that protecting ourselves will take priority (more than before) in all procedures we pursue. Thus we can conclude that new generations should incorporate self-protecting behavior and techniques to benefit the patients in the most fruitful ways.

High-quality CPR cardiopulmonary resuscitation is among the most prominent issues to save humanity from the high burden of cardiac events. Relatively novel techniques such as mechanized devices for CPR, extracorporeal membrane oxygenation (ECMO), and therapeutic temperature management promise the highest possible solution to improve survival rates, in conjunction with urgent coronary angiography with revascularization.

Pandemics can be overcome not by the heroic behaviors of a few people but by the solidarity of society. The medical community should find the best solutions to help those in need with cardiac diseases even in pandemic conditions since this pandemic will not go away like magic. The aim of this book is to support patients and their next of kin, as well as health care workers, those who have dedicated themselves to healthy well-being with their relentless endeavor.

Keywords: Cardiac arrest, Cardiac arrhythmias, Cardiopulmonary resuscitation, COVID-19 pandemics, Defibrillation, Treatment.

INTRODUCTION

As an ageless phenomenon of life, medicine has been viewed as an art of recognizing and relieving human sufferings, treating diseases and wounds for ages. The last centuries have witnessed warfare, socioeconomic crises, and many other threats which had a great impact on the medical database used and practicing ways in cardiac resuscitation.

Cardiovascular disease (CVD) is the leading cause of death for adults. Expedient diagnosis and prompt institution of treatment can save lives, especially during the deadliest cardiac emergencies, including sudden cardiac death, acute pulmonary edema, lethal arrhythmias, and acute pericarditis.

In order to establish an easier recognition and a more holistic, systematic approach to cardiac emergencies, revolutionary steps forward and developments in cardiac markers, monitoring, defibrillation, therapeutic hypothermia or temperature management (TTM), capnographic recordings, and the like were developed after 60's and 70's. Now we can postulate that these innovations must have mitigated the hazards of cardiac diseases globally. Maybe this is why cancer and infectious diseases are championing on the morbidity and death list in most parts of the world in the last decades.

The most prominent death scenario comprises **out-of-hospital cardiac arrest (OHCA)** in the middle-aged population globally. Lethal dysrhythmias can be divided into four types: ventricular fibrillation-VF, pulseless ventricular tachycardia (PVT), asystole, and pulseless electrical activity, which are responsible for impaired cardiac functioning and even sudden cardiac death.

VF is one of the most deadly cardiac arrhythmias and certainly the most common one. It can be described as the erratic, disorganized firing of impulses from the ventricles, producing no palpable pulses in the periphery. Literature data have shown that the earlier defibrillation and bystander cardiopulmonary resuscitation (CPR) are commenced, the lower is the patient mortality. Since considerable differences can affect people's lives in this context, the role of medical command bears utmost importance to direct these patients to facilities with discrete capabilities

VF is among the most common and fatal cardiac arrhythmias. Literature findings demonstrated that patient mortality could be much lower when defibrillation is performed early and when laypeople initiate cardiopulmonary resuscitation (CPR). As important differences in this process can have an impact on our lives, the role of the EMS medical command is of great significance in directing these patients to facilities with adequate levels of resources (Stoecklein, 2018).

EMERGENT CORONARY REVASCULARIZATION

Emergent Coronary Revascularization is an outstanding life-saving intervention in patients with acute coronary syndromes, mostly AMI.

ALTERNATIVE APPROACHES TO THE MANAGEMENT OF VF

Most patients with refractory VF are resistant to conventional treatment strategies. Nonetheless, some new techniques produced promising outcomes (Bell, 2018). Of note, double sequential defibrillation can represent an option for the conventional approach for the treatment of PVT or refractory VF (Simon, 2018).

Recently, procedures like extracorporeal life support and bedside ultrasound have been launched. These may represent a logical and practical way to manage patients with refractory arrest rhythms, both in-hospital and out-of-hospital milieu. Likewise, drones have been introduced as one of the contemporary advances, to bring automated external defibrillators (AED) to the patient with OHCA. Also, digital and mobile technology have launched new apps to optimize interventions carried out by laypeople, to increase survival in this group of patients with poor expectancy for return of spontaneous circulation (ROSC) (Latimer *et al.*, 2018).

A major challenge for contemporary medicine as a whole is operating a system focused on the optimized outcomes of patients with OHCA. This challenge can only be overcome with a flexible and resourceful approach that comprises various teams, from call receivers, monitors, to emergency medical service (EMS) staff and the healthcare workers in the receiving center (McCoy *et al.*, 2018). The application of these techniques for OHCA in a healthcare system will yield the most favorable outcomes for survivors without sequelae among well-known or 'classical' approaches.

A majority of the current management guidelines to improve survival following arrest situations are the result of efforts to improve CPR quality, increasing the chances of ROSC and the like. The emphasis on the delivery of proven techniques and the reliable implementation of these strategies through the measurement and audit of quality improvement strategies will create a foundation so that innovations in resuscitation could be designed and planned (Reed-Schrader, 2018). After all those above mentioned important developments, post-cardiac arrest interventions have aroused more curiosity. Therapeutic hypothermia or TTM, which has become the state-of-art in most hospitals, will produce the best probability of relief after the ROSC without remarkable sequelae (Walker, 2018).

THE PANDEMICS

This catastrophic change had its impact on almost every aspect of our lives, including how we should manage cardiac arrest patients, how to perform CPR, ACLS, *etc.* Bugger *et al.* investigated the net effect of the pandemic restrictions on certain major cardiovascular emergencies (myocardial infarction, pulmonary thromboembolism, and aortic dissection) in Austria (Bugger *et al.* 2020). Although it was a retrospective registry-based study, the authors highlighted the reductions of admission rates related to these three entities. The total numbers of admissions due to the three major emergency conditions during the pandemic restrictions were below the corresponding figures in the previous years (RR 0.77, p<0.001). This decrease has been postulated to be mainly caused by lower acute coronary syndrome admissions (RR 0.77, p = 0.004).

COVID-19 has killed more than 1.600.000 people worldwide – and the total of officially reported cases has surpassed 70 million. However, we should all realize that COVID-19 is not the last epidemic. It is obvious that there will be new generations and our long years to spend with masks, sanitizers and hand disinfectants. In the long run, it is important to organize efforts to perform selective admissions to health institutions, in order to overcome overcrowdedness.

To be more specific, the education of pre-school and school children and women plays a key role to increase family awareness. The threat of the pandemic disease should be concretized, so that the lifestyles of the peoples will adapt to the "new normal". Such a great breakthrough will mandate organized efforts, both by the governments and civil society (Fig. **1**).

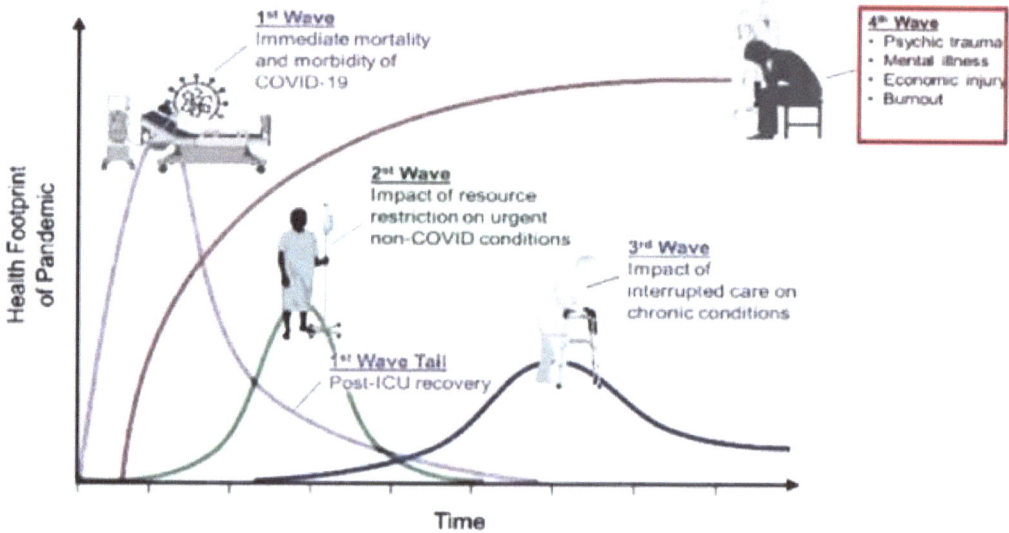

Fig. (1). Immediately after the first phase reflecting sudden illness and mortality resulting from COVID-19, the lack of resources and the consequences of the restrictions for the patients with non-COVID serious illnesses. The 3rd wave depicts the long-term consequences of the lack of care of chronic diseases, and finally, the individual and social psychological effects and related trauma are described in the fourth phase.

CONCLUSION

Cardiac disease, both developed *de novo* and acute exacerbations of chronic conditions remain the most prominent death cause for the middle-aged and elderly, mostly in the developed, industrialized countries. Medical community should find the best solutions to help those in need with cardiac diseases even in the pandemic conditions, since this pandemic will not go away like a magic.

The objective of this manuscript is to enlighten ways to recognize and devise interventions for acute cardiac diseases, along with creating novel techniques for state-of-the-art resuscitative measures.

REFERENCES

Bell, S.M., Lam, D.H., Kearney, K., Hira, R.S. (2018). Management of refractory ventricular fibrillation (prehospital and emergency department). *Cardiol. Clin., 36*(3), 395-408.
[http://dx.doi.org/10.1016/j.ccl.2018.03.007] [PMID: 30293606]

Bugger, H., Gollmer, J., Pregartner, G. (2020). Complications and mortality of cardiovascular emergency admissions during COVID-19 associated restrictive measures. *PLoS One.*15(9):e0239801. *Published, 2020*(Sep), 24.

Latimer, A.J., McCoy, A.M., Sayre, M.R. (2018). Emerging and future technologies in out-of-hospital cardiac arrest care. *Cardiol. Clin., 36*(3), 429-441.
[http://dx.doi.org/10.1016/j.ccl.2018.03.010] [PMID: 30293609]

McCoy, A.M. (2018). Ten steps to improve cardiac arrest survival in your community. *Cardiol. Clin., 36*(3), 335-342.
[http://dx.doi.org/10.1016/j.ccl.2018.03.011] [PMID: 30293599]

Reed-Schrader, E., Rivers, W.T., White, L.J., Clemency, B.M. (2018). Cardiopulmonary resuscitation quality issues. *Cardiol. Clin., 36*(3), 351-356.
[http://dx.doi.org/10.1016/j.ccl.2018.03.002] [PMID: 30293601]

Simon, E.M., Tanaka, K. (2018). Double sequential defibrillation. *Cardiol. Clin., 36*(3), 387-393.
[http://dx.doi.org/10.1016/j.ccl.2018.03.006] [PMID: 30293605]

Stoecklein, H.H., Youngquist, S.T. (2018). The role of medical direction in systems of out-of-hospital cardiac arrest. *Cardiol. Clin., 36*(3), 409-417.
[http://dx.doi.org/10.1016/j.ccl.2018.03.008] [PMID: 30293607]

Walker, A.C., Johnson, N.J. (2018). Critical care of the post-cardiac arrest patient. *Cardiol. Clin., 36*(3), 419-428.
[http://dx.doi.org/10.1016/j.ccl.2018.03.009] [PMID: 30293608]

CHAPTER 2

Cardiovascular Disease and COVID-19

Abstract: Cardiovascular disease (CVD) has long been the leading cause of global morbidity and mortality. However, with the COVID-19 pandemic, which has been the focus of attention all over the world since the end of 2019, this issue has gained different importance. The presence of CVD leads to more severe COVID-19 and an increased probability of mortality. In addition, both CVD and COVID-19 pave the way to myocardial injury, which also boosts the morbidity and death toll. Another point is the possible deprivation of usual healthcare received by cardiac patients (CVD and others) because of the shifted emphasis of the hospital and prehospital medical services on COVID-19. As the public can foresee that the pandemic will not disappear rapidly soon, healthcare organization faces a challenge to be redesigned radically. The objective of this chapter is to analyze CVD, myocardial injury, and other cardiac diseases resulting from COVID-19 itself, together with the impact of the pandemics on the usual healthcare of cardiac patients.

Keywords: Acute myocardial infarction, Cardiovascular disease, Coronavirus, COVID-19, Diagnosis, Treatment.

INTRODUCTION

"Acute coronary syndromes" (ACS) is a general term for conditions that occur as a result of a sudden blockage of the blood flow to the heart. These syndromes range from potentially reversible unstable angina (UA) phase to irreversible cell death from myocardial infarction (MI), including non-ST elevation myocardial infarction (NSTEMI) or ST-elevation myocardial infarction (STEMI).

DISTINGUISHING FEATURES OF ACUTE CORONARY SYNDROMES

UA, NSTEMI, and STEMI have a common pathophysiological origin of atherosclerotic coronary artery disease (CAD), which is characterized by plaque formation on the walls of arteries that supply blood flow to the heart. Erosion or rupture of the plaque leads to a blood clot (thrombosis) that blocks blood flow to the heart, depriving the heart of oxygen and consequently leading to myocardial necrosis (tissue death in the heart muscle).

Ozgur KARCIOGLU

Cardiovascular disease (CVD) has been associated with viral infections or outbreaks for decades. It has been reported that approximately half of COVID-19 patients have CVD, and this rate increases to 70% in intensive care units (ICU) (Zhou *et al.*, 2020, Wang *et al.*, 2020). It is known that 50% of the cases with Middle-East Respiratory Syndrome (MERS) infection in 2012 had DM and HT, and 30% had CVD (Badawi *et al.*, 2016). Meanwhile, certain CV risk factors have been thought to affect the clinical course of COVID-19 (Table 1).

Table 1. CV risk factors that are thought to affect the clinical course of COVID-19.

• Male gender
• Advanced age
• DM
• Hypertension
• Obesity
• A history of cardiovascular or cerebrovascular disease

FINDINGS FROM DIFFERENT DATABASE STUDIES

In the study which analyzed 5700 patients in New York, frequency of hypertension (HT) was reported as 56.6%, obesity 41.7%, DM 33.8%, CAD 11.1%, and congestive heart failure (CHF) 6.9% (Richardson *et al.*, 2020). In the study that included more than 72,000 patients in China, 12.8% HT, 5.3% DM, 4.2% CVD were found. The frequency of comorbidity is similar in industrialized countries, except that the HT, metabolic disorders, and obesity rates are significantly higher than in the far east, but the prevalence varies considerably.

When analyzing 22,254 patients who were screened with PCR tests between 5 March and 9 April in NYC, at least one comorbid disease was reported in about half of those with positive tests (46%) (Kalyanaraman Marcello, 2020). In the sample, 33% diabetes, 37% HT, 24% CVD, 11% chronic renal failure (CRF) were noted. Among the hospitalized patients, 28% died. Male gender, age, DM, history of heart disease, presence of CRF are risk factors for both test positivity and death.

In a case series from Detroit, Suleyman *et al.* searched for independent risk factors for admission to intensive care units: being over the age of 60, male sex, HT, DM, CRF, severe obesity (BMI>= 40), and cancer were reported to be the ones (Suleyman *et al.*, 2020). Smoking was also higher in hospitalized patients. Admissions due to dyspnea, tachypnea, or hypoxia also increases the risk of hospitalization. Fever increases the likelihood of hospitalization but does not predict poor outcomes in patients with COVID-19. Inflammatory markers were also found higher in those hospitalized in ED when compared to those discharged from ED.

Respiratory failure developed in 74% of those hospitalized in ICU, and MV was required in 81% of these. 25% of those hospitalized had to be transferred to ED. The majority of those who received MV under 40 years of age (62.5%) had severe obesity, while only 26% of those who did not need MV had the condition. Mortality in ICU was 40%, and 7% in all those hospitalized. 45.6% of those who require MV died of severe complications.

ARE ETHNIC DIFFERENCES IMPORTANT FOR COVID-19?

Marcello *et al.* conducted a study that analyzed more than 22,000 patients in NYC and reported that 26% of COVID-19s were black, and 34% were Hispanic (Marcello *et al.*, 2020). They reported that comorbidities are more common in ethnic groups than others, but being black or Hispanic after adjustments is not directly related to positive PCR testing or death.

In another cohort reported from Louisiana, it is stated that blacks, which make up only 31% of the population, constitute 77% of the COVID-19 patients who are admitted into the hospital, but being black is not an independent risk factor when confounding factors are excluded (Price-Haywood *et al.*, 2020). 70.6% of the dead are black.

Mechanisms that trigger myocardial damage in COVID-19:
Severe systemic inflammatory stimulus - cytokine storm
Ischemia due to increased consumption or demand
Plaque rupture
Vascular inflammation

MYOCARDIAL INJURY SEVERITY AND MORTALITY

Autopsy showed interstitial mononuclear inflammatory cell infiltration in the myocardium (Xu, 2020). Also, markers showing myocardial damage increase with COVID-19 (Xu 2020, Guo 2020, Shi, 2020). Shi *et al.* reported that myocardial damage was close to 20% in patients who died (Shi, 2020). Moreover, cardiac damage is the risk factor that affects mortality most strongly and independently (hazard ratio: 4.26). Guo *et al.* reported that high troponin levels accompanied significantly increased mortality (Guo, 2020).

In the series of Guo *et al.*, which included 187 patients with COVID-19, they stated that there was a better clinical course in patients with CVD and no acute myocardial injury compared to those with both. For example, mortality in patients with fulminant myocarditis is between 40% and 70% (Caforio 2013. Ammirati 2019).

How Much Myocardial Damage Occurs in COVID-19?

In many studies, the myocardial damage has been reported to increase in parallel with the severity of the COVID-19 infection. He *et al*. demonstrated that more than half of the patients diagnosed with COVID-19 hospitalized in China in February 2020 had myocardial damage (He *et al.*, 2020). This has been shown to have a direct affect in-hospital mortality (61% *vs*. 25%). In the study, levels of CRP and BNP were significantly higher (3 times or more) in those with myocardial damage than those of the others.

Chen *et al*. revealed that the disease is closely related to myocardial damage in their analysis on 150 COVID-19 cases (Chen *et al*, 2020). High levels of cTnI and the development of CHF have been disclosed as independent risk factors for myocardial damage.

In Whom does Myocardial Damage Occur and How do we Identify it?

Myocardial damage is more common in older people with COVID-19 and those with increased TnT levels (Shi *et al*. 2020, Guo *et al*. 2020). Although TnT levels are normal in these patients, HT, CAD, CHF and DM are more common than others.

While COVID-19 infects the alveoli in the lung and triggers obstruction in the small airways, it can also affect the vessels, causing damage to the heart, kidney and nervous system, intestines and liver. For example, protein or blood cells may be detected in the urine in every second patient. It was also stated that hemodialysis was performed in 14% to 30% of the intensive care patients with COVID-19 in Wuhan. It is postulated that all this damage cannot be explained only by 'storming cytokines'.

In patients with COVID-19, death usually occurs from multiple organ failure, and it can be difficult to distinguish between myocardial damage and other organ failure syndromes. Myocardial damage occurs in patients with cardiac dysfunction and ventricular dysrhythmias.

Guo *et al*. reported that 28% of 187 COVID-19 patients had myocardial damage (Guo *et al.*, 2020). He *et al*. raised the bar, and showed that 50% of 54 patients with COVID-19 diagnosed in China in February 2020 had myocardial damage (He, *et al.* 2020).

Bansal *et al*. reported that acute cardiac damage was present in 8% to 12% of all COVID-19 cases as a result of the literature review (Bansal, *et al*. 2020). Systemic inflammation and direct viral involvement contribute to cardiac injury. Presence of CVD and acute cardiac damage significantly accompany significant deterioration.

PATHOLOGICAL FINDINGS

SARS-CoV-2 positivity in cardiac tissue as well as CD3+, CD45+, and CD68+ cells in the myocardium and gene expression of tumor necrosis growth factor α, interferon γ, chemokine ligand 5, as well as interleukin-6, -8, and -18 were identified in autopsy cases died of COVID-19 (Lindner *et al*., 2020). Cardiac tissue from 39 consecutive autopsy cases were analyzed (median age: 85) SARS-CoV-2 could be documented in 24 of 39 patients (61.5%). Of note, there was no significant difference regarding inflammatory cell infiltrates or leukocyte numbers per high power field between those with a diagnosis of COVID-19 and those without. These findings suggest that among individuals with COVID-19, overt myocarditis may not be identified in the acute phase, but the long-term consequences of this cardiac infection needs to be elucidated.

GLOBAL VIEW OF MYOCARDIAL INFARCTION (STEMI/NSTEMI) AFTER COVID-19

Due to the serious increase in COVID-19 cases all over the world, the health system is concerned that the "other" (non-COVID-19) patients will be ignored when its focus has shifted while the whole system faces a serious healthcare burden.

Very interesting data were obtained from the world in this regard. In Hong Kong, Tam *et al*. shared data which indicated that the 'speed of care' was severely affected after COVID-19 in STEMI cases (Tam, *et al*. 2020). In Hong Kong, there was a rapid increase in the duration of the ambulance reaching to the patient (Symptom onset to first medical contact) from 80-90 minutes to 318 minutes after the call. This raises a concern that healthcare system in the COVID-19 era may not be able to care for cardiac emergencies adequately due to the burden and chaos it brings to most institutions.

Diagnostic Strategies

In the pandemic period, invasive procedures necessitating close contact with the patient carry a high risk for disease transmission. Thus, additional non-invasive evaluation is required in the ED to verify the diagnosis, as STEMI cases can also be admitted with atypical symptoms and signs. In this way, both COVID-19 risk classification is made and the diagnosis is tried to be clarified in terms of STEMI. Myocardial wall movement deficits are evaluated by POCUS or bedside echocardiography. The diagnosis is clarified by clinical examination, ECG, laboratory (enzyme elevation), and imaging data. Coronary CT-angiography can be considered, for example, where ECG and echocardiography are vague and the patient is stable. Activation of the catheterization laboratory should be considered immediately thereafter.

Myocarditis, which is more common in viral infections such that in the COVID-19 period, may also mimic STEMI. Among patients with COVID-19, death was found to be significantly more common in patients diagnosed with myocarditis.

TREATMENT STRATEGY: PCI OR FIBRINOLYSIS?

The standard method for STEMI patients during the pandemic period will be the primary PCI within the appropriate time frame (Mahmud *et al.*, 2020). In all cases, catheterization should be considered as a priority in the management of hemodynamic unstable patients. For this procedure, PPE should be fully worn and the intervention applied in a specially designed and adapted catheter laboratory.

On the other hand, some centers advocate that fibrinolysis can represent a reasonable alternative for patients with STEMI during the COVID-19 pandemic, especially because of the agents' considerable efficacy and safety and advantages in conserving medical resources (Wang, 2020). In this small but well-designed comparison study, fibrinolysis achieved a comparable in-hospital and 30-day primary composite end point in those with STEMI, as compared with those who underwent PPCI during the COVID-19 pandemic. No major bleeding episode was recorded in either group. In the USA, the consensus document published with associations of cardiologists and emergency physicians stated that fibrinolytic-based strategies will be developed in cases where PCI cannot be implemented or the timing will not be correct (Mahmud, 2020) (Fig. **1**).

Respiratory decompensation in intubated cases with severe COVID-19 in whom ARDS is also in the differential diagnosis should be evaluated on a case-by-case basis. There should be a critical assessment as to whether the patient will benefit from an invasive approach to have an impact on life expectancy.

DID THE PANDEMIC PROCESS AFFECT HEART ATTACKS?

Yes, a lot. Italian researchers reported that the number of patients with STEMI or NSTEMI admitted to the catheter laboratory during the COVID-19 epidemic period decreased significantly, compared to the same period of the previous year (De Rosa, 2020). They found a total reduction of 48.4%, (26.5% in STEMI and

65% in NSTEMI) (P <0.001). The decrease in female patients with STEMI was more pronounced than in men (41.2% *vs.* 17.8%). Although the pandemic primarily affected Northern Italy, a similar decrease occurred in Southern and central Italy in a few weeks. STEMI case fatality rate boosted significantly with the pandemic compared to last year [risk ratio (RR) = 3.3, P <0.001]. Complications also increased (RR = 1.8, P = 0.009). This is an alarm finding in terms of public health and must be dealt with robust interventions (Tables **2** and **3**).

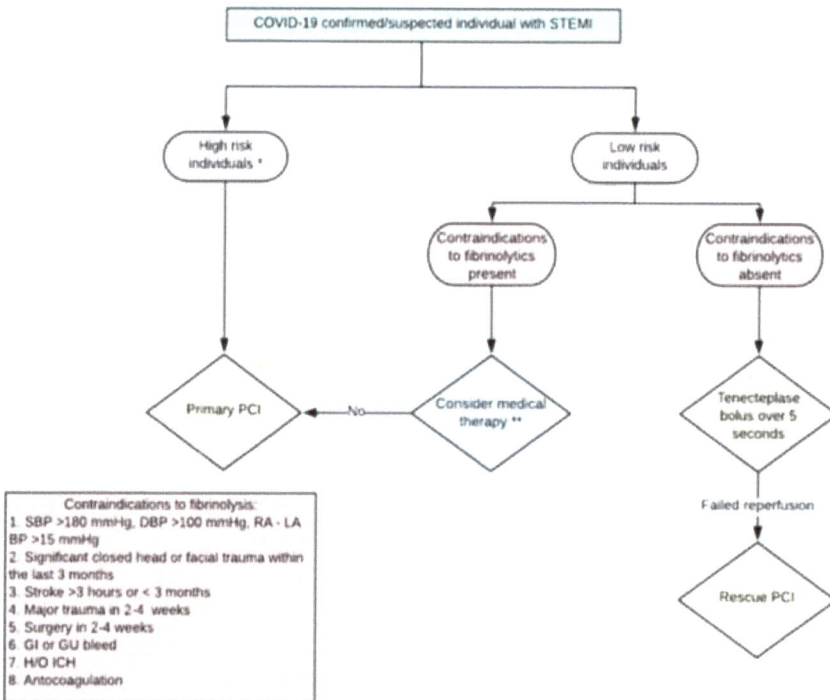

Fig. (1). Management of STEMI in COVID-19 period.

Table 2. COVID-19 is associated with CVD in 5 different ways.

1. People who have previously been diagnosed with CVD have an increased risk of more severe disease and death when they are infected with COVID-19.
2. COVID-19 directly or indirectly causes CV complications. These are AMI, arrhythmias, myocarditis and VTE.
3. Medicines and other treatments for COVID-19 can damage CVS, as in hydroxychloroquine.
4. Patients may become susceptible to disease transmission for reasons such as going out to hospital for CV care, breaking a quarantine, *etc.*
5. The management, diagnosis and treatment of CVD may be delayed and the clinical course may deteriorate due to the treatments and other problems in the pandemic environment.

Table 3. The problems encountered in the pandemic process in the care of CVD emergencies and similar cases.

Problem source	Description
Reasons arising from the patient	Drug use and disruptions in follow-ups
	Inability to go to the hospital with the fear of COVID-19
	Difficulties getting an appointment for examination or follow-up
	Difficulties in asking questions, consulting in urgent situations
	COVID-19-related problems experienced by the patients' caregiver or next of kin
Causes arising from the hospital/physician	Disruptions such as changing the patient's permanent physician and care team, getting sick, death
	Material supply and problems in the arrangement of the catheter lab team
	Changes in interpretations in diagnosis and treatment protocols due to COVID-19 contamination concerns (such as fibrinolytic administration rather than PCI, keeping the patient free from interventions)
System-related problems	Failure to adequately protect the physician and the patient due to shortages in providing PPE
	Failure to provide the system organization and materials to initiate procedures/interventions safely
	Insufficiency in online systems to facilitate counseling, asking questions, *etc.*
	Underdeveloped home care systems

Case example: Fig. (**2**) depicts a patient with concurrent COVID-19 and mycocardial infarction.

Case report: An obese black American woman in her 60s was admitted to ED with chief complaint of chest pain. She gives a medical history of coronary artery disease (had multiple stents), COPD (and smoking actively), pulmonary hypertension, and uncontrolled diabetes. Echocardiogram showed moderately reduced ejection fraction (EF) of 30-35%. Emergent left heart catheterization showed subtotal occlusion of her previous stent in the right coronary artery (RCA). She was treated with aspiration thrombectomy and a drug eluting stent placement. The patient was transferred to ICU after the stent placement and was initially placed on BIPAP followed by intubation due to worsening hypoxia. X-ray repeated at that time showed bilateral ground glass opacities (GGO) consistent with ARDS. She was started on HCQ along with azithromycin immediately and continued on MV with ARDS protocol. Her troponins peaked to 18 and then started to trend down (Adapted from Siddamreddy *et al.*, 2020) (Figs. **3** and **4**).

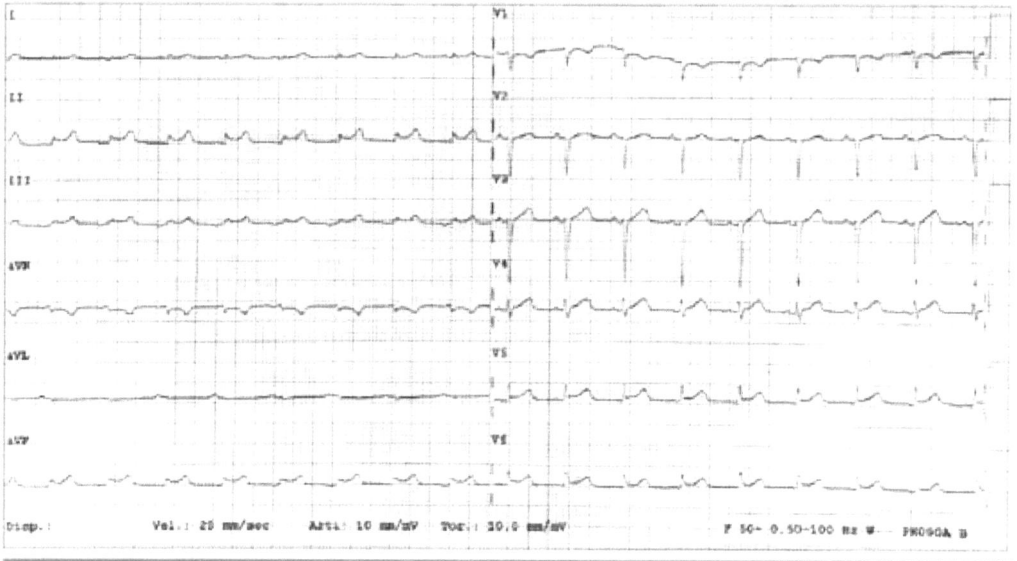

Fig. (2). ECG tracing of 53-years old woman with cardiac involvement during COVID-19 pandemics. There is a marked low voltage in the limb leads. ST elevation is notable in inferolateral leads, T inversion and ST depression are seen in V1 and aVR. It is also remarkable that the cardiac pulse is recorded over 100.

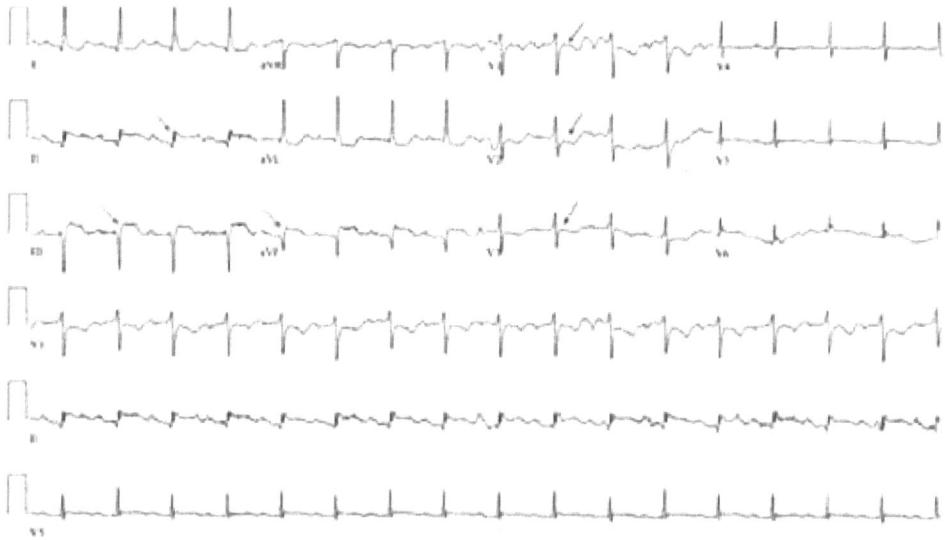

Fig. (3). A. ECG revealed ST elevations (red arrow) in leads II, III, aVF with reciprocal changes in V1, V2, V3 (blue arrow) which are interpreted to indicate acute inferior wall STEMI. **B.** Chest X-ray suggesting bilateral pulmonary edema, secondary to STEMI.

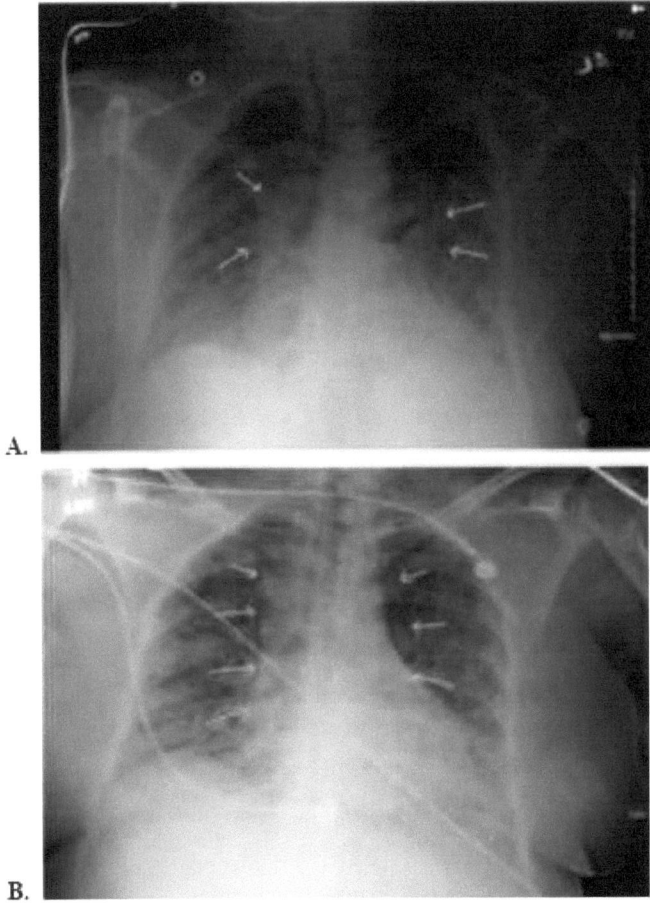

Fig. (4). Chest X-ray showing bilateral GGO with worsening aeration suggestive of ARDS (arrows).

SUMMARY AND CONCLUSIONS

What should be done to Mitigate Pandemic Effects on CVD?

Cardiac injury in COVID-19 is mostly included in multi-organ system failure with acute respiratory syndrome, albeit it represents a deadly disease per se. COVID-19 may result in various overlapping CVD-related manifestations, such as cardiac arrest, myocarditis, AMI, stress-induced cardiomyopathy, cardiogenic shock, arrhythmias and HF. Expedient recognition and management of cardiac damage is warranted. Patients report a constellation of unpredictable symptoms which worsen with advancing age, malnutrition, and cardiorespiratory and metabolic comorbidities. COVID-19 is shown to be associated with cardiac involvement, even after the resolution of the upper respiratory tract infection. Treatment for *de novo* heart failure, arrhythmias, ACS, thromboses and/or prothrombotic state should be tailored for each individual.

Although it is understandable and necessary for the ambulance and emergency care system to pay special attention to suspected COVID cases, it is also vital that other patients in need of emergency care are not left behind. While adapting to the new challenging pandemic milieu, this point should be emphasized in training healthcare workers- EMS personnel, physicians and nurses.

REFERENCES

Ammirati, E., Veronese, G., Brambatti, M., Merlo, M., Cipriani, M., Potena, L., Sormani, P., Aoki, T., Sugimura, K., Sawamura, A., Okumura, T., Pinney, S., Hong, K., Shah, P., Braun, Ö., Van de Heyning, C.M., Montero, S., Petrella, D., Huang, F., Schmidt, M., Raineri, C., Lala, A., Varrenti, M., Foà, A., Leone, O., Gentile, P., Artico, J., Agostini, V., Patel, R., Garascia, A., Van Craenenbroeck, E.M., Hirose, K., Isotani, A., Murohara, T., Arita, Y., Sionis, A., Fabris, E., Hashem, S., Garcia-Hernando, V., Oliva, F., Greenberg, B., Shimokawa, H., Sinagra, G., Adler, E.D., Frigerio, M., Camici, P.G. (2019). Fulminant *versus* acute nonfulminant myocarditis in patients with left ventricular systolic dysfunction. *J. Am. Coll. Cardiol., 74*(3), 299-311.
[http://dx.doi.org/10.1016/j.jacc.2019.04.063] [PMID: 31319912]

Badawi, A., Ryoo, S.G. (2016). Prevalence of comorbidities in the Middle East respiratory syndrome coronavirus (MERS-CoV): a systematic review and meta-analysis. *Int. J. Infect. Dis., 49*, 129-133.
[http://dx.doi.org/10.1016/j.ijid.2016.06.015] [PMID: 27352628]

Bansal, M. (2020). Cardiovascular disease and COVID-19. *Diabetes Metab. Syndr., 14*(3), 247-250.
[http://dx.doi.org/10.1016/j.dsx.2020.03.013] [PMID: 32247212]

Bravi, F., Flacco, M.E., Carradori, T., Volta, C.A., Cosenza, G., De Togni, A., Acuti Martellucci, C., Parruti, G., Mantovani, L., Manzoli, L. (2020). Predictors of severe or lethal COVID-19, including angiotensin converting Enzyme inhibitors and angiotensin II receptor blockers, in a sample of infected Italian citizens. *PLoS One, 15*(6), e0235248.
[http://dx.doi.org/10.1371/journal.pone.0235248] [PMID: 32579597]

Caforio, A.L., Pankuweit, S., Arbustini, E., Basso, C., Gimeno-Blanes, J., Felix, S.B., Fu, M., Heliö, T., Heymans, S., Jahns, R., Klingel, K., Linhart, A., Maisch, B., McKenna, W., Mogensen, J., Pinto, Y.M., Ristic, A., Schultheiss, H.P., Seggewiss, H., Tavazzi, L., Thiene, G., Yilmaz, A., Charron, P., Elliott, P.M. European society of cardiology working group on myocardial and pericardial diseases. (2013). Current state of knowledge on aetiology, diagnosis, management, and therapy of myocarditis: a position statement of the European Society of Cardiology Working Group on Myocardial and Pericardial Diseases. *Eur. Heart J., 34*(33), 2636-2648, 2648a-2648d.
[http://dx.doi.org/10.1093/eurheartj/eht210] [PMID: 23824828]

Chen, Q., Xu, L., Dai, Y., Ling, Y., Mao, J., Qian, J., Zhu, W., Di, W., Ge, J. (2020). Cardiovascular manifestations in severe and critical patients with COVID-19. *Clin. Cardiol., 43*(7), 796-802.
[http://dx.doi.org/10.1002/clc.23384] [PMID: 32562427]

De Rosa, S., Spaccarotella, C., Basso, C., Calabrò, M.P., Curcio, A., Filardi, P.P., Mancone, M., Mercuro, G., Muscoli, S., Nodari, S., Pedrinelli, R., Sinagra, G., Indolfi, C. Società italiana di cardiologia and the CCU academy investigators group. (2020). Reduction of hospitalizations for myocardial infarction in Italy in the COVID-19 era. *Eur. Heart J., 41*(22), 2083-2088.
[http://dx.doi.org/10.1093/eurheartj/ehaa409] [PMID: 32412631]

Guo, T., Fan, Y., Chen, M., Wu, X., Zhang, L., He, T., Wang, H., Wan, J., Wang, X., Lu, Z. (2020). Cardiovascular implications of fatal outcomes of patients with coronavirus disease 2019 (COVID-19). *JAMA Cardiol., 5*(7), 811-818. [published online ahead of print, 2020 Mar 27].
[http://dx.doi.org/10.1001/jamacardio.2020.1017] [PMID: 32219356]

He, X.W., Lai, J.S., Cheng, J., Wang, M.W., Liu, Y.J., Xiao, Z.C., Xu, C., Li, S.S., Zeng, H.S. (2020). Impact of complicated myocardial injury on the clinical outcome of severe or critically ill COVID-19 patients. *Zhonghua Xin Xue Guan Bing Za Zhi, 48*(6), 456-460.

[PMID: 32171190]

Hoffmann, M., Kleine-Weber, H., Schroeder, S., Krüger, N., Herrler, T., Erichsen, S., Schiergens, T.S., Herrler, G., Wu, N.H., Nitsche, A., Müller, M.A., Drosten, C., Pöhlmann, S. (2020). SARS-CoV-2 cell entry depends on ace2 and tmprss2 and is blocked by a clinically proven protease inhibitor. *Cell, 181*(2), 271-280.e8.
[http://dx.doi.org/10.1016/j.cell.2020.02.052] [PMID: 32142651]

Hu, H., Yao, N., Qiu, Y. (2020). Comparing rapid scoring systems in mortality prediction of critically ill patients with novel coronavirus disease. *Acad. Emerg. Med., 27*(6), 461-468.
[http://dx.doi.org/10.1111/acem.13992] [PMID: 32311790]

Kalyanaraman Marcello, R, Dolle, J, Grami, S (2020). Characteristics and outcomes of COVID-19 patients in new york city's public hospital system. *Preprint. medRxiv, 2020*, 05.29.20086645.
[http://dx.doi.org/10.1101/2020.05.29.20086645]

Kühl, U., Pauschinger, M., Noutsias, M., Seeberg, B., Bock, T., Lassner, D., Poller, W., Kandolf, R., Schultheiss, H.P. (2005). High prevalence of viral genomes and multiple viral infections in the myocardium of adults with "idiopathic" left ventricular dysfunction. *Circulation, 111*(7), 887-893.
[http://dx.doi.org/10.1161/01.CIR.0000155616.07901.35] [PMID: 15699250]

Lindner, D., Fitzek, A., Bräuninger, H., Aleshcheva, G., Edler, C., Meissner, K., Scherschel, K., Kirchhof, P., Escher, F., Schultheiss, H.P., Blankenberg, S., Püschel, K., Westermann, D. (2020). Association of cardiac infection with SARS-CoV-2 in confirmed COVID-19 autopsy cases. *JAMA Cardiol., 5*(11), 1281-1285.
[http://dx.doi.org/10.1001/jamacardio.2020.3551] [PMID: 32730555]

Mahmud, E., Dauerman, H.L., Welt, F.G.P., Messenger, J.C., Rao, S.V., Grines, C., Mattu, A., Kirtane, A.J., Jauhar, R., Meraj, P., Rokos, I.C., Rumsfeld, J.S., Henry, T.D. (2020). Management of acute myocardial infarction during the COVID-19 pandemic: A Consensus Statement from the Society for Cardiovascular Angiography and Interventions (SCAI), the American college of cardiology (ACC), and the American college of emergency physicians (ACEP). *Catheter. Cardiovasc. Interv., 96*(2), 336-345.
[http://dx.doi.org/10.1002/ccd.28946] [PMID: 32311816]

Pankuweit, S., Moll, R., Baandrup, U., Portig, I., Hufnagel, G., Maisch, B. (2003). Prevalence of the parvovirus B19 genome in endomyocardial biopsy specimens. *Hum. Pathol., 34*(5), 497-503.
[http://dx.doi.org/10.1016/S0046-8177(03)00078-9] [PMID: 12792925]

Peng, YD, Meng, K, Guan, HQ (2020). Clinical characteristics and outcomes of 112 cardiovascular disease patients infected by 2019-nCoV. *Zhonghua Xin Xue Guan Bing Za Zhi, 48*, E004.
[http://dx.doi.org/10.3760/cma.j.cn112148-20200220-00105]

Price-Haywood, E.G., Burton, J., Fort, D., Seoane, L. (2020). Hospitalization and mortality among black patients and white patients with COVID-19. *N. Engl. J. Med., 382*(26), 2534-2543.
[http://dx.doi.org/10.1056/NEJMsa2011686] [PMID: 32459916]

Puntmann, V.O., Carerj, M.L., Wieters, I., Fahim, M., Arendt, C., Hoffmann, J., Shchendrygina, A., Escher, F., Vasa-Nicotera, M., Zeiher, A.M., Vehreschild, M., Nagel, E. (2020). Outcomes of cardiovascular magnetic resonance imaging in patients recently recovered from coronavirus disease 2019 (COVID-19). *JAMA Cardiol., 5*(11), 1265-1273.
[http://dx.doi.org/10.1001/jamacardio.2020.3557] [PMID: 32730619]

Richardson, S, Hirsch, JS, Narasimhan, M (2020). Presenting characteristics, comorbidities, and outcomes among 5700 patients hospitalized with COVID-19 in the New York city area. *JAMA, 323*(20), 2052-2059.
[http://dx.doi.org/10.1001/jama.2020.7681]

Robinson, J., Hartling, L., Vandermeer, B., Klassen, T.P. (2015). Intravenous immunoglobulin for presumed viral myocarditis in children and adults. *Cochrane Database Syst. Rev., 5*(5), CD004370.
[http://dx.doi.org/10.1002/14651858.CD004370.pub3] [PMID: 25992494]

Shi, S, Qin, M, Shen, B (2020). Association of cardiac injury with mortality in hospitalized patients with COVID-19 in Wuhan, China. *JAMA Cardiol,* March;25.

[http://dx.doi.org/10.1001/jamacardio.2020.0950]

Siddamreddy, S., Thotakura, R., Dandu, V., Kanuru, S., Meegada, S. (2020). Corona virus disease 2019 (COVID-19) presenting as acute st elevation myocardial infarction. *Cureus, 12*(4), e7782. [http://dx.doi.org/10.7759/cureus.7782] [PMID: 32337148]

Suleyman, G., Fadel, R.A., Malette, K.M., Hammond, C., Abdulla, H., Entz, A., Demertzis, Z., Hanna, Z., Failla, A., Dagher, C., Chaudhry, Z., Vahia, A., Abreu Lanfranco, O., Ramesh, M., Zervos, M.J., Alangaden, G., Miller, J., Brar, I. (2020). Clinical characteristics and morbidity associated with coronavirus disease 2019 in a series of patients in metropolitan detroit. *JAMA Netw. Open, 3*(6), e2012270. [http://dx.doi.org/10.1001/jamanetworkopen.2020.12270] [PMID: 32543702]

Tam, C.F., Cheung, K.S., Lam, S. (2020 Apr). Impact of coronavirus disease 2019 (COVID-19) outbreak on ST segment-elevation myocardial infarction care in Hong Kong, China. *Circ Cardiovasc Qual Outcomes, 13*(4), e006661.

Tikellis, C., Thomas, M.C. (2012). Angiotensin-converting enzyme 2 (ACE2) is a key modulator of the renin angiotensin system in health and disease. *Int. J. Pept., 2012*, 256294-256294. [http://dx.doi.org/10.1155/2012/256294] [PMID: 22536270]

Wang, D., Hu, B., Hu, C., Zhu, F., Liu, X., Zhang, J., Wang, B., Xiang, H., Cheng, Z., Xiong, Y., Zhao, Y., Li, Y., Wang, X., Peng, Z. (2020). Clinical characteristics of 138 hospitalized patients with 2019 novel coronavirus-infected pneumonia in Wuhan, China. *JAMA, 323*(11), 1061-1069. [http://dx.doi.org/10.1001/jama.2020.1585] [PMID: 32031570]

Wang, N., Zhang, M., Su, H., Huang, Z., Lin, Y., Zhang, M. (2020). Fibrinolysis is a reasonable alternative for STEMI care during the COVID-19 pandemic. *J. Int. Med. Res., 48*(10), 300060520966151. [PMID: 33108941]

Xu, Z., Shi, L., Wang, Y., Zhang, J., Huang, L., Zhang, C., Liu, S., Zhao, P., Liu, H., Zhu, L., Tai, Y., Bai, C., Gao, T., Song, J., Xia, P., Dong, J., Zhao, J., Wang, F.S. (2020). Pathological findings of COVID-19 associated with acute respiratory distress syndrome. *Lancet Respir. Med., 8*(4), 420-422. [http://dx.doi.org/10.1016/S2213-2600(20)30076-X] [PMID: 32085846]

Zeng, J.H., Liu, Y.X., Yuan, J., Wang, F.X., Wu, W.B., Li, J.X., Wang, L.F., Gao, H., Wang, Y., Dong, C.F., Li, Y.J., Xie, X.J., Feng, C., Liu, L. (2020). First case of COVID-19 complicated with fulminant myocarditis: a case report and insights. *Infection, 48*(5), 773-777. [http://dx.doi.org/10.1007/s15010-020-01424-5] [PMID: 32277408]

Zhang, H., Penninger, J.M., Li, Y., Zhong, N., Slutsky, A.S. (2020). Angiotensin-converting enzyme 2 (ACE2) as a SARS-CoV-2 receptor: molecular mechanisms and potential therapeutic target. *Intensive Care Med., 46*(4), 586-590. [http://dx.doi.org/10.1007/s00134-020-05985-9] [PMID: 32125455]

Zhao, Y., Zhao, Z., Wang, Y. (2020). Single-cell RNA expression profiling of ACE2, the putative receptor of Wuhan 2019-nCov. *bioRxiv, 26*(January). [http://dx.doi.org/10.1101/2020.01.26.919985]

Zhou, F., Yu, T., Du, R., Fan, G., Liu, Y., Liu, Z., Xiang, J., Wang, Y., Song, B., Gu, X., Guan, L., Wei, Y., Li, H., Wu, X., Xu, J., Tu, S., Zhang, Y., Chen, H., Cao, B. (2020). Clinical course and risk factors for mortality of adult inpatients with COVID-19 in Wuhan, China: a retrospective cohort study. *Lancet, 395*(10229), 1054-1062. [http://dx.doi.org/10.1016/S0140-6736(20)30566-3] [PMID: 32171076]

CHAPTER 3

Myocardial Damage, Myocarditis, and COVID-19

Abstract: For centuries, complications of cardiovascular disease (CVD) have been documented as the prominent cause of mortality and morbidity worldwide. CVD and pandemic disease precipitate different kinds of damage in the myocardium, which also contribute to the death rates in the vulnerable population.

Almost all viral infections, including COVID-19 and influenza species, have the potential to inflict damage to the myocardial tissue, which also contributes to the severity of the disease itself. For instance, COVID-19 can trigger multiple organ failures with remarkable end results on cardiovascular functions. Its damage to the CVD like myocarditis, myocardial injury, *de novo* heart failure, acute coronary syndromes including STEMI, and various kinds of fatal and non-fatal dysrhythmias can be mentioned. Although most cases with myocarditis are asymptomatic or exhibit a mild course, it can precipitate acute heart failure and fatal respiratory failure.

Clinicians should be alert in patients with signs and symptoms compatible with myocarditis, pericarditis and/or endocarditis in the pandemic period and routine care because expedient diagnosis and management can prevent adverse outcomes in selected cases.

Keywords: Cardiovascular disease, COVID-19, Diagnosis, Endocarditis, Management, Myocardial damage, Myocarditis, Pericarditis.

MYOCARDIAL INJURY INFLICTED BY COVID-19

Although COVID-19 has been recognized to cause pneumonia, respiratory failure, and ARDS as the mainstays of its pathophysiology, myocarditis can also be detected in a substantial percentage of cases with COVID-19.

Acute cardiac injury (ACI) is among the most important complications of COVID-19. Zuin *et al.* published a meta-analytic study to enlighten the interactions between ACI and risks of death in these vulnerable populations (Zuin *et al.*, 2020). They included 8 articles, which recruited 1686 patients (mean age 60 years) in the final analysis. Rates of ACI was recorded higher among fatalities than it was in survivors (62% *vs.* 7%, P<0.0001). The analysis verified an increased mortality risk in those complicated with ACI within the course of the pandemic disease (P<0.0001).

Ozgur KARCIOGLU

There are some other studies that demonstrated that ACI is detected frequently in those with COVID-19 (Shi S, 2020). Greater proportions of patients with ACI needed noninvasive mechanical ventilation (MV) (46% *vs.* 4%; P < .001) or invasive MV (22% *vs.* 4%; P<.001) than those without ACI.

COVID-19 patients with severe myocardial damage have been shown to be exposed to a significantly higher risk of severe disease course, need for intensive care, and mortality (Li X, 2020). In this meta-analytic study, high levels of CK, CK-MB, LDH, and IL-6, and *de novo* dysrhythmias are linked with poor outcomes and the need for ICU admission, and the death rates are higher in patients with supranormal LDH and IL-6 readings. Of note, newly occurring arrhythmias have also been associated with an increased risk of grave outcome and/or need for intensive care (P<0.001).

Mechanisms of how SARS-CoV-2 Induces Inflammation and Disease

The suggested mechanisms of ACI are the viral entry of the virus to the myocardial cells and injury to the myocardium, systemic inflammation, hypoxia, cytokine storm, the immune response mediated by interferons, and plaque destabilization. The SARS-CoV-2 is an immunogenic virus that activates the innate immune system, particularly macrophages. In other disease conditions, activated macrophages produce interferons that trigger the destruction of the virus. However, in the case of SARS-CoV-2, macrophageal activation results in the release of interleukin 1 beta, which induces systemic inflammation. The pathological findings in cardiac tissue involved in COVID-19 infection exhibited only minor changes to interstitial inflammatory infiltration to the hyperactivation of inflammation, cytokine storm, myocyte necrosis, myocarditis, MI, and HF (Fig. **1**). Microthrombi and vascular inflammation have been noted in the vessels. The infection also induces systemic complications like sepsis and DIC.

COVID-19 can induce ACI other than ischemia, including broken heart syndrome or stress cardiomyopathy, acute and fulminant myocarditis (Chen C, 2020, Chen L, 2020).

Mechanisms of myocardial injury can involve discrete pathways with resultant pathophysiological effects (Table **1**).

Table 1. Mechanisms of myocardial injury.

	Hypothesized Mechanism of Injury
Myocarditis	Systemic inflammatory response; direct myocardial cell injury *via* viral entry using ACE-2 receptor; T-cell–mediated immune response

(Table 1) cont.....

	Hypothesized Mechanism of Injury
Myocardial infarction	Plaque rupture (Type I MI); myocardial oxygen supply/demand mismatch (Type II MI) from increased cardiometabolic demand
Microangiopathy/cytokine storm	Cytokine-induced activation of microvasculature predisposing to vasomotor abnormalities; augmented thrombosis and other aspects of dysfunction
Arrhythmia	Hypoxia-mediated; coronary perfusion impairment; direct tissue injury; scar-mediated injury, inflammatory response; medication-induced electrolyte abnormality

Recommended approach to COVID-19 patients with cardiogenic or mixed circulatory shock involves both the clinical status of the patient and the capabilities of the institution.

MYOCARDITIS

is the general term for the inflammatory state or disease of the myocardium. It can be precipitated by a variety of infectious and noninfectious causes (*i.e.*, toxic effects or autoimmunity). Pharmacological agents can also cause myocarditis. Time from inciting cause to the manifestation of symptoms can be as short as hours in some cases, while some are delayed to months. Young people are reported to have myocarditis more frequently than the elderly.

Cardiotropic Viruses as the Causes

Many different viruses have been accused in human myocarditis so far. The most common viral genetic material reported in myocarditis are human herpes virus 6 and parvovirus B19. Enteroviridae cause myocarditis in some regions. H1N1 influenza A infection has been recorded to precipitate fulminant myocarditis. Other injurious agents of myocardium have been reported as electric shock, hyperpyrexia, radiation (Table **2**).

Different researchers reported viruses as the etiological agents at rates between 37% and 77% in patients with myocarditis (Pankuweit 2003, Kuhl 2005). In patients with ejection fraction below 45%, viral etiology was found to be 42% (Marburg registry). Cardiac MRI revealed myocardial involvement following COVID-19 infection in 78 patients (78%) and myocardial inflammation in 60 (60%) (Puntmann, 2020).

Fulminant Myocarditis (FM)

FM is characterized by sudden and severe diffuse myocardial inflammation often leading to death. Cardiogenic shock, ventricular arrhythmias, or multiorgan system failure are the final common pathways to death. Patients with FM have a death rate of 40% to 70%.

Table 2. Known and documented causes of myocarditis, (*some of them regional).

Infections	Viruses	adenovirus, coxsackie B virus, cytomegalovirus, dengue*, echovirus, Epstein-Barr virus, hepatitis (B and C), herpesvirus, HIV, influenza A and B, mumps, parvovirus, poliomyelitis*, rabies*, rubella, rubeola, varicella
	Bacteria	actinomycosis, brucellosis, chlamydia, cholera*, clostridia, diphtheria*, gonococcal, haemophilus, legionella, meningococcal, mycoplasma, pneumococcal, salmonella, staphylococcal, streptococcal, tetanus*, tuberculosis*, tularemia*,
	Spirochets*	Leptospirosis, Lyme disease, Treponema pallidum (Syphilis), Tick-borne **relapsing fever**, Louse-borne **relapsing fever**,
	Rickettsia*	Q fever, Rocky mountain spotted fever, typhus
	Others*	**Protozoal (*e.g.*,** Amebiasis, Malaria, Toxoplasmosis), **Mycotic (*e.g.*,** Candidiasis, Mucormycosis), **Helminthic (*e.g.*,** Schistosomiasis, Echinococcosis),
Noninfectious causes	Radiation	-
	Systemic disorders	Kawasaki disease, celiac disease, inflammatory bowel disease (Crohn's disease, ulcerative colitis), thyrotoxicosis
	Exposure to cardiotoxic agents	alcohol, antibiotics, lithium, snake bites,* cocaine

Patients can present very differently, depending on the predominance of systemic signs and symptoms of an infectious or inflammatory disorder. The ECG may disclose low QRS voltage as a sign of myocardial edema; with or without left ventricular (LV) hypertrophy (Nakashima, 1994).

Hyperinflammataory state or "cytokine storm" is the main physiopathological pathway in patients with multiple organ failure after COVID-19 (Chen 2020, Wang 2020).

Diagnosis

Acute myocarditis should be included in the differential diagnosis in young patients with

• Patient presenting with hypotension, tachycardia, narrow arterial pulse pressure, shocky appearance unexplained by hemorrhage, with or without fever.

• Acute conduction abnormalities *e.g.*, marked with wide QRS or prolonged PR interval.

• Deliberate acutely appeared CV signs and symptoms often mistaken for conditions like AMI or acute HF.

• Manifestations of elevated right heart pressure: Pain on the right upper quadrant (liver zone), acutely elevated liver enzymes, jaundice, distended neck veins, pretibial edema, *etc.* (Kociol, 2020).

• An endomyocardial biopsy can be warranted for diagnosis.

A major problem is that acute myocarditis can be overlapping with sepsis. Both myocarditis can create an infectious focus for sepsis and sepsis can affect and depress myocardium to precipitate signs and symptoms of myocarditis. It can be difficult to distinguish which one is the dominant diagnosis.

In a meta-analytic study, Li *et al.* reported that elevated levels of troponin, creatine kinase–MB, myoglobin, and NT-proBNP were linked with a worse outcome of COVID-19 infection, with a similar trend for (Li JW, 2020).

USG/POCUS/ECHOCARDIOGRAPHY

Duke criteria are an important guide in this regard (Table **3**).

Table 3. Modified Duke criteria.

Definitive infective endocarditis
+ Pathological criteria
- Demonstration of microorganisms in vegetative debris, intracardiac abscess or embolism by culture or histological examination
- Pathological confirmation of the presence of vegetation or intracardiac abscess with a histology indicative of active endocarditis
+ Clinical criteria
2 major criteria or 1 major and 3 minor criteria or 5 minor criteria
Possible infective endocarditis
+ 1 major + 1 minor criterion *or* + 3 minor criteria
Rule out criteria:
+ A strong alternative diagnosis which can explain the signs and symptoms that are thought to be related to endocarditis, or
+ Endocarditis symptoms and signs disappear with antibiotic treatment lasted for four days or less; or
+ No finding in favor of infective endocarditis in surgical or autopsy material in patients receiving antibiotic therapy

INITIAL MANAGEMENT

Patients who are considered to have myocarditis should be hospitalized. They should be closely monitored with regard to HF, DCMP, arrhythmias, conduction disorders and TTEE. Table depicts dos and don'ts of the initial management (Table 4).

Table 4. Dos and don'ts of the initial management.

Do:	Supportive management needs to be instituted as soon as possible once FM is highly suspected. Rehydrate patients as guided by the ultrasonographic evaluation of inferior/superior vena cavae for filling pressures.
	Fever should be treated, if any.
	Additional oxygen can be given in accord with the patient's condition.
Don't:	Administration of negative inotropic agents such as beta-1 blockers and calcium channel blockers. Because heart rate is increased as a compensatory measure to stabilize organ perfusion.
	Exertion should be avoided during recovery.
	Be careful when using NSAIDs for potential Na retention and kidney injury.

Fluid treatment may be required, but in case of HF, monitoring CVP and prevention of hypervolemia should be considered. Water and salt restrictions are applied if needed.

Treatment Strategies for Myocarditis

IVIG, CST and VAD/mechanical circulatory support can be employed as last-chance maneuvers in severe cases when necessary (Veldtman, 2020). Myocardial damage can result in HF which should be diagnosed and managed immediately. Therapeutic anticoagulation is indicated in patients with depressed myocardium and/or visualized thrombi in the chambers *via* echo or POCUS.

Specific treatments are to be performed should specific myocarditis agents (Chagas, Lyme, Diphtheria, AIDS, echinococci or fungi) be identifed in selected cases.

In the presence of influenza epidemic, oseltamivir and similar antivirals should be commenced at the earliest period in case of a suspicion of myocarditis.

IV Immune Globulins (IVIG)

These should not be used routinely, instead, need to be reserved for carefully selected cases (Robinson, 2015).

Hemodynamic Maneuvers

Extracorporeal devices; ECMO/IABP could be life-saving should they be commenced expediently (Figs. **1** and **2**).

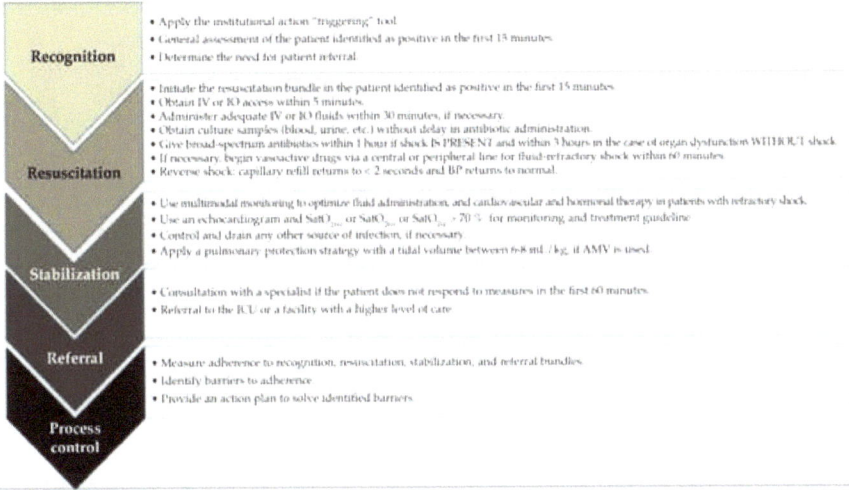

Fig. (1). Bundles of measures for multisystem inflammatory syndrome temporally related to COVID-19 and recognition, resuscitation, stabilization, referral, and process measurement elements (Adapted from Kohn Loncarica *et al.* 2019).

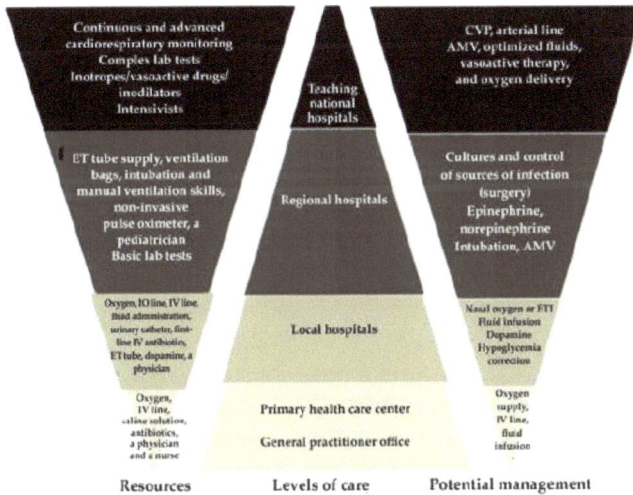

Fig. (2). Levels of care, resources, and potential management (Adapted from Singh *et al.* 2020).

CONCLUSIONS

For more than a year, COVID-19 outbreak has caused CVD in greater numbers of patients, when compared to the past. Injury to the cardiomyocytes is encountered commonly in documented cases with COVID-19, which gives rise to death toll attributed to CVD-linked pathophysiology. This phenomenon is explained partly with a boost in metabolic stress. Markers of injured myocardium (cardiac enzymes, LDH, BNP, IL-6 and others) increase in related to the extent of the myocardial damage incurred by the disease.

Although most cases with myocarditis are asymptomatic or exhibit a mild course, it can precipitate acute heart failure, and fatal respiratory failure.

Clinicians should be alert in patients with signs and symptoms compatible with myocarditis, pericarditis and/or endocarditis in the pandemic period and routine care because expedient diagnosis and management can prevent adverse outcomes and death.

Management of acute myocarditis, especially FM should be elaborated with a multidisciplinary approach. Expedient commencement of supportive treatment for the "ABC"s (*i.e.*, fluid replacement, adequate oxygenation, circulatory support) constitutes the essentials of the management, albeit individual differences should not be overlooked. Patients with FM may prompt inotropic agents or mechanical circulatory assist to keep vital organ perfusion at optimal levels while awaiting transplantation.

REFERENCES

Ammirati, E., Veronese, G., Brambatti, M., Merlo, M., Cipriani, M., Potena, L., Sormani, P., Aoki, T., Sugimura, K., Sawamura, A., Okumura, T., Pinney, S., Hong, K., Shah, P., Braun, Ö., Van de Heyning, C.M., Montero, S., Petrella, D., Huang, F., Schmidt, M., Raineri, C., Lala, A., Varrenti, M., Foà, A., Leone, O., Gentile, P., Artico, J., Agostini, V., Patel, R., Garascia, A., Van Craenenbroeck, E.M., Hirose, K., Isotani, A., Murohara, T., Arita, Y., Sionis, A., Fabris, E., Hashem, S., Garcia-Hernando, V., Oliva, F., Greenberg, B., Shimokawa, H., Sinagra, G., Adler, E.D., Frigerio, M., Camici, P.G. (2019). Fulminant *versus* acute nonfulminant myocarditis in patients with left ventricular systolic dysfunction. *J. Am. Coll. Cardiol., 74*(3), 299-311.
[http://dx.doi.org/10.1016/j.jacc.2019.04.063] [PMID: 31319912]

Badawi, A., Ryoo, S.G. (2016). Prevalence of comorbidities in the Middle East respiratory syndrome coronavirus (MERS-CoV): a systematic review and meta-analysis. *Int. J. Infect. Dis., 49*, 129-133.
[http://dx.doi.org/10.1016/j.ijid.2016.06.015] [PMID: 27352628]

Bansal, M. (2020). Cardiovascular disease and COVID-19. *Diabetes Metab. Syndr., 14*(3), 247-250.
[http://dx.doi.org/10.1016/j.dsx.2020.03.013] [PMID: 32247212]

Bemtgen, X., Krüger, K., Supady, A., Duerschmied, D., Schibilsky, D., Bamberg, F., Bode, C., Wengenmayer, T., Staudacher, D.L. (2020). First successful treatment of coronavirus disease 2019 induced refractory cardiogenic plus vasoplegic shock by combination of percutaneous ventricular assist device and extracorporeal membrane oxygenation: a case report. *ASAIO J., 66*(6), 607-609.
[http://dx.doi.org/10.1097/MAT.0000000000001178] [PMID: 32472827]

Bravi, F., Flacco, M.E., Carradori, T., Volta, C.A., Cosenza, G., De Togni, A., Acuti Martellucci, C., Parruti, G., Mantovani, L., Manzoli, L. (2020). Predictors of severe or lethal COVID-19, including Angiotensin Converting Enzyme inhibitors and Angiotensin II Receptor Blockers, in a sample of infected Italian citizens. *PLoS One, 15*(6), e0235248.

[http://dx.doi.org/10.1371/journal.pone.0235248] [PMID: 32579597]

Caforio, A.L., Pankuweit, S., Arbustini, E., Basso, C., Gimeno-Blanes, J., Felix, S.B., Fu, M., Heliö, T., Heymans, S., Jahns, R., Klingel, K., Linhart, A., Maisch, B., McKenna, W., Mogensen, J., Pinto, Y.M., Ristic, A., Schultheiss, H.P., Seggewiss, H., Tavazzi, L., Thiene, G., Yilmaz, A., Charron, P., Elliott, P.M. (2013). Current state of knowledge on aetiology, diagnosis, management, and therapy of myocarditis: a position statement of the European Society of Cardiology Working Group on Myocardial and Pericardial Diseases. *Eur. Heart J., 34*(33), 2636-2648, 2648a-2648d.
[http://dx.doi.org/10.1093/eurheartj/eht210] [PMID: 23824828]

Chen, Q., Xu, L., Dai, Y., Ling, Y., Mao, J., Qian, J., Zhu, W., Di, W., Ge, J. (2020). Cardiovascular manifestations in severe and critical patients with COVID-19. *Clin. Cardiol., 43*(7), 796-802.
[http://dx.doi.org/10.1002/clc.23384] [PMID: 32562427]

Chen, C., Zhou, Y., Wang, D.W. (2020). SARS-CoV-2: a potential novel etiology of fulminant myocarditis. *Herz, 45*(3), 230-232.
[http://dx.doi.org/10.1007/s00059-020-04909-z] [PMID: 32140732]

Chen, L., Li, X., Chen, M., Feng, Y., Xiong, C. (2020). The ACE2 expression in human heart indicates new potential mechanism of heart injury among patients infected with SARS-CoV-2. *Cardiovasc. Res., 116*(6), 1097-1100.
[http://dx.doi.org/10.1093/cvr/cvaa078] [PMID: 32227090]

De Rosa, S., Spaccarotella, C., Basso, C., Calabrò, M.P., Curcio, A., Filardi, P.P., Mancone, M., Mercuro, G., Muscoli, S., Nodari, S., Pedrinelli, R., Sinagra, G., Indolfi, C. (2020). Reduction of hospitalizations for myocardial infarction in Italy in the COVID-19 era. *Eur. Heart J., 41*(22), 2083-2088.
[PMID: 32412631]

Guo, T., Fan, Y., Chen, M., Wu, X., Zhang, L., He, T., Wang, H., Wan, J., Wang, X., Lu, Z. (2020). Cardiovascular implications of fatal outcomes of patients with coronavirus disease 2019 (COVID-19). *JAMA Cardiol., 5*(7), 811-818.
[http://dx.doi.org/10.1001/jamacardio.2020.1017] [PMID: 32219356]

He, X.W., Lai, J.S., Cheng, J., Wang, M.W., Liu, Y.J., Xiao, Z.C., Xu, C., Li, S.S., Zeng, H.S. (2020). Impact of complicated myocardial injury on the clinical outcome of severe or critically ill COVID-19 patients. *Zhonghua Xin Xue Guan Bing Za Zhi, 48*(6), 456-460.
[http://dx.doi.org/10.3760/cma.j.cn112148-20200228-00137] [PMID: 32171190]

Hoffmann, M., Kleine-Weber, H., Schroeder, S., Krüger, N., Herrler, T., Erichsen, S., Schiergens, T.S., Herrler, G., Wu, N.H., Nitsche, A., Müller, M.A., Drosten, C., Pöhlmann, S. (2020). SARS-CoV-2 cell entry depends on ACE2 and TMPRSS2 and is blocked by a clinically proven protease inhibitor. *Cell, 181*(2), 271-280.e8.
[http://dx.doi.org/10.1016/j.cell.2020.02.052] [PMID: 32142651]

Hu, H., Yao, N., Qiu, Y. (2020). Comparing rapid scoring systems in mortality prediction of critically ill patients with novel coronavirus disease. *Acad. Emerg. Med., 27*(6), 461-468.
[http://dx.doi.org/10.1111/acem.13992] [PMID: 32311790]

Kalyanaraman Marcello, R., Dolle, J., Grami, S., Adule, R., Li, Z., Tatem, K., Anyaogu, C., Apfelroth, S., Ayinla, R., Boma, N., Brady, T., Cosme-Thormann, B.F., Costarella, R., Ford, K., Gaither, K., Jacobson, J., Kanter, M., Kessler, S., Kristal, R.B., Lieber, J.J., Mukherjee, V., Rizzo, V., Jr, Rowell, M., Stevens, D., Sydney, E., Wallach, A., Chokshi, D.A., Davis, N. New York City Health + Hospitals COVID-19 Population Health Data Team. (2020). Characteristics and outcomes of COVID-19 patients in New York City's public hospital system. *PLoS One, 15*(12), e0243027.
[http://dx.doi.org/10.1371/journal.pone.0243027] [PMID: 33332356]

Kociol, R.D., Cooper, L.T., Fang, J.C., Moslehi, J.J., Pang, P.S., Sabe, M.A., Shah, R.V., Sims, D.B., Thiene, G., Vardeny, O. American Heart Association Heart Failure and Transplantation Committee of the Council on Clinical Cardiology. (2020). Recognition and initial management of fulminant myocarditis: a scientific statement from the american heart association. *Circulation, 141*(6), e69-e92.

[http://dx.doi.org/10.1161/CIR.0000000000000745] [PMID: 31902242]

Kohn Loncarica, G., Fustiñana, A., Jabornisky, R. (2019). Recomendaciones para el manejo del shock séptico en niños durante la primera hora (segunda parte). *Arch. Argent. Pediatr., 117*(1), e24-e33.
[PMID: 30652451]

Krittanawong, C., Kumar, A., Hahn, J., Wang, Z., Zhang, H.J., Sun, T., Bozkurt, B., Ballantyne, C.M., Virani, S.S., Halperin, J.L., Jneid, H. (2020). Cardiovascular risk and complications associated with COVID-19. *Am. J. Cardiovasc. Dis., 10*(4), 479-489.
[PMID: 33224599]

Kühl, U., Pauschinger, M., Noutsias, M., Seeberg, B., Bock, T., Lassner, D., Poller, W., Kandolf, R., Schultheiss, H.P. (2005). High prevalence of viral genomes and multiple viral infections in the myocardium of adults with "idiopathic" left ventricular dysfunction. *Circulation, 111*(7), 887-893.
[http://dx.doi.org/10.1161/01.CIR.0000155616.07901.35] [PMID: 15699250]

Li, J.W., Han, T.W., Woodward, M., Anderson, C.S., Zhou, H., Chen, Y.D., Neal, B. (2020). The impact of 2019 novel coronavirus on heart injury: A Systematic review and Meta-analysis. *Prog. Cardiovasc. Dis., 63*(4), 518-524.
[http://dx.doi.org/10.1016/j.pcad.2020.04.008] [PMID: 32305557]

Li, X., Pan, X., Li, Y., An, N., Xing, Y., Yang, F., Tian, L., Sun, J., Gao, Y., Shang, H., Xing, Y. (2020). Cardiac injury associated with severe disease or ICU admission and death in hospitalized patients with COVID-19: a meta-analysis and systematic review. *Crit. Care, 24*(1), 468.
[http://dx.doi.org/10.1186/s13054-020-03183-z] [PMID: 32723362]

Lindner, D., Fitzek, A., Bräuninger, H., Aleshcheva, G., Edler, C., Meissner, K., Scherschel, K., Kirchhof, P., Escher, F., Schultheiss, H.P., Blankenberg, S., Püschel, K., Westermann, D. (2020). Association of cardiac infection with SARS-CoV-2 in confirmed COVID-19 autopsy cases. *JAMA Cardiol., 5*(11), 1281-1285.
[http://dx.doi.org/10.1001/jamacardio.2020.3551] [PMID: 32730555]

Mahmud, E., Dauerman, H.L., Welt, F.G.P., Messenger, J.C., Rao, S.V., Grines, C., Mattu, A., Kirtane, A.J., Jauhar, R., Meraj, P., Rokos, I.C., Rumsfeld, J.S., Henry, T.D. (2020). Management of acute myocardial infarction during the COVID-19 pandemic: A Consensus Statement from the Society for Cardiovascular Angiography and Interventions (SCAI), the American College of Cardiology (ACC), and the American College of Emergency Physicians (ACEP). *Catheter. Cardiovasc. Interv., 96*(2), 336-345.
[http://dx.doi.org/10.1002/ccd.28946] [PMID: 32311816]

Nakashima, H., Honda, Y., Katayama, T. (1994). Serial electrocardiographic findings in acute myocarditis. *Intern. Med., 33*(11), 659-666.
[http://dx.doi.org/10.2169/internalmedicine.33.659] [PMID: 7849377]

Pankuweit, S., Moll, R., Baandrup, U., Portig, I., Hufnagel, G., Maisch, B. (2003). Prevalence of the parvovirus B19 genome in endomyocardial biopsy specimens. *Hum. Pathol., 34*(5), 497-503.
[http://dx.doi.org/10.1016/S0046-8177(03)00078-9] [PMID: 12792925]

Peng, Y.D., Meng, K., Guan, H.Q., Leng, L., Zhu, R.R., Wang, B.Y., He, M.A., Cheng, L.X., Huang, K., Zeng, Q.T. (2020). [Clinical characteristics and outcomes of 112 cardiovascular disease patients infected by 2019-nCoV]. *Zhonghua Xin Xue Guan Bing Za Zhi, 48*(6), 450-455.
[PMID: 32120458]

Price-Haywood, E.G., Burton, J., Fort, D., Seoane, L. (2020). Hospitalization and mortality among black patients and white patients with COVID-19. *N. Engl. J. Med., 382*(26), 2534-2543.
[http://dx.doi.org/10.1056/NEJMsa2011686] [PMID: 32459916]

Puntmann, V.O., Carerj, M.L., Wieters, I., Fahim, M., Arendt, C., Hoffmann, J., Shchendrygina, A., Escher, F., Vasa-Nicotera, M., Zeiher, A.M., Vehreschild, M., Nagel, E. (2020). Outcomes of cardiovascular magnetic resonance imaging in patients recently recovered from coronavirus disease 2019 (COVID-19). *JAMA Cardiol., 5*(11), 1265-1273.
[http://dx.doi.org/10.1001/jamacardio.2020.3557] [PMID: 32730619]

Ranard, L.S., Fried, J.A., Abdalla, M., Anstey, D.E., Givens, R.C., Kumaraiah, D., Kodali, S.K., Takeda, K.,

Karmpaliotis, D., Rabbani, L.E., Sayer, G., Kirtane, A.J., Leon, M.B., Schwartz, A., Uriel, N., Masoumi, A. (2020). Approach to acute cardiovascular complications in COVID-19 infection. *Circ Heart Fail, 13*(7), e007220.
[http://dx.doi.org/10.1161/CIRCHEARTFAILURE.120.007220] [PMID: 32500721]

Richardson, S., Hirsch, J.S., Narasimhan, M., Crawford, J.M., McGinn, T., Davidson, K.W., Barnaby, D.P., Becker, L.B., Chelico, J.D., Cohen, S.L., Cookingham, J., Coppa, K., Diefenbach, M.A., Dominello, A.J., Duer-Hefele, J., Falzon, L., Gitlin, J., Hajizadeh, N., Harvin, T.G., Hirschwerk, D.A., Kim, E.J., Kozel, Z.M., Marrast, L.M., Mogavero, J.N., Osorio, G.A., Qiu, M., Zanos, T.P. The northwell COVID-19 research consortium. (2020). Presenting characteristics, comorbidities, and outcomes among 5700 patients hospitalized with COVID-19 in the new york city area. *JAMA, 323*(20), 2052-2059.
[http://dx.doi.org/10.1001/jama.2020.6775] [PMID: 32320003]

Robinson, J., Hartling, L., Vandermeer, B., Klassen, T.P. (2015). Intravenous immunoglobulin for presumed viral myocarditis in children and adults. *Cochrane Database Syst. Rev., 5*(5), CD004370.
[http://dx.doi.org/10.1002/14651858.CD004370.pub3] [PMID: 25992494]

Shi, S., Qin, M., Shen, B., Cai, Y., Liu, T., Yang, F., Gong, W., Liu, X., Liang, J., Zhao, Q., Huang, H., Yang, B., Huang, C. (2020). Association of cardiac injury with mortality in hospitalized patients with COVID-19 in Wuhan, China. *JAMA Cardiol., 5*(7), 802-810.
[http://dx.doi.org/10.1001/jamacardio.2020.0950] [PMID: 32211816]

Siddamreddy, S., Thotakura, R., Dandu, V., Kanuru, S., Meegada, S. (2020). Corona virus disease 2019 (COVID-19) presenting as acute ST elevation myocardial infarction. *Cureus, 12*(4), e7782.
[http://dx.doi.org/10.7759/cureus.7782] [PMID: 32337148]

Singh, D.D., Han, I., Choi, E.H., Yadav, D.K. (2020). Recent advances in pathophysiology, drug development and future perspectives of SARS-CoV-2. *Front. Cell Dev. Biol., 8*, 580202.
[http://dx.doi.org/10.3389/fcell.2020.580202] [PMID: 33240881]

Suleyman, G., Fadel, R.A., Malette, K.M., Hammond, C., Abdulla, H., Entz, A., Demertzis, Z., Hanna, Z., Failla, A., Dagher, C., Chaudhry, Z., Vahia, A., Abreu Lanfranco, O., Ramesh, M., Zervos, M.J., Alangaden, G., Miller, J., Brar, I. (2020). Clinical characteristics and morbidity associated with coronavirus disease 2019 in a series of patients in metropolitan detroit. *JAMA Netw. Open, 3*(6), e2012270.
[http://dx.doi.org/10.1001/jamanetworkopen.2020.12270] [PMID: 32543702]

Tam, C.F., Cheung, K.S., Lam, S., Wong, A., Yung, A., Sze, M., Lam, Y.M., Chan, C., Tsang, T.C., Tsui, M., Tse, H.F., Siu, C.W. (2020). Impact of coronavirus disease 2019 (COVID-19) outbreak on st-segmen--elevation myocardial infarction care in Hong Kong, China. *Circ. Cardiovasc. Qual. Outcomes, 13*(4), e006631.
[http://dx.doi.org/10.1161/CIRCOUTCOMES.120.006631] [PMID: 32182131]

Tikellis, C., Thomas, M.C. (2012). Angiotensin-converting enzyme 2 (ACE2) is a key modulator of the renin angiotensin system in health and disease. *Int. J. Pept., 2012*, 256294-256294.
[http://dx.doi.org/10.1155/2012/256294] [PMID: 22536270]

Van Linthout, S., Klingel, K., Tschöpe, C. (2020). SARS-CoV-2-related myocarditis-like syndromes Shakespeare's question: what's in a name? *Eur. J. Heart Fail., 22*(6), 922-925.
[http://dx.doi.org/10.1002/ejhf.1899] [PMID: 32430971]

Veldtman, G.R., Pirisi, M., Storti, E., Roomi, A., Fadl-Elmula, F.E.M., Vriz, O., Bokhari, S., Ammash, N., Salam, Y., Liu, G.Z., Spinelli, S., Barbieri, G., Hashmi, S. (2020). Management principles in patients with COVID-19: perspectives from a growing global experience with emphasis on cardiovascular surveillance. *Open Heart, 7*(2), e001357.
[http://dx.doi.org/10.1136/openhrt-2020-001357] [PMID: 33168640]

Wang, D., Hu, B., Hu, C., Zhu, F., Liu, X., Zhang, J., Wang, B., Xiang, H., Cheng, Z., Xiong, Y., Zhao, Y., Li, Y., Wang, X., Peng, Z. (2020). Clinical characteristics of 138 hospitalized patients with 2019 novel coronavirus-infected pneumonia in Wuhan, China. *JAMA, 323*(11), 1061-1069.
[http://dx.doi.org/10.1001/jama.2020.1585] [PMID: 32031570]

Xu, Z., Shi, L., Wang, Y., Zhang, J., Huang, L., Zhang, C., Liu, S., Zhao, P., Liu, H., Zhu, L., Tai, Y., Bai, C., Gao, T., Song, J., Xia, P., Dong, J., Zhao, J., Wang, F.S. (2020). Pathological findings of COVID-19 associated with acute respiratory distress syndrome. *Lancet Respir. Med.,* 8(4), 420-422. [published correction appears in Lancet Respir Med. 2020 Feb 25;].
[http://dx.doi.org/10.1016/S2213-2600(20)30076-X] [PMID: 32085846]

Zeng, J.H., Liu, Y.X., Yuan, J., Wang, F.X., Wu, W.B., Li, J.X., Wang, L.F., Gao, H., Wang, Y., Dong, C.F., Li, Y.J., Xie, X.J., Feng, C., Liu, L. (2020). First case of COVID-19 complicated with fulminant myocarditis: a case report and insights. *Infection, 48*(5), 773-777. [published online ahead of print, 2020 Apr 10].
[http://dx.doi.org/10.1007/s15010-020-01424-5] [PMID: 32277408]

Zhang, H., Penninger, J.M., Li, Y., Zhong, N., Slutsky, A.S. (2020). Angiotensin-converting enzyme 2 (ACE2) as a SARS-CoV-2 receptor: molecular mechanisms and potential therapeutic target. *Intensive Care Med., 46*(4), 586-590.
[http://dx.doi.org/10.1007/s00134-020-05985-9] [PMID: 32125455]

Zhao, Y., Zhao, Z., Wang, Y. (2020). Single-cell RNA expression profiling of ACE2, the putative receptor of Wuhan 2019-nCov. *bioRxiv.*
[http://dx.doi.org/10.1101/2020.01.26.919985]

Zhou, F., Yu, T., Du, R., Fan, G., Liu, Y., Liu, Z., Xiang, J., Wang, Y., Song, B., Gu, X., Guan, L., Wei, Y., Li, H., Wu, X., Xu, J., Tu, S., Zhang, Y., Chen, H., Cao, B. (2020). Clinical course and risk factors for mortality of adult inpatients with COVID-19 in Wuhan, China: a retrospective cohort study. *Lancet, 395*(10229), 1054-1062.
[http://dx.doi.org/10.1016/S0140-6736(20)30566-3] [PMID: 32171076]

Zuin, M., Rigatelli, G., Zuliani, G., Bilato, C., Zonzin, P., Roncon, L. (2020). Incidence and mortality risk in coronavirus disease 2019 patients complicated by acute cardiac injury: systematic review and meta-analysis. *J. Cardiovasc. Med. (Hagerstown), 21*(10), 759-764.
[http://dx.doi.org/10.2459/JCM.0000000000001064] [PMID: 32740433]

CHAPTER 4

Coagulopathies, Prothrombotic State, Thromboembolism, Bleeding, and COVID-19

Abstract: COVID-19 is known to trigger a prothrombotic state, causing thromboses and thromboembolic events (TTEE) in patients with COVID-19. Both bleeding and thrombosis can result in significant morbidity in COVID-19. The entity paves the way to arterial TTEE (*i.e.*, stroke and/or extremity ischemia) as well as small vessel thrombosis, which are commonly recorded at autopsy in the pulmonary vasculature. Elevated D-dimer is associated with a higher risk for TTEE, hemorrhage, critical illness, and mortality. Likewise, levels of fibrinogen, ferritin, procalcitonin are also higher in patients with thrombosis. There is also a propensity to develop pulmonary thromboembolism (PTE) in cases with COVID-19. Treatment with anticoagulant prophylaxis (*i.e.*, heparin and/or aspirin) is recommended in many researches, but robust evidence is still warranted to draw firm conclusions on the benefit-to-harm ratio of the agents in most patients.

Keywords: Anticoagulant prophylaxis, Cardiovascular disease, Coagulopathy, COVID-19, D-dimer, Thromboembolic events, Thrombosis.

INTRODUCTION

Bleeding diathesis, coagulopathy, and TTEE are ominous factors that predict a severe course and send the patients to intensive care units. Many studies noted that high levels of fibrin degradation products such as D-dimer are directly linked with death rates, which is suggestive of a coagulopathy associated with COVID-19 (Zhou, 2020, Samkari,2020). However, there is still scarce evidence of coagulopathy and thrombotic risk in COVID-19 patients. Paradoxically, both thromboses and bleeding diathesis are reported from samples of patients in the pandemic era. For example, intracranial hemorrhage as well as thrombotic ischemic lesions were reported in different series of COVID-19 (Helms, 2020).

Although rare, DIC, low platelet count, and hypofibrinogenemia were associated with important bleeding in those with COVID-19 (Samkari *et al.*, 2020). However, Tang *et al.* pointed out that 71% of those who died of COVID-19 had the criteria of disseminated intravascular coagulation (DIC), while only 0.6% of survivors did (Tang, 2020).

The high number of arterial and/or venous TTEE diagnosed within 24 h of admission and the high rate of positive TTEE imaging in cases with COVID-19 suggest that there is a need to improve specific algorithms to recognize TTEE and investigate the efficacy and safety of thromboprophylaxis in ambulatory patients (Lodigiani, 2020).

SARS-COV-2 involvement of the epithelial tissue of the lung precipitates the process of inflammation, which activates neutrophils and starts the construction of a neutrophil extracellular trap (NET) (Fig. **1**).

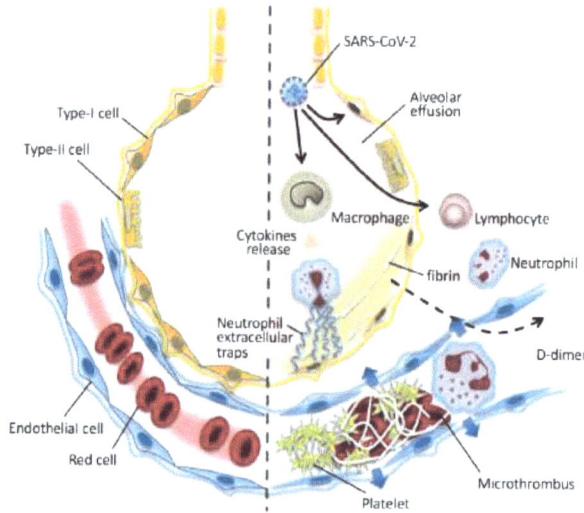

Fig. (1). Inflammatory cascade in the alveoli triggered by cytokines initiates microthrombi in the lung vessels that turn into thromboembolism in some cases.

An algorithm is developed as a workflow in patients suspected to have VTE, in the setting of COVID-19 (Aryal *et al*. 2020).

Microvascular thromboses can also ensue during COVID-19. Some patients who died of COVID-19 underwent autopsies which revealed pulmonary microvascular thrombosis (Menter, 2020, Ackermann, 2020).

COVID-19 infection precipitates a marked increase in fibrinogen and D-dimer. This phenomenon is postulated to represent systemic hypercoagulability which gives rise to venous TTEE. This is the rationale behind the fact that the extent of D-dimer increases correlates with death rates in patients with confirmed COVID-19.

LABORATORY VARIABLES

Thrombocytopenia and high d-dimer are the two parameters which suggest high risk of need for intensive care and mortality (Lippi, 2020).

In-hospital mortality has been linked with advanced age, high D-dimer (> 1000 µg/L), and high SOFA score on admission (Zhou, 2020).

High levels of D-dimer obtained on admission is suggestive for hemorrhage, VTE/TTEE, and grave outcome.

Mouhat *et al.* reported that D-dimer levels above 2590 ng/mL can predict PTE in COVID-19 patients with clinical deterioration (Mouhat, 2020).

COVID-19 cases have mostly been shown to exhibit low platelet count probably resulting from high turnover of platelets (Wool, 2020) (Table **1**). Nonetheless, disseminated intravascular coagulopathy (DIC) and hemorrhage are infrequent in cases with COVID-19.

ESR, CRP, fibrinogen, ferritin, and procalcitonin were higher in patients with thrombotic complications than in those without.

Elevated NLR, and PLR have been postulated as prognostic and risk stratifying factor of severe form of disease (Chan 2020, Rokni, 2020).

Laboratory data showing increased risk for thrombosis were summarized in Table **2**.

Table 1. Platelet variables in cases with COVID-19 (Adapted from Wool, 2020).

-	COVID-19 patients Mean (SD)		Non-COVID-19 ICU patients Mean (SD)		Normal range
Platelet count, x10^9/L	234.1	151.1	250.3	152.7	150–450
MPV, fL	11.58*	1.04	10.49	1	9.0–12.4
-	median	range	median	range	
IPF x10^9/L		42.57	12.2–99.5	4.25	3.3–5.2	1.25–7.02
IPF %		14.63	4.2–25.0	7.05	6.4–7.7	3.3–8.6

N = 20, *i.e.*, 10 pairs of patients matched for platelet count.
* p = 0.013, paired Student's *t* test (compared to non-COVID-19 patients). MPV, mean platelet volume; IPF, immature platelet fraction.

Table 2. Laboratory variables representing enhanced risk for thromboembolic events.

D-dimer> 2,500 ng / mL [aOR, 6.79 (2.39-19.30)],
D-dimer> 1000 ng / mL and <2,500 ng / mL [(aOR, 3.04 (1.26-7.31)],
PLT> 450 × 109 / L [aOR, 3.56 (1.27-9.97)],
CRP> 100 mg / L [aOR, 2.71 (1.26-5.86)],
ESR> 40 mm / h [aOR, 2.64 (1.07-6.51)].

Can we prescribe antiplatelet agents in the pandemic era? Yes and no. antiplatelet agents have been suggested to be useful in COVID-19 cases, but currently there is no robust data to be used as a proof for this. Such an approach can impose a higher risk of bleeding in patients with low platelet counts (Iba *et al.*, 2020).

TROPONIN AND BNP CAN PREDICT THE SEVERITY OF COVID-19

This relationship has been disclosed in many studies (Lippi, 2020). However, troponin levels are elevated not only in COVID-19, but also in many diseases such as myocarditis, PTE, and AMI (Januzzi, 2020). Similarly, natriuretic peptides, such as BNP, are elevated in many entities, such as heart failure.

Inflammatory markers and CRP as a marker of severity and occurences of TTEE Blood markers of hyperinflammatory state including ESR, CRP, fibrinogen, ferritin, and procalcitonin were found to be increased in those with thrombotic complications (Samkari, 2020).

In a study from Iran on 233 consecutive cases with laboratory-confirmed COVID-19, Rokni *et al.* reported that mean CRP levels of patients deceased and survived from COVID-19 were 15 and 13.2 mg/L, respectively (p=0.15) (Rokni, 2020). On the other hand, in a meta-analytic study, Amiri-Dashatan *et al.* disclosed that those with severe COVID-19 had higher levels of CRP [standardized mean difference (SMD)= 3.26 mg/L; (95% CI 2.5, 3.9); p<0.05; I2 = 98.02%], TNFα [SMD = 1.78 ng/mL; (95% CI 0.39, 3.1); p=0.012; I2 = 98.2%], and IL-6 [SMD = 3.67 ng/mL; (95% CI 2.4, 4.8); p<0.05; I2 = 97.8%] than those with the mild form of the disease (Amiri-Dashatan, 2020). Likewise, another study found that CRP values higher than 100 mg/dL and D-dimer > 500 ng/ml can predict in-hospital death (Ullah, 2020). Some other authors investigated the incidence, time course, blood chemistry data, and prognoses of cases with COVID-19 suspected to have TTEE (Thondapu, 2020). They reported that male sex, high levels of CRP, and platelet count on presentation were linked to VTE. In brief, evidence-based medicine supports that CRP appears to be a test of high accuracy to predict both severe course of the disease and TTEE.

Sepsis-induced coagulopathy (SIC) score was also postulated to have considerable predictive power (Zheng, 2021) (Table **3**).

Table 3. Sepsis-induced coagulopathy (SIC) score.

Variable	Score	Range
Platelet count (x10^9/L)	1	100 to 150
	2	<100
PT-INR	1	1,2 to 1,4
	2	>1,4
SOFA	1	1
	2	>2
SIC-total score	<100	-

Viscoelastic tests to assess hypercoagulability: Some researchers advocated that hypercoagulability and hypofibrinolysis exist together and are identified correctly by viscoelastic tests (VET). A majority of patients had coagulopathy and bleeding tendency on viscoelastic tests missed by standard coagulation tests (Rodrigues, 2020).

PULMONARY THROMBOEMBOLISM (PTE) AND COVID-19

It is a vital problem which cannot be underestimated in the management of COVID-19 patients. Mouhat *et al.* reported that D-dimer levels above 2590 ng/mL can predict PTE in COVID-19 patients with clinical deterioration (Mouhat, 2020).

COVID-19 patients were compared with Influenza patients admitted with respiratory insufficiency before the pandemics (2019) respecting PTE. They have written that the rate of PTE influenza patients was found to be lower than that of cases with COVID-19 (Poissy, 2020).

In a multicentric study, the percentages of VTE visualized in CTPA or USG was 27% and arterial TTEE were 4% in patients admitted into intensive care (Klok, 2020). In this study, PTE was the most frequently reported thrombotic event (n = 25, 81%).

Wang *et al.* cited that up to two-fifths of cases admitted with COVID-19 have been assigned in the high-risk group for thromboembolism (Wang, 2020).

Case example: Three patients with PTE concomitant with COVID-19 were depicted.

Management principles: VTE prophylaxis *via* heparinization is indicated for all patients with severe course of COVID-19 (Algorithm). Heparin can be administered as low molecular weight heparin (LMWH) or unfractioned heparin (UFH). Contraindications or this scheme include active, ongoing or recent hemorrhage or a history/diagnosis of heparin-induced thrombocytopenia. These situations mandate use of another option like fondaparinux.

In a retrospective study, Daughety *et al.* reported a VTE rate of 7% and an overall TTEE rate of 12% in hospital sample of patients admitted with COVID-19 (Daughety *et al.* 2020). They have employed a high-dose heparin thromboprophylaxis strategy for cases with elevated D-dimer (> 2.5 mg/L) and severe disease course was associated with a 6% percentage of major bleeding (Fig. **2**). They concluded that it is still unfounded whether high-dose thromboprophylaxis improves the course of cases with COVID-19.

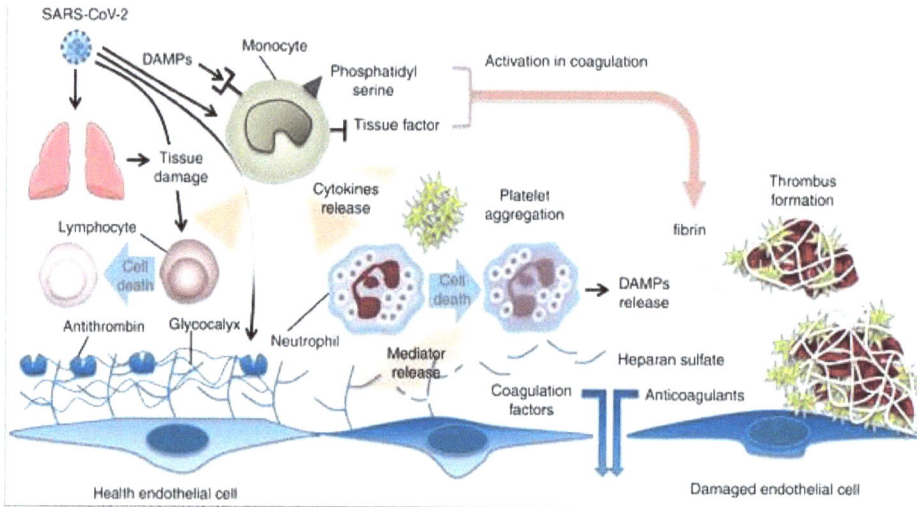

Fig. (2). Heparin can reverse the pathological process precipitated by procoagulant activity.

SHOULD WE HEPARINIZE THE PATIENTS WITH COVID-19?

Yes. In a Spanish multicentric broad-based study, heparin was given in conjunction to the treatment of more than 1700 patients treated in 17 hospitals, whilst 285 patients served as controls. (Ayerbe, 2020). Heparin treatment was linked with lower death rate in those with COVID-19. In another study by Tang *et al.* the death rate of 99 patients who received heparin and had a sepsis-induced coagulopathy (SIC) index> 4 was below that of the patients in the control group (Tang N, *et al.*2020). Enoxaparin can be administered at a dose of 1 mg/kg/12 h or 1,5 mg/kg/d (not to exceed 180 mg/d).

Aspirin: In an observational multicentric study of patients presented with

COVID-19 between March 2020 and July 2020 disclosed that decreased risk of mechanical ventilation was attributed to aspirin use (p=0.007), ICU admission (p=0.005), and death rate (p=0.02) (Chow *et al.* 2020).

CONCLUSION

Pathologically increased bleeding diathesis or tendency to coagulation and TTEE is a risk factor for transfer to intensive care unit, severe clinical course and poor prognosis. Unacceptably high rates of cases with severe clinical course and respiratory failure due to COVID-19 had deadly TTEE. Patients suspected to have TTEE can be more easily detected using sensitive markers such as D-dimer, fibrinogen, BNP and others, depending on the clinical presentation. Finally, many researchers pointed out that clinicians should set anticoagulation targets higher than its current position in critically ill patients.

REFERENCES

Ackermann, M., Verleden, S.E., Kuehnel, M., Haverich, A., Welte, T., Laenger, F., Vanstapel, A., Werlein, C., Stark, H., Tzankov, A., Li, W.W., Li, V.W., Mentzer, S.J., Jonigk, D. (2020). Pulmonary vascular endothelialitis, thrombosis, and angiogenesis in Covid-19. *N. Engl. J. Med., 383*(2), 120-128.
[http://dx.doi.org/10.1056/NEJMoa2015432] [PMID: 32437596]

Al-Samkari, H., Karp Leaf, R.S., Dzik, W.H., Carlson, J.C.T., Fogerty, A.E., Waheed, A., Goodarzi, K., Bendapudi, P.K., Bornikova, L., Gupta, S., Leaf, D.E., Kuter, D.J., Rosovsky, R.P. (2020). COVID-19 and coagulation: bleeding and thrombotic manifestations of SARS-CoV-2 infection. *Blood, 136*(4), 489-500.
[http://dx.doi.org/10.1182/blood.2020006520] [PMID: 32492712]

Amiri-Dashatan, N., Koushki, M., Ghorbani, F., Naderi, N. (2020). Increased inflammatory markers correlate with liver damage and predict severe COVID-19: a systematic review and meta-analysis. *Gastroenterol. Hepatol. Bed Bench, 13*(4), 282-291.
[PMID: 33244370]

Aryal, M.R., Gosain, R., Donato, A., Pathak, R., Bhatt, V.R., Katel, A., Kouides, P. (2020). Venous thromboembolism in COVID-19: towards an ideal approach to thromboprophylaxis, screening, and treatment. *Curr. Cardiol. Rep., 22*(7), 52.
[http://dx.doi.org/10.1007/s11886-020-01327-9] [PMID: 32529517]

Ayerbe, L., Risco, C., Ayis, S. (2020). The association between treatment with heparin and survival in patients with Covid-19. *J. Thromb. Thrombolysis, 50*(2), 298-301.
[http://dx.doi.org/10.1007/s11239-020-02162-z] [PMID: 32476080]

Bikdeli, B., Madhavan, M.V., Jimenez, D., Chuich, T., Dreyfus, I., Driggin, E., Nigoghossian, C., Ageno, W., Madjid, M., Guo, Y., Tang, L.V., Hu, Y., Giri, J., Cushman, M., Quéré, I., Dimakakos, E.P., Gibson, C.M., Lippi, G., Favaloro, E.J., Fareed, J., Caprini, J.A., Tafur, A.J., Burton, J.R., Francese, D.P., Wang, E.Y., Falanga, A., McLintock, C., Hunt, B.J., Spyropoulos, A.C., Barnes, G.D., Eikelboom, J.W., Weinberg, I., Schulman, S., Carrier, M., Piazza, G., Beckman, J.A., Steg, P.G., Stone, G.W., Rosenkranz, S., Goldhaber, S.Z., Parikh, S.A., Monreal, M., Krumholz, H.M., Konstantinides, S.V., Weitz, J.I., Lip, G.Y.H. Global COVID-19 Thrombosis Collaborative Group, Endorsed by the ISTH, NATF, ESVM, and the IUA, Supported by the ESC Working Group on Pulmonary Circulation and Right Ventricular Function. (2020). COVID-19 and thrombotic or thromboembolic disease: implications for prevention, antithrombotic therapy, and follow-up: JACC state-of-the-art review. *J. Am. Coll. Cardiol., 75*(23), 2950-2973.
[http://dx.doi.org/10.1016/j.jacc.2020.04.031] [PMID: 32311448]

Casini, A., Alberio, L., Angelillo-Scherrer, A., Fontana, P., Gerber, B., Graf, L., Hegemann, I., Korte, W., Kremer Hovinga, J., Lecompte, T., Martinez, M., Nagler, M., Studt, J.D., Tsakiris, D., Wuillemin, W., Asmis,

L. (2020). Thromboprophylaxis and laboratory monitoring for in-hospital patients with COVID-19 - a Swiss consensus statement by the Working Party Hemostasis. *Swiss Med. Wkly.,* *150*, w20247.
[http://dx.doi.org/10.4414/smw.2020.20247] [PMID: 32277760]

Chan, A.S., Rout, A. (2020). Use of neutrophil-to-lymphocyte and platelet-tolymphocyte ratios in COVID-19. *J. Clin. Med. Res.,* *12*(7), 448-453.
[http://dx.doi.org/10.14740/jocmr4240] [PMID: 32655740]

Giorgi-Pierfranceschi, M., Khanna, A.K., Kethireddy, S. (2020). Is aspirin effective in preventing ICU admission in patients with COVID-19 pneumonia? A comment to "Aspirin Use is Associated with Decreased Mechanical Ventilation, ICU Admission, and In-Hospital Mortality in Hospitalized Patients with COVID-19". *Anesth. Analg., Publish Ahead of Print*(Oct), 21. Epub ahead of print
[http://dx.doi.org/10.1213/ANE.0000000000005292] [PMID: 33369927]

Cui, S., Chen, S., Li, X., Liu, S., Wang, F. (2020). Prevalence of venous thromboembolism in patients with severe novel coronavirus pneumonia. *J. Thromb. Haemost.,* *18*(6), 1421-1424.
[http://dx.doi.org/10.1111/jth.14830] [PMID: 32271988]

Cuker, A., Peyvandi, F. (2020). https://www.uptodate.com/contents/coronavirus-disease-2019-covi--19-hypercoagulability?search=covid-19&source=machineLearning&graphicRef=128045#graphicRef128045

Daughety, M.M., Morgan, A., Frost, E., Kao, C., Hwang, J., Tobin, R., Patel, B., Fuller, M., Welsby, I., Ortel, T.L. (2020). COVID-19 associated coagulopathy: Thrombosis, hemorrhage and mortality rates with an escalated-dose thromboprophylaxis strategy. *Thromb. Res.,* *196*, 483-485.
[http://dx.doi.org/10.1016/j.thromres.2020.10.004] [PMID: 33091700]

Gupta, N., Zhao, Y.Y., Evans, C.E. (2019). The stimulation of thrombosis by hypoxia. *Thromb. Res.,* *181*, 77-83.
[http://dx.doi.org/10.1016/j.thromres.2019.07.013] [PMID: 31376606]

Helms, J., Tacquard, C., Severac, F., Leonard-Lorant, I., Ohana, M., Delabranche, X., Merdji, H., Clere-Jehl, R., Schenck, M., Fagot Gandet, F., Fafi-Kremer, S., Castelain, V., Schneider, F., Grunebaum, L., Anglés-Cano, E., Sattler, L., Mertes, P.M., Meziani, F. CRICS TRIGGERSEP Group (Clinical Research in Intensive Care and Sepsis Trial Group for Global Evaluation and Research in Sepsis). (2020). High risk of thrombosis in patients with severe SARS-CoV-2 infection: a multicenter prospective cohort study. *Intensive Care Med.,* *46*(6), 1089-1098.
[http://dx.doi.org/10.1007/s00134-020-06062-x] [PMID: 32367170]

Iba, T., Levy, J.H., Levi, M., Connors, J.M., Thachil, J. (2020). Coagulopathy of coronavirus disease 2019. *Crit. Care Med.,* *48*(9), 1358-1364.
[PMID: 32467443]

Klok, F.A., Kruip, M.J.H.A., van der Meer, N.J.M., Arbous, M.S., Gommers, D.A.M.P.J., Kant, K.M., Kaptein, F.H.J., van Paassen, J., Stals, M.A.M., Huisman, M.V., Endeman, H. (2020). Incidence of thrombotic complications in critically ill ICU patients with COVID-19. *Thromb. Res.,* *191*, 145-147.
[http://dx.doi.org/10.1016/j.thromres.2020.04.013] [PMID: 32291094]

Levi, M., van der Poll, T. (2017). Coagulation and sepsis. *Thromb. Res.,* *149*, 38-44.
[http://dx.doi.org/10.1016/j.thromres.2016.11.007] [PMID: 27886531]

Lippi, G., Favaloro, E.J. (2020). D-dimer is associated with severity of coronavirus disease 2019: a pooled analysis. *Thromb. Haemost.,* *120*(5), 876-878.
[http://dx.doi.org/10.1055/s-0040-1709650] [PMID: 32246450]

Lippi, G., Lavie, C.J., Sanchis-Gomar, F. (2020). Cardiac troponin I in patients with coronavirus disease 2019 (COVID-19): Evidence from a meta-analysis. *Prog. Cardiovasc. Dis.,* *63*(3), 390-391.
[http://dx.doi.org/10.1016/j.pcad.2020.03.001] [PMID: 32169400]

Lippi, G., Plebani, M., Henry, B.M. (2020). Thrombocytopenia is associated with severe coronavirus disease 2019 (COVID-19) infections: A meta-analysis. *Clin. Chim. Acta,* *506*, 145-148.
[http://dx.doi.org/10.1016/j.cca.2020.03.022] [PMID: 32178975]

Lodigiani, C., Iapichino, G., Carenzo, L., Cecconi, M., Ferrazzi, P., Sebastian, T., Kucher, N., Studt, J.D., Sacco, C., Bertuzzi, A., Sandri, M.T., Barco, S. (2020). Venous and arterial thromboembolic complications in COVID-19 patients admitted to an academic hospital in Milan, Italy. *Thromb. Res., 191*, 9-14. [http://dx.doi.org/10.1016/j.thromres.2020.04.024] [PMID: 32353746]

Lorenzo, C., Francesca, B., Francesco, P., Elena, C., Luca, S., Paolo, S. (2020). Acute pulmonary embolism in COVID-19 related hypercoagulability. *J. Thromb. Thrombolysis, 50*(1), 223-226. [http://dx.doi.org/10.1007/s11239-020-02160-1] [PMID: 32474757]

Luo, W.R., Yu, H., Gou, J.Z., Li, X.X., Sun, Y., Li, J.X., He, J.X., Liu, L. (2020). Histopathologic findings in the explant lungs of a patient with COVID-19 treated with bilateral orthotopic lung transplant. *Transplantation, 104*(11), e329-e331. [http://dx.doi.org/10.1097/TP.0000000000003412] [PMID: 33122591]

Maxwell, A.J., Ding, J., You, Y., Dong, Z., Chehade, H., Alvero, A., Mor, Y., Draghici, S., Mor, G. (2021). Identification of key signaling pathways induced by SARS-CoV2 that underlie thrombosis and vascular injury in COVID-19 patients. *J. Leukoc. Biol., 109*(1), 35-47. [http://dx.doi.org/10.1002/JLB.4COVR0920-552RR] [PMID: 33242368]

Menter, T., Haslbauer, J.D., Nienhold, R., Savic, S., Hopfer, H., Deigendesch, N., Frank, S., Turek, D., Willi, N., Pargger, H., Bassetti, S., Leuppi, J.D., Cathomas, G., Tolnay, M., Mertz, K.D., Tzankov, A. (2020). Postmortem examination of COVID-19 patients reveals diffuse alveolar damage with severe capillary congestion and variegated findings in lungs and other organs suggesting vascular dysfunction. *Histopathology, 77*(2), 198-209. [http://dx.doi.org/10.1111/his.14134] [PMID: 32364264]

Mouhat, B., Besutti, M., Bouiller, K., Grillet, F., Monnin, C., Ecarnot, F., Behr, J., Capellier, G., Soumagne, T., Pili-Floury, S., Besch, G., Mourey, G., Lepiller, Q., Chirouze, C., Schiele, F., Chopard, R., Meneveau, N. (2020). Elevated D-dimers and lack of anticoagulation predict PE in severe COVID-19 patients. *Eur. Respir. J., 56*(4), 2001811. [http://dx.doi.org/10.1183/13993003.01811-2020] [PMID: 32907890]

Osakwe, N., Hart, D. (2020). Clinical presentation of acute pulmonary embolism in patients with coronavirus disease 2019 (COVID-19). *Case Rep. Hematol.,* Nov 16; *2020*, 8855957. [http://dx.doi.org/10.1155/2020/8855957] [PMID: 33224540]

Poissy, J., Goutay, J., Caplan, M., Parmentier, E., Duburcq, T., Lassalle, F., Jeanpierre, E., Rauch, A., Labreuche, J., Susen, S. Lille ICU Haemostasis COVID-19 Group. (2020). Pulmonary embolism in patients With COVID-19: awareness of an increased prevalence. *Circulation, 142*(2), 184-186. [http://dx.doi.org/10.1161/CIRCULATIONAHA.120.047430] [PMID: 32330083]

Rodrigues, A., Seara Sevivas, T., Leal Pereira, C., Caiado, A., Robalo Nunes, A. (2021). Viscoelastic tests in the evaluation of haemostasis disturbances in SARS-CoV2 infection. *Acta Med. Port., 34*(1), 44-55. [http://dx.doi.org/10.20344/amp.14784] [PMID: 33159728]

Rokni, M., Ahmadikia, K., Asghari, S., Mashaei, S., Hassanali, F. (2020). Comparison of clinical, para-clinical and laboratory findings in survived and deceased patients with COVID-19: diagnostic role of inflammatory indications in determining the severity of illness. *BMC Infect. Dis., 20*(1), 869. [http://dx.doi.org/10.1186/s12879-020-05540-3] [PMID: 33225909]

Tang, N., Bai, H., Chen, X., Gong, J., Li, D., Sun, Z. (2020). Anticoagulant treatment is associated with decreased mortality in severe coronavirus disease 2019 patients with coagulopathy. *J. Thromb. Haemost., 18*(5), 1094-1099. [http://dx.doi.org/10.1111/jth.14817] [PMID: 32220112]

Tang, N., Li, D., Wang, X., Sun, Z. (2020). Abnormal coagulation parameters are associated with poor prognosis in patients with novel coronavirus pneumonia. *J. Thromb. Haemost., 18*(4), 844-847. [http://dx.doi.org/10.1111/jth.14768] [PMID: 32073213]

Thondapu, V, Montes, D, Rosovsky, R (2020). Venous thrombosis, thromboembolism, biomarkers of inflammation, and coagulation in coronavirus disease 2019. *J. Vasc Surg Venous Lymphat Disord,* Nov

12;*S2213-333X*(20), 30627-2.
[http://dx.doi.org/1016/j.jvsv.2020.11.006] [PMID: 33188961]

Ullah, W., Thalambedu, N., Haq, S., Saeed, R., Khanal, S., Tariq, S., Roomi, S., Madara, J., Boigon, M., Haas, D.C., Fischman, D.L. (2020). Predictability of CRP and D-Dimer levels for in-hospital outcomes and mortality of COVID-19. *J. Community Hosp. Intern. Med. Perspect., 10*(5), 402-408.
[http://dx.doi.org/10.1080/20009666.2020.1798141] [PMID: 33235672]

Wang, T., Chen, R., Liu, C., Liang, W., Guan, W., Tang, R., Tang, C., Zhang, N., Zhong, N., Li, S. (2020). Attention should be paid to venous thromboembolism prophylaxis in the management of COVID-19. *Lancet Haematol., 7*(5), e362-e363.
[http://dx.doi.org/10.1016/S2352-3026(20)30109-5] [PMID: 32278361]

Wool, G.D., Miller, J.L. (2021). The impact of COVID-19 disease on platelets and coagulation. *Pathobiology, 88*(1), 15-27.
[http://dx.doi.org/10.1159/000512007] [PMID: 33049751]

Zheng, R., Zhou, J., Song, B., Zheng, X., Zhong, M., Jiang, L., Pan, C., Zhang, W., Xia, J., Chen, N., Wu, W., Zhang, D., Xi, Y., Lin, Z., Pan, Y., Liu, X., Li, S., Xu, Y., Li, Y., Tan, H., Zhong, N., Luo, X., Sang, L. (2021). COVID-19-associated coagulopathy: thromboembolism prophylaxis and poor prognosis in ICU. *Exp. Hematol. Oncol., 10*(1), 6.
[http://dx.doi.org/10.1186/s40164-021-00202-9] [PMID: 33522958]

Zhou, F., Yu, T., Du, R., Fan, G., Liu, Y., Liu, Z., Xiang, J., Wang, Y., Song, B., Gu, X., Guan, L., Wei, Y., Li, H., Wu, X., Xu, J., Tu, S., Zhang, Y., Chen, H., Cao, B. (2020). Clinical course and risk factors for mortality of adult inpatients with COVID-19 in Wuhan, China: a retrospective cohort study. *Lancet, 395*(10229), 1054-1062.
[http://dx.doi.org/10.1016/S0140-6736(20)30566-3] [PMID: 32171076]

CHAPTER 5

Chest Pain and Acute Coronary Syndromes (ACS)

Abstract: Acute coronary syndromes (ACS), especially acute myocardial infarction (AMI), is the leading cause of death in the world. These represent damage to the cardiac myocytes in the setting of acute cessation of blood supply. Chest pain is a common presentation in patients with AMI; however, there are multiple non-cardiac causes of chest pain. The diagnosis cannot always be made based on the initial presentation. The emergent evaluation of a patient with probable ACS includes a careful assessment of history, risk factors and presenting signs and symptoms, *de novo* ECG abnormalities, and workup of cardiac troponins. Validated risk scores, such as HEART, TIMI, and GRACE, can be helpful in predicting outcomes and the likelihood of ACS in a patient with chest pain. ECG should be performed within 10 minutes of presentation. ST elevation MI (STEMI) is diagnosed with elevated ST segments in two consecutive leads on ECG. Likewise, elevated levels of cardiac troponins in the first hours of presentation are mostly a prerequisite for diagnosis.

Although cardiac catheterization is viewed as the standard diagnostic modality for coronary artery disease, exercise testing, stress studies, echocardiography, and coronary computed tomography angiography (CCTA) may be important adjuncts. Cardiac catheterization laboratory (CCL), coronary care units, EDs, EMS, and primary care institutions need to cooperate in unison to produce the best results for public health.

This chapter gives a brief outline of the diagnosis and management of ACS in the pandemic period.

Keywords: Acute coronary syndrome, Acute myocardial infarction, Cardiac catheterization, COVID-19, ST elevation myocardial infarction.

INTRODUCTION

Cardiovascular disease is the most common cause of death among adults in most parts of the world. These may be deaths in a short time following Acute Myocardial Infarction (AMI) or may develop as a result of other acute coronary syndromes (ACS). Approximately half of the patients with out-of-hospital cardiac arrest with the first rhythm identified as VF and who survive hospital admission have evidence of acute MI. Of all out-of-hospital cardiac arrests, .50% will have significant coronary artery lesions on acute coronary angiography (Al-Khatib SM, 2018). Sudden cardiac death (SCD) constitutes major public health problems, accounting for approximately 50% of all cardiovascular deaths. For this reason, a great economic resource is allocated for the prevention of cardiovascular diseases (CVD) in the world, especially in developed countries. In developing countries, on the other hand, larger bills are faced because therapeutic approaches are prominent rather than preventive medicine.

ETIOLOGY

The inability to meet the oxygen requirement of the heart with the supplied blood for a certain period of time and the accumulation of substances such as lactic acid and free radicals in the myocardial tissue precipitates chest pain (CP). In other words, it is acute ischemia of myocardial cells that directly triggers the pain.

The amount of blood passing through a vein is proportional to the diameter of the vein. When atherosclerosis reduces the vessel diameter by half, there is a serious decrease in the blood carried by vessel. As a rule, reduced blood flow to the coronary arteries is caused by atherosclerosis. However, sometimes abnormal spasm of the arteries can also cause insufficient blood flow, which is called vasospastic angina or "Prinzmetal's angina".

CP is the most common complaint of AMI. However, CP has many causes other than AMI or CVD. History is an important aid in distinguishing them. Pain or discomfort radiating to the shoulder, arm, neck, or jaw may indicate heart disease. Since ischemia afflicts dermatomes between C8 and T4, this kind of spreading pain occurs. In many cases, pain can be defined in the areas listed in addition to CP, or in some cases, only these pains can be noted. For example, an AMI case may present with neck or arm pain without CP.

PATHOGENESIS

CP is divided into visceral or somatic, in accord with the mechanism. Visceral pain is pain caused by internal organs such as the heart, blood vessels, esophagus, and visceral pleura. Somatic pain is easily identified, its location is well-defined and indicated (*e.g.*, by the finger), and it is a sharp pain, while visceral pain is not well localized due to pain fibers entering the spinal cord at different levels, difficult to describe, vaguely defined, unclear and blunt. There is also a psychological component in vital diseases such as ACS, DAA, and PE. This consists of fear of death (*angor animi*, severe anguish, nonspecific fear, and anxiety).

Noncardiac Chest Pain

NCCP is also a common presentation encountered in routine practice. Most of them are classified in the 'pleuritic' CP and are of the nature of "somatic pain" (Table **1**). Well-defined, sharply circumscribed area of pain is generally in this category, but it should be noted that there may be exceptions. In other words, a pain that appears to be precisely somatic may, in fact, be a harbinger of severe visceral pain, for example, ACS or aortic dissection.

Table 1. Causes of pleuritic or somatic CP include.

• Pulmonary embolism (PE).
• Pneumothorax.
• Pneumonia.
• Pericarditis.
• Serositis/connective tissue disease.
• Malignancies involving the pleura.
• Pathologies below the diaphragm.
• Musculoskeletal disorders

Angina pectoris is examined under two headings: **Stable angina and unstable angina pectoris (USAP).** Stable angina pectoris (SAP) is the feeling of pain with ischemia as the oxygen requirement of the heart increases during effort without coronary thrombus. SAP attacks always begin with physical or emotional stress, and often the patient recognizes and predicts this pain. SAP usually resolves when the patient is at rest or with the use of agents such as isosorbide dinitrate or with oxygen. USAP is not so easily relieved. USAP can start at rest, even while asleep. It is also called preinfarction angina because it often represents underlying severe atherosclerosis (Table **2**). Fig. (**1**) illustrates the advancement of coronary arterial atherosclerotic process and its reflections on ECG.

Table 2. The criteria sought for the definition of USAP.

- anginal pain that started for the first time in the last 1.5 months
- the change in the duration and characteristics of the pain (*e.g.*, it used to last 3 minutes but now it is 15 minutes, or it used to be start while running but now walking)
- Pain within the first 2 weeks after AMI
- Pain precipitated in the early period after PTCA
- Pain concurrent with changes in ECG findings.

A   B   C

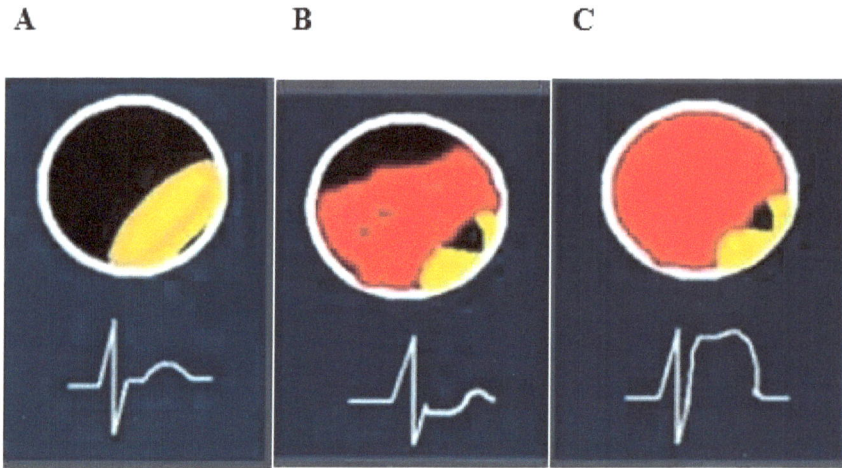

Fig. (1). Schematization of the progression of coronary artery disease. **A** . Patient with stable angina, **B**. Patient with USAP, who can progress to AMI at any time. **C**. Patient with hyperacute STEMI and transmural infarction. The findings accompanying this are also seen in ECG traces.

MEDICAL HISTORY

In the case of CP, the "targeted medical history" can not be overemphasized, and should be obtained expediently. The treatment of the patient is guided by the symptoms consistent with the history, although in patients with SCD there may be no history consistent with CVD.

Pain in angina pectoris is caused by the accumulation of lactic acid and CO_2 in the ischemic myocardial tissue. The patient usually complains of CP under the sternum and epigastric discomfort. The patient may describe his/her discomfort as pain, pressure, compression or crushing sensation. Pain is often mistaken for indigestion. In other patients, the pain spreads to the shoulder, arm, neck, jaw or back. Some patients experience distress, dyspnea or sweating.

Pearl: "Typical" or "coronary" CP is expected to last 2 to 20 minutes, and pain in USAP and AMI is expected to last from 20 minutes to 2 hours. It is likely that CP, which is reported to last for 'a few seconds' or 12 - 24 hours, may be caused by a non-ACS cause, from costochondritis to aortic dissection. "Typical" pain often increases with pronounced exertion, such as climbing stairs, walking in cold, stress, heavy eating, and resolves with rest or use of nitrates. On the contrary, pain that can be indicated precisely with a finger, pain that is precipitated by turning left and right, tilting or standing up, or induction *via* certain positions increase the likelihood of another diagnosis.

Many specialty associations put forward classifications of angina to categorize patients in regards to the severity of the clinical picture. Angina Classification of Canadian Cardiovascular Society (CCS) is among the most commonly used schemes (Table **3**).

Table 3. Angina Classification of Canadian Cardiovascular Society (CCS).

Class I: Angina: occurs only with compulsive, rapid, or prolonged effort. No angina is seen with daily activity
Class II: Daily activity is slightly restricted. Angina occurs with rapid climbing stairs, walking uphill, walking after meals, cold, wind, or stress
Class III: Daily activity is significantly restricted. Angina by walking one or two blocks or climbing a flight of stairs at normal speed
Class IV: Can't do almost any activity without discomfort. There may also be anginal complaints at rest.

ATYPICAL PRESENTATIONS

Only 1/3 of the patients have a sole complaint of CP on presentation. In large studies, it was reported that almost half of the AMI cases did not have CP when they were admitted to the hospital. Patients with CP can define classical angina, angina equivalents (*i.e.*, palpitation, dyspnea, syncope, altered mental status, hypotension *etc.*) and atypical CP. Atypical and painless presentations are more common in women and the elderly. The risk of wrong-incomplete treatment is higher in AMI cases presenting with atypical complaints and history.

When the patient complains of CP, the following important items of the history should be questioned

- exact location of chest pain
- spread of pain, if any (*e.g.* lower jaw, back, shoulders)
- duration of pain
- the causes of pain (exercise, stress, *etc.*)
- the nature of the pain (blunt or sharp)
- accompanying complaints
- factors that increase and decrease pain
- similar previous pain episodes
- Are there any drugs -especially cardiac ones- that the patient uses regularly and what are they?
- Examples; nitrates, propranolol or other beta blockers, diuretics, antihypertensives, antidysrhythmics (amiodarone, propafenone *etc.*), digitalis,
- Is the patient still receiving treatment for a serious illness?
- Previous AMI or angina, heart failure, hypertension, diabetes, chronic lung disease. any diseases like?

- Is the patient allergic to anything?
- Briefly learn the risk factors (hypertension, smoking, family history, *etc.*) and try to have an idea about the severity of the patient.

Pearl: It is a great danger to establish diagnoses such as noncardiac CP, anxiety and/or conversion disorder very quickly in a patient presenting with CP. Musculoskeletal triggering, such as neither sharp pain, nor relief with antacids, or turning left or right, can definitely rule out cardiac etiology.

DIAGNOSIS (PHYSICAL EXAMINATION AND LABORATORY EXAMINATION)

The differential diagnosis of chest pain and its triage according to urgency (Table 4):

Table 4. Some life-threatening and semi-urgent entities presenting mostly with chest pain and their distinguishing features.

Diagnosis	Location	Characteristic	Spread	Some Associated Symptoms
Cardiac CP (Angina pectoris)	Mid-chest, may be widespread, or epigastric	Crushing, pressure-like	Shoulder, R or L arm, chin, neck, back	Perspiration, nausea, dyspnea, syncope or agitation
Pericarditis	Mid-chest	Sharp, somatic, pleuritic	Shoulder, neck, back	Fever, pericardial rub
Aortic dissection- DAA	Mostly mid-back and mid-chest, may also involve legs	Tearing, crushing pain	Varies with the involvement	Leg pain, neurologic deficit, findings of peripheral arterial occlusion, stroke
Pulmonary embolism (massive)	Mostly widespread	May be in different forms, can masquerade angina pectoris or pneumothorax	Unexpected	Dyspnea, hypotension, tachycardia, hypoxemia, anxiety-agitation, altered mental status
Pulmonary embolism (segmental)	Sharp/pleuritic pain in a well-defined area of the chest (right or left)	somatic, pleuritic	Unexpected	Tachycardia (half of the patients), tachypnea, dyspnea, rarely syncope or altered mental status

Diagnosis	Location	Characteristic	Spread	Some Associated Symptoms
Spontaneous pneumothorax	Sharp/pleuritic pain in a well-defined area of the chest (right or left)	Sudden-onset, sharp, somatic, pleuritic	Shoulder, back	Dyspnea, rarely perspiration, syncope
Pneumonia	A part of the chest, mostly lateral	sharp, somatic, pleuritic	Unexpected	Fever, signs of sepsis
Perforated duodenal/peptic ulcer	Mid-upper abdomen - epigastric	Severe, sharp	Shoulder, lower chest	Severe abdominal pain, rigidity/ guarding, perspiration, nausea/vomiting
Esophageal rupture (Boerhaave syndrome)	Mid-chest	Severe, sharp, usually follows a heavy meal or forceful vomiting	Mid-chest, back	Dyspnea, subcutaneous crepitation (emphysema), fever: if untreated: sepsis/septic shock
MVP- Mitral valve prolapse	Mostly mid-chest	Sharp, somatic, pleuritic	Unexpected	Pain is mostly accompanied by palpitation/tachycardia. Lightheadedness or anxiety may be noted with pain.
Costochondritis/costochondral syndromes	Pain in involved area	Sharp, somatic, pleuritic and/or widespread, can increase with inspiration and decrease with rest	Unexpected	Unexpected

Emergency Conditions

Acute MI, Unstable angina, dissecting aortic aneurysm (DAA), acute PE, esophageal rupture, spontaneous pneumothorax, pericarditis with tamponade.

Less Urgent Conditions

Heart valve diseases, esophageal spasm, esophagitis, pain reflected from the abdomen (gastritis, perforated ulcer, pancreatitis, cholecystitis), pneumonia, pleuritis.

Benign (Non-emergency) Diseases

Chest wall pain unrelated to heart and internal organs, costochondritis, Tietze's syndrome, hyperventilation, anxiety, slipping rib syndrome, fibrositis, thoracic spinal disease, thoracic zona zoster.

PHYSICAL EXAMINATION

Evaluation of the patient presenting with CP starts with the primary survey like all other patients. Life-threatening problems are detected and resuscitated at the first examination. Special attention needs are blood pressure, respiratory rate, pulse rate, regularity (the presence of irregular pulse suggests dysrhythmia) and the level of consciousness. The slightest deviation from the normal level of consciousness should primarily suggest insufficient cerebral perfusion due to low cardiac stroke volume.

Pearl: In cardiac patients unresponsive to external stimuli, 'CAB sequence' is applied, respectively, in the context of CPR protocol; while ABCDE sequence can be performed in responsive and stable patients. The sequence of ABCDE is also followed in cases with definite or suspect trauma (ATLS 10th Edition, 2018).

The secondary survey of the cardiac patient should be systematic and complete. Physical examination of most ACS cases is generally normal. However, a full systemic exam is necessary because important information in details can be obtained. For example, DVT finding in the lower extremity (Homans' sign) may suggest PE, rales in the lungs and peripheral (pretibial) edema may suggest HF. Inaudible breathing sounds on auscultation in a lung area and eliciting hyperresonance with percussion lead to the diagnosis of spontaneous pneumothorax. Since hyper- or hypotension can be seen in AMI, compensated or decompensated HF, DAA and PE, it should be noted and treatment should be started.

Pearl: Physical examination and evaluation of the case with ACS is not for the diagnosis of ACS, but for finding accompanying pathologies and acute complications. Among these are chorda tendinea rupture in the setting of AMI, acute heart failure, papillary muscle rupture, pericardial rub, aortic dissection that may cause AMI, Homans' sign suggesting DVT and/ or PE, and pneumothorax.

Pulses: While sinus tachycardia can be encountered in almost every cardiac and/or noncardiac emergency, bradycardia may be present especially in inferior wall ischemia with right coronary artery (RCA) occlusion. In some cases, bradycardia may occur with vagal stimulation triggered by the actual event. An audible S3 is very valuable as a sign of HF. Although not typically expected, one in 6 or 7 MI cases may have tenderness on palpation of the chest wall.

Clues to the secondary survey summarized by the words "look", "listen" and "feel" are given below:

Look

Inspection

Look for signs that indicate that the patient is being treated for heart disease. Scar tissues of cardiac surgery (*e.g.* sternal incision), pacemaker or nitrate patch are among these. It is also noted that conditions such as marked scoliosis, kyphoscoliosis, pectus excavatus may also lead to CP.

Skin Color

shows oxygenation of red blood cells, as well as pump function. Since vital organs will be protected as much as possible in pump failure, peripheral perfusion is sacrificed first. In advanced cases, a skin lesion called cutis marmoratus can be seen, which is a sign of severe shock or even prearrest. The petechiae may represent endocarditis, while red and hot skin may indicate sepsis.

Capillary Refill

The fingernails, kept at heart level, are pressed strongly for a few seconds and then released. If it takes more than 2 to 3 seconds for the healthy pink color to regain, it may be a sign of arterial circulatory failure or shock. If it takes over 4-5 seconds, it can be evaluated as advanced shock and pre-exitus. All these findings should be consistent with the general condition of the patient and accompanying pathologies.

Neck (jugular) Vein Distention (JVD)

Internal-external jugular veins are distended when central venous pressure increases, this is called JVD. The patient should be examined while sitting at an angle of 45 degrees, not lying flat. Evaluation can be difficult in obese, short-necked patients. In pump failure, backward pressure increase in the systemic circulation and JVD occur. On the other hand, significant JVD may not be seen in hypovolemic patients despite presence of CHF.

Peripheral/Presacral Edema

It suggests right heart failure and/or some kidney diseases. Peripheral and presacral edema occurs due to chronic backward pressure in the systemic circulation. It is more prominent in the ankles and pretibial area. When investigating edema in bedridden patients, the presacral region should be particularly examined and palpated. It is generally classified as mild or pitting edema. For this separation, the edematous area is pressed tightly. If there is a significant depression when we pull our finger, it is considered as pitting edema. Edema seen in hypothyroidism or hypoproteinemia caused by nephrotic syndrome is not a "pitting" one.

Listen

Breathing Sounds

Lung areas should be auscultated regarding equal aeration and pathological sounds (rales, wheezing, rhonchi) that are signs of pulmonary congestion and/or bronchospasm.

Pearl: Although most physicians suppose that rales = HF; wheezing = asthma; rhonchus = pneumonia or COPD, there is not always a one-to-one relationship. For example, all three can be found in COPD, both rales and wheezing can be heard in HF, and even wheezing may be dominant in a patient with pulmonary edema. In cases of severe asthma, "silent chest", in which a typical wheezing cannot be heard, is an ominous finding reflecting very severe attack.

Heart Sounds

While S1 and S2 are normal sounds, S3 (gallop rhythm) is heard in patients with CHF. Sometimes, with a careful examination, the fourth heart sound called S4 can be heard just before S1. S4 is found in increased atrial contraction, *e.g.* left ventricular hypertrophy due to chronic hypertension.

Carotid Artery Murmur

Murmur is the sound of turbulence, fluctuation, vortexing of blood passing through a vessel. Murmur indicates that the vessel is partially occluded, the most common cause of which is atherosclerotic plaques. If the patient has a newly emerged carotid murmur, for example, in cases of supraventricular tachycardia, massaging the carotid artery is contraindicated. However, it can be disregarded because it is not a sensitive examination method in chaotic and noisy environments in the ED or ICU.

Abdominal Auscultation and Palpation

In cases of DAA and AAA that may be confused with or accompanying ACS, a *de novo* murmur may be heard in the abdomen or a markedly pulsating mass may be palpated. If there is such a suspicion in routine palpation, it should be investigated by avoiding brutal movements and repeat palpation because one can cause the rupture of the structure by escalating the intra-aortic pressure.

Feel

Pulse

Look at the rate and regularity of the pulse. It is also important that the pulses are equal on both sides/four limbs (both arms and both legs). The unequal pulses on both sides suggests underlying peripheral vascular disease or aortic disease. Since angina pectoris may be together with dysrhythmias triggered by ischemia, it is important to note the rhythm disturbance.

Pulse Deficit

Pulse Deficitis the difference between the pulse rate elicited from the patient's peripheral artery and that of the cardiac apex, which is most recorded in atrial fibrillation.

Pulsus Alternans

The force of a beat hitting our finger that changes from beat to beat, typically heard in pericardial tamponade.

Pulsus Parvus Et Tardus

It is the type of heartbeats that feel weak and late in those with aortic stenosis.

Skin

Various skin changes can occur in cardiovascular disease. Pale, sweaty skin shows peripheral vascular constriction and sympathetic stimuli. This can be seen in heart disease or some other conditions such as GI hemorrhage, mechanical bowel obstruction (blood or fluid losses, shocky states). A mottled, rash appearance is often a sign of chronic heart failure and, in advanced cases, cardiogenic shock.

Clubbing

It is seen in patients with chronic heart failure, lung cancer or COPD. It occurs because of chronic hypoxemia (Fig. **2**).

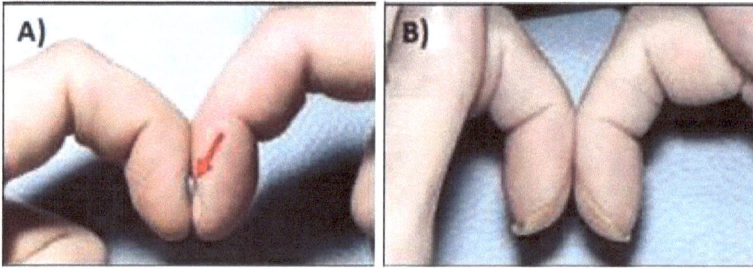

Fig. (2). Clubbing is one of the specific findings indicating chronic hypoxemia.

ECG: Key Points

The ECG, which is required to be obtained and interpreted in the first 10 minutes in most guidelines, is one of the most important tools in the diagnosis of ACS/AMI. ECG provides vital information not only for ischemic changes, but also for many different issues such as rhythm disturbances, electrolyte imbalance, pacemaker dysfunction and valve diseases. Additional information such as the extent of infarct tissue and the axis of the heart can be obtained from the ECG trace. One of the important points here is that a single ECG taken should not be considered sufficient in establishing the diagnosis of the patient and ruling out life-threatening diagnoses. For example, in a case presenting with CP, the sensitivity of the first ECG in detection of AMI is around 40-60%, when the same patient is followed up with repeated ECG scans within hours, this rate can reach up to 95%. For this reason, we should learn to say, "I took the first ECG which seems normal", not "There's nothing abnormal with the patient's ECG" and that this is the beginning of a realistic follow-up.

Pearl: Requirements for the diagnosis of STEMI:

De novo ST elevation; In at least two consecutive leads from the J point in V2 – V3 ≥2 mm (0.2 mV) in men or ≥1.5 mm (0.15 mV) in women; ≥1 mm (0.1 mV) in other precordial and consecutive limb leads

Treatment

Patients with angina pectoris are often in fear of a catastrophe (*angor animi*). In order to reduce the myocardial oxygen requirement, it is necessary to put the patient in a state of rest, both physically and emotionally (Table **5**).

Table 5. Maneuvers and drugs recommended during the initial management.

A B C
- Safety circle: Continuous rhythm monitoring, wide-bore (12-16 G) and bilateral vascular access, oxygen supply (if SpO_2 <94%)
- 12-lead ECG (should be taken and interpreted in the first 10 minutes)
- Acetyl salicylic acid *; 165 to 325 mg PO
- Pain relief - Morphine Sulphate* 3 to 5 mg IV
- Antiischemic therapy: Beta blockade – Metoprolol* 5 to 15 mg IV

* Drugs are administered unless there are contraindications.

High-flow Nasal Oxygen Therapy (HFNOT)

HFNOT can be given to increase the oxygen delivery in the myocardium. However, since many studies in recent years have shown that excessive oxygenation is not beneficial but harmful, it should be administered with caution.

Nitroglycerin

Reduces the work of the myocardium while dilating the coronary arteries to a lesser extent. If the pain does not go away with one or two doses of nitroglycerin, you should consider that this may not be a "simple/stable angina pectoris", but a more serious event such as AMI or USAP.

Beta blockers are also among the main agents known to improve prognosis in non-AMI ACS. Agents such as metoprolol, atenolol, acebutolol can be chosen. It is recommended to start oral treatment within the first 24 hours, as the intravenous route has no distinct advantage. It is one of the agents that do not need to be given within the first hour in new guidelines. It can be administered *via* nasogastric tube in unconscious, intubated patients. These agents should be avoided in those with hypotension, marked bradycardia, shock state, decompensated CHF, and Raynaud's phenomenon. Although the history of asthma is not an absolute contraindication, it should be given carefully in selected patients with asthma. Sildenafil and derivatives can cause uncontrollable hypotension and vasodilation especially when used in conjunction with nitrates. Therefore, every middle-aged and elderly men should be questioned about consumption of these agents in the recent two or three days before administration of nitrates.

Acute Myocardial Infarction (AMI)

It is estimated that the number of people who died due to AMI in 2013 in the world is 8.5 million. It is one of the most common causes of death.

AMI is the death of a part of the muscle tissue as a result of long-term insufficiency of arterial blood flow to the myocardial cells. AMI is most commonly associated with atherosclerotic heart disease. The initiation of the event is the occlusion of the already atherosclerotic vessel with thrombus. Other predisposing factors of AMI; hypoglycemia, hypovolemia (GI bleeding), trauma, burns, coronary artery spasm, microembolism, acute volume overload, hypotension and acute hypoxia.

The location and size of AMI depends on the artery involved and the location of the occlusion. Most infarcts involve the left ventricle. Occlusion of the left coronary artery leads to an anterior, lateral or septal infarction. Inferior wall infarction occurs with occlusion of the right coronary artery. Infarctions are usually divided into transmural or subendocardial. In ST elevation-transmural infarctions (STEMI) all layers of the myocardium are damaged. It is also called "Q wave infarction" because it is seen together with apparent Q waves on the ECG. In non-ST elevation infarctions (NSTEMI) only the subendocardial layer is damaged. Since Q waves are not seen in ECG, it was previously called non-Q wave infarction.

Tissues affected by AMI are damaged to varying degrees. If the obstruction is not eliminated and collateral circulation is insufficient, it causes tissue ischemia, infarction and death. Dead tissue turns into scar tissue over time. Dead myocardium is surrounded by ischemic tissue. This tissue can survive through collateral circulation. This ischemic tissue is often the source of dysrhythmias.

Among the many complications of AMI, dysrhythmias are the most common. Life-threatening dysrhythmias can occur immediately and cause death within a short time from the onset of symptoms, this is called sudden cardiac death (SCD). SCD is the most common form of death caused by AMI. By definition, death occurs within one hour after the onset of symptoms in cases with sudden cardiac death and within 24 hours in cases not witnessed. 60% of all cardiovascular deaths are in this class, so it can be the most common form of death in the world (Adabag, 2010).

Congestive Heart Failure

May also occur due to myocardial damage. The patient may have right HF, left HF, or both - global insufficiency. HF occurs when the pump ability of the heart has been damaged but is able to meet the body's basic needs. If the heart cannot meet the body's basic oxygen demand, inadequate tissue perfusion occurs, leading to cardiogenic shock. The heart is ineffective and inadequate in cardiogenic shock, leading to both hypotension and respiratory failure.

Another cause of death in AMI is ventricular aneurysm in the myocardial wall. The damaged part of the wall is weakened. Sometimes a tear can occur here, which can also cause SCD.

Signs and Symptoms

The most common complaint of AMI is pain under the sternum or epigastrium. The nature or description of the pain is usually completely resembling "stable" angina pectoris. The pain can be severe and often expressed as constricting, sometimes mild. It mostly spreads to shoulders, arms, neck, chin or back. Contrary to stable angina, the pain can begin while resting, and does not relieve with rest. It does not improve with sublingual (SL) nitrates and other simple treatments. Often, morphine or IV nitrates are required for pain relief. Some MI patients, especially the elderly and diabetics, may not feel chest pain at all. Instead, they may complain of shoulder, arm, neck, jaw or back pain. Some MI patients have no pain or complaints. The diagnosis of MI in these patients is established by ECG changes and the level of cardiac enzymes. Some patients with MI can experience adjunctive symptoms (those apart from chest pain) which can distract the physician from the essential diagnosis of ACS (Table **6**). On the other hand, some elements in the history can increase the likelihood of AMI as opposed to other diagnoses (Table **7**).

Table 6. Other symptoms commonly seen in patients with MI (apart from chest pain).

sweating
feeling of distress and fear- *angor animi*
dyspnea and air hunger, orthopnea
nausea and vomiting, hiccups,
indigestion, loss of appetite
paleness
altered mental status, dizziness
general weakness, fatigue.

Table 7. Some elements in the history that increase the likelihood of AMI.

Pain spreads to the right arm or shoulder
It spreads to both arms or shoulders
Pain is related to effort
It spreads to the left arm
Pain is accompanied by sweating, nausea or vomiting

(Table 7) cont.....

Pain is more severe than previous angina or looks like previous AMI
It is defined as pressure

Some patients, especially the elderly and those with diabetes or kidney failure may not have pain at all. Autonomic neuropathy, debility, and inadequate function of neurons are the reasons for this. Instead, there is a history of dyspnea, general malaise, illness or syncope. Besides, many AMI patients underestimate their condition. For this reason, some patients do not seek medical care in the first hours, which is the most critical time, and cell death occurs in the myocardium due to delay.

Vital signs in AMI depend on the pump damage in the patient and how severely the autonomic nervous system responds to the event. Blood pressure may be normal, increased or decreased due to pump failure and parasympathetic tone. Pulse rate varies depending on dysrhythmias. The pulse is fast or slow; regular or irregular; it can be weak or strong. Breathing may be normal or accelerated.

Dysrhythmias are the most common complication of myocardial infarction. Some dysrhythmias are the harbinger of life-threatening dysrhythmias and require emergent intervention. Life-threatening dysrhythmias such as ventricular fibrillation can lead to sudden death. Non-life-threatening dysrhythmias do not require intervention, they will resolve after treatment of the ACS.

All patients with CP should be admitted to the hospital and investigated thoroughly. All patients who complain of CP and have a compatible history should be considered as AMI until proven otherwise. Age and other factors are not helpful in differential diagnosis.

Approach to ACS in Pregnancy

Few patients with CP in pregnancy are associated with ACS. Pulmonary, GI, musculoskeletal causes are prominent. 6 AMIs are detected in 100,000 pregnancies, and the mortality rate is between 5% to 11%.

38% of pregnancy-related AMIs are seen in antepartum, 21% intrapartum, and 41% in postpartum 6 weeks. In pregnancy, it is accepted that last trimester pregnant women are at higher risk. Physiological anemia, increase in metabolic demand of the growing fetus and uterus, decrease in diastolic blood pressure, increase in stroke volume and pulse are the explanations. With the difficulty of all these factors in labor, the O_2 demand of the myocardium increases and the frequency of AMI increases. The flow of large amounts of blood from the uterus to the systemic circulation immediately after birth also creates an unprecedented stress on the myocardium, which underlies AMIs in the early puerperal period.

It was found that anterior coronary vessels were involved more than all others (69%). In a large autopsy study, coronary artery dissection was found in 28% of these patients, and thrombosis without atherosclerosis was recorded in 8%. Pregnancy-related hypercoagulability is also considered to play a role. It is known that vasospasm tendency increases during pregnancy.

Pearl: In addition to coronary risk factors for ACS in pregnant women, eclampsia-preeclampsia, anemia, migraine and thrombophilia increase the risk of ACS in pregnancy.

Although there are no fundamental differences in management compared to other ACS/AMI patients, certain points should be known. Of AMIs in pregnancy, ¾ are STEMI and ¼ are NSTEMI. There are also studies that give different rates.

Pearl: Since the radiation dose given during coronary angiography and PCI will remain within safe limits (<5 rad) during pregnancy, it is not harmful in the presence of indication.

A Cochrane review suggested that the use of beta blockers for continuous hypertension control during pregnancy may lead to low birth weight, but the results were controversial. The use of ASA is also controversial because it has been associated with some malformations. Chronic and high dose ASA use is harmful.

Pearl: Heparinization can be administered safely in pregnancy. However, it is recommended to stop just before labor. There are reservations about nitroglycerin infusion. Nitrates can be left to the back of queue in the treatment of ischemia, as they can lead to hypotension and uterine malperfusion. Metoprolol administration is generally considered safe. Low-dose ASA appears to be safe compared to other antiplatelet agents.

ACE inhibitors and ARBs are contraindicated during pregnancy. Statins should also be avoided as they are Class X. There is no fundamental difference in invasive interventions and PCI. Data are safer and more positive for bare metal stents. Since it will require clopidogrel for a long time after DESs, it should be avoided. The most important point here is to evaluate the risks to be taken in terms of urgent and vital treatments required by the clinical condition of the patient and teratogenicity.

A. Approach Steps to the Patient with Chest Pain in Nature/Outdoor Activities

Should be planned emergently by lay rescuers or professionals on the scene, if available. Austere conditions will definitely restrict the capabilities of the rescuer, but basic principles should be followed (Table **8**).

Table 8. Steps to be taken in case of a patient with chest pain in nature/outdoor activities.

1. To oxygenate/bring to fresh air, loosening clothes
2. Calling 911 to explain the situation and ask for help (none of the other interventions should delay seeking help).
3. To learn about medications (aspirin, nitroglycerin) and allergies, previous heart disease history
4. Understanding pulse and respiratory rate and regularity, consciousness as much as possible. Checking blood pressure with a manual sphygmomanometer, if available. Applications on some smartphones detect and report them.
5. To get information about chest pain, to note additional symptoms such as nausea, pallor of the skin, cold sweat, loss of appetite.
6. Since similar findings can be seen with the decrease in blood sugar level (hypoglycemia) in diabetic patients, to measure blood sugar if it is easily accessible. If the level is below 60 mg/dL, 100-200 mL of sugar in water can be given to conscious patients.
7. Keeping the patient in the most comfortable position, preventing additional movement (walking, *etc.*)
8. Talking to the patient in a calming way, reducing excitement
9. Administering nitroglycerin in tablet or spray form sublingually, if available. It should not be tried more than 3 times, it may cause excessive drop in blood pressure. Intake of sildenafil and similar (Viagra and equivalents) within the last 48 hours prior to administration in men should be ruled out.
10. If there is a health center nearby, a 12-lead ECG should be obtained.

B. Prehospital Approach To The Patient Suspected of ACS (911/112)

For the patient with AMI, prehospital intervention is as important as the distinction between life and death. Approximately half of the patients who die after AMI die within the first hour, in the prehospital period.

Pre-hospital Intervention Aims

- To prevent pain and fear, to give the most comfortable position
- To reverse severe dysrhythmias
- To manage acute heart failure
- To limit the infarct size - inhibit its growth
- If pre-diagnosis ACS is to be transferred to a center with a catheter laboratory, contact EMS command control center (CCC).

• To initiate thrombolytic therapy if the transport time will be long.

Time is the main factor. Complete the primary survey quickly and start the secondary survey. Take the focused medical history during the physical exam whilst starting treatment. The patient should be in the position he/she is comfortable with, ideally with his head raised by 30 degrees. Make reassuring statements to the patient. This will reduce anxiety and fear, and reduce heart rate and oxygen utilization of the myocardium. Do not let the patient stand up or walk.

Pearl: SpO$_2$ below 94%, start supplemental O$_2$ in dyspneic and tachypneic patient without known COPD diagnosis. Give high flow oxygen to patients with clear indication to start.

Supplemental O$_2$

May limit infarct size by increasing myocardial oxygen delivery. Vital signs should be repeated at frequent intervals. Establish a wide vascular access as early as possible and keep the vascular access open. Stick the ECG electrodes and take the first ECG. Cardiac monitoring should continue throughout the entire examination and transport. Record dysrhythmias and add to patient report. Complete the exam, including history and lung auscultation. Audible rales in lung bases are an early harbinger of HF.

Give medication according to written protocols after evaluating the patient. Usually prescribed medications for pain;

Nitroglycerin

It reduces preload, afterload and myocardial oxygen consumption by dilating peripheral arteries and veins. By expanding the coronary arteries, collateral vessels increase blood flow. One can mostly distinguish angina pectoris and myocardial infarction by administering nitroglycerin. AMI symptoms usually do not go away with nitroglycerin. It should not be administered in men without taking a history of sildenafil. Should be avoided in case of persistent bradycardia and hypotension.

Morphine Sulfate

It reduces myocardial oxygen requirement by reducing venous return to the heart (preload) and systemic arterial resistance (afterload). It relieves pain also by directly affecting the central nervous system. Morphine also reduces myocardial oxygen requirement in this way by preventing sympathetic discharge of the nervous system.

Beta Blockers

(By asking CCC): Metoprolol, which selectively blocks beta-1 receptors, has a mortality-reducing effect. It should be avoided in patients with hypotension, bradycardia, decompensated HF, asthma and peripheral artery disease.

Nitrous Oxide

It is useful to give a mixture of nitrous oxide and oxygen in a certain ratio in the treatment of ACS/AMI. It is a fixed combination of nitrous oxide and oxygen in 1/1 ratio. 50% oxygen will be given with this. It has a pure analgesic effect without affecting hemodynamics. The effect ends after 2-5 minutes after stopping the administration.

Benzodiazepines (Diazepam, Midazolam)

May be given if the patient is extremely distressed and agitated. It is not an analgesic, instead, it only helps to relax the patient. When morphine is given, diazepam may not be needed in most cases. Intramuscular administration should not be performed.

Lidocaine

It is the drug of choice in most situations for ventricular dysrhythmias with pulse. It is effective in most dysrhythmias associated with AMI. It has approximately similar potency to amiodarone.

Procainamide

It can be used in dysrhythmias unresponsive to lidocaine or in patients allergic to lidocaine.

Atropine Sulphate

It is parasympatholytic and is especially recommended for sinus bradycardia. Caution should be exercised and avoided as much as possible in ACS and AMI. It is not effective in transplanted and denervated heart. An effect should not be expected in total AV block, either.

Epinephrine (Adrenaline)

Used in the case of cardiovascular collapse and life-threatening dysrhythmias such as ventricular fibrillation and asystole.

Adenosine

It is useful to stop symptomatic supraventricular tachyarrhythmias, especially PSVT. In recent guidelines, it is also recommended as the first line treatment in tachycardias with wide QRS.

Verapamil

It is used in supraventricular tachyarrhythmias, especially when increased heart rate decreases cardiac output. Its effect triggering AV block is more pronounced than diltiazem. Its use should be avoided in the case of CP/ACS.

Diltiazem

Used in supraventricular tachyarrhythmias. Since its side effects are not as severe and severe as verapamil, it is increasingly preferred.

How was the EMS Management of ACS Changed in The COVID-19 Era?

It was changed substantially. For example, in the very heart of the outbreak in the first months of 2020, Lombardy, Italy modified the regional network concerning time-dependent emergencies, including ACS (Carugo S, *et al*. 2020). Specifically, 13 Macro-Hubs were identified to deliver timely optimal care to patients with ACS (Fig. **3**).

They concluded that the redefinition of ACS network according to enlarged Macro-Hubs allowed to continue with timely ACS management, while reserving a high number of intensive care beds for the pandemic. Patients with ACS and COVID-19 presented a worst outcome, particularly in case of STEMI.

Thrombolytic Therapy in the Field

It has been shown that the thrombolytic administration initiated by a doctor or paramedic in the field is safe and effective, and does not increase complications. It has been shown in the field that the combination of tissue plasminogen activator (t-PA) infusion or single dose thrombolytic (tenecteplase) and low molecular weight heparin facilitates reperfusion and improves AMI outcomes. This combination has been routinely recommended for the pharmacological reperfusion treatment of AMI in the pre-hospital period.

Studies have shown that Tenecteplase treatment (6000-10.000 U) is beneficial and effective in submassive and massive PE which are the other major causes of sudden collapse of a patient.

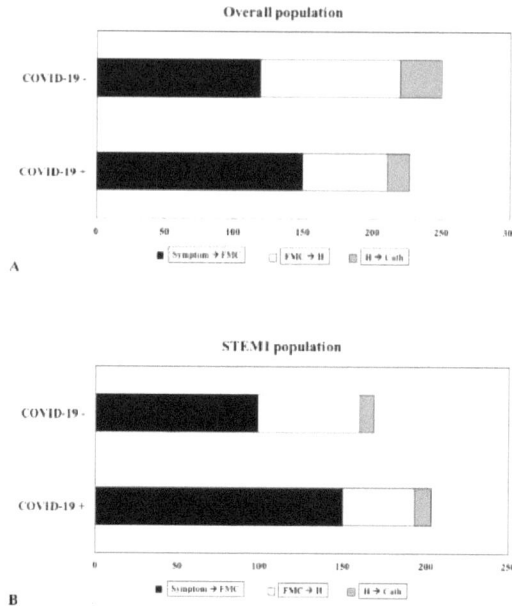

Fig. (3). The time interval from FMC to CCL was significantly shorter in patients with COVID-19, both in the overall population and in STEMI patients (87 (IQR 41–310) *versus* 160 (IQR 67–1220) minutes, P = 0.001, and 61 (IQR 23–98) *versus* 80 (IQR 47–126) minutes, P = 0.01, respectively). In-hospital mortality and cardiogenic shock rates were higher among patients with COVID-19 than those without (32% *vs* 6%, P < 0.0001, and 16.8% *vs* 6.7%, P < 0.0003, respectively).

Reperfusion is critical in treating patients with AMI. The Door-to-Drug range can be shortened by taking ECG in the field, recognizing that the pain represents the high-risk ischemic CP with a short targeted history, providing the contraindications and indications of fibrinolytic therapy with history, and using CP checklists (Table **9**).

Table 9. Requirements for thrombolytic administration by paramedics in the field.

1. 12-lead ECG
2. Sending the ECG to the command control center, to a physician authorized in this regard.
3. Completing the reperfusion checklist-excluding contraindications
4. Standard STEMI drug therapy (nitrate, ASA, O_2, heparin *etc.*)
5. Destination plan (which hospital to go to?)
6. Quality improvement plan
7. Developing common policies with the participation of all parties (accepting hospital, community stakeholders and caregivers)

In the Cochrane review and meta-analysis published by McCaul *et al.* in 2014, it was revealed that prehospital thrombolytic administration saves time and provides more effective treatment. Nevertheless, it was stated that this decision should be made by taking local characteristics into consideration.

SUMMARY: Important points in approaching a patient with chest pain in the field/hospital are summarized in Table **10**.

Table 10. Important steps in approaching a patient with chest pain in the field and/or early hospital period.

1- Recognizing acute ischemic CP and providing information before arriving at the hospital
2- Taking history about CP,
3- Providing ECG (12-lead) and sending ECG to the hospital *via* fax or other means
4- To evaluate the patient's conditions for fibrinolytic therapy
5- Venous access,
6- Recording vital signs and pulse O_2 saturation
7- Administering O_2: Hypoxia and respiratory failure may worsen the existing coronary occlusion in these patients.
8- Starting MONA-B treatment - Oxygen 4 L/min - Nitroglycerin (before starting the infusion of men should be asked sildenafil use, if any doubt should not be infused) 0.4 mg SL or spray (a 2-5 minutes, repeated 3 times, improvement or IV should be initiated at a dose 10-20 mg/min) ® (Perlinganit 10 mg ampoule) can be titrated (repeatable) according to the result after 2 mg IV push - Morphine 2-4 mg IV can be given every 5-15 minutes. - Aspirin 160-325 mg PO will be chewed and swallowed with water. - If ischemic pain is suspected, the beta-blocking agent metoprolol 5 mg IV can be given in 2 minutes and a total of 15 mg every 5 minutes.
9- To record the initial rhythm and to recognize it early, to start the treatment of arrhythmias (esp. VF/VT)
10- To apply transcutaneous pads for transcutaneous pacing in patients with symptomatic sinus bradycardia or high-grade AV block.
11- Decide with the emergency medicine or cardiology specialist for primary PTCA or fibrinolytic and transport the patient to the suitable institution. If the transport time will exceed 60 minutes, to start fibrinolytic treatment with the appropriate protocol.

In brief, it will be for the benefit of the patient and the society if the necessary interventions are performed by paramedics in the ambulance or in the field as soon as possible so that the prolonged transport time does not cause delay in effective treatment. Necessary interventions should be performed in the most accurate and fastest way in coordination with the CCC, including thrombolytic administration.

C. Approach to the Patient with ACS in the Hospital

ACS/AMI is often diagnosed in the hospital with typical CP complaints, ECG changes and changes in enzyme levels.

With 12-lead ECG, it is tried to understand whether the patient has had ACS/AMI, its location and severity (ST Segment Elevated Myocardial Infarction -STEMI or NSTEMI). ECG is not a perfect test in this regard. In the first 24 hours, only 60% of the patients are diagnosed with AMI *via* ECG, 25% of them are non-specific and 15% are normal. When ECG serial monitoring is done, the accuracy rate rises to 95%, but it can never reach 100% in demonstrating ACS.

Pearl: ECG provides vital information for ACS, but AMI can never be ruled out by looking at the ECG. It just becomes less likely.

It is known that AMI cases are missed by 2-5% in the world. This situation is independent from the physician branch. Considering that "typical" cases are seen only 5% of all cases, this is not very surprising. Ultimately, the clinician should prepare himself for the "deceptive, atypical" phenomenon, not the "book-like" phenomenon.

Pearl: It has been demonstrated that women, very young and old cases, cases with autonomic neuropathy due to diabetes and renal failure are more often missed or misdiagnosed. The fact that they present with atypical complaints and findings also has a role in this. Serial ECG monitoring, careful evaluation of the clinical situation, correct interpretation of enzymes, and requesting consultation at the required point will minimize the risk of overlooking ACS/AMI.

Determination of the ACS subtype; It is important for the correct planning of emergency treatment.

There are 4 subtypes of ACS:

STEMI

ST elevation or newly developed left bundle branch block (LBBB) is detected in the ECG of a patient presenting with typical complaints. In the presence of these two criteria, it is not necessary to wait for cardiac enzyme results in order to initiate emergency medical and interventional treatment.

NSTEMI

Patients with significant increases in cardiac enzymes but no diagnostic ECG findings are defined as NSTEMI and are monitored and treated accordingly.

Unstable Angina Pectoris (USAP)

These are conditions without specific ECG findings, no cardiac enzyme elevation, but due to the character of the pain, they are monitored and treated in the ACS category. Diagnosis is mostly empirical and made clinically.

Sudden Cardiac Death

Death due to ACS and its complications in a previously undiagnosed patient, within 1 hour if witnessed after the onset of symptoms, and within 24 hours if not known or unknown.

Is additional testing required in the diagnosis of ACS?

Both yes and no. Yes, additional tests are required for both exclusion of differential diagnoses, how ACS damages the myocardium, how myocardial dysfunction will affect the prognosis, and technical preparations of the intervention (such as stent, by-pass surgery). However, typical pain, history characteristics, risk factors, vital and other physical examination findings make us very close to a pre-diagnosis to consider ACS in a patient.

Pearl: Until proven otherwise, the patient with a presumptive diagnosis of ACS is ACS and should be treated accordingly.

How about ACS?

Chronic stable angina pectoris (SAP) is one of the most common chronic diseases in the world and is the first among coronary artery diseases. Basically, it is known that oxygen delivery in the myocardium enters a negative balance with the onset of atherosclerotic heart disease in the very young, for example in the 20s (Table **11**) (Fig. **4**).

Table 11. The main factors determining myocardial oxygen delivery in chronic stable angina pectoris (SAP) are.

Arterial oxygen content
Coronary blood flow
Coronary perfusion pressure
Perfusion time
Degree of coronary artery stenosis

(Table 11) cont.....

| Coronary vascular resistance |
| Coronary sinus venous pressure |
| Ventricular diastolic pressure |
| Coronary collateral blood flow |

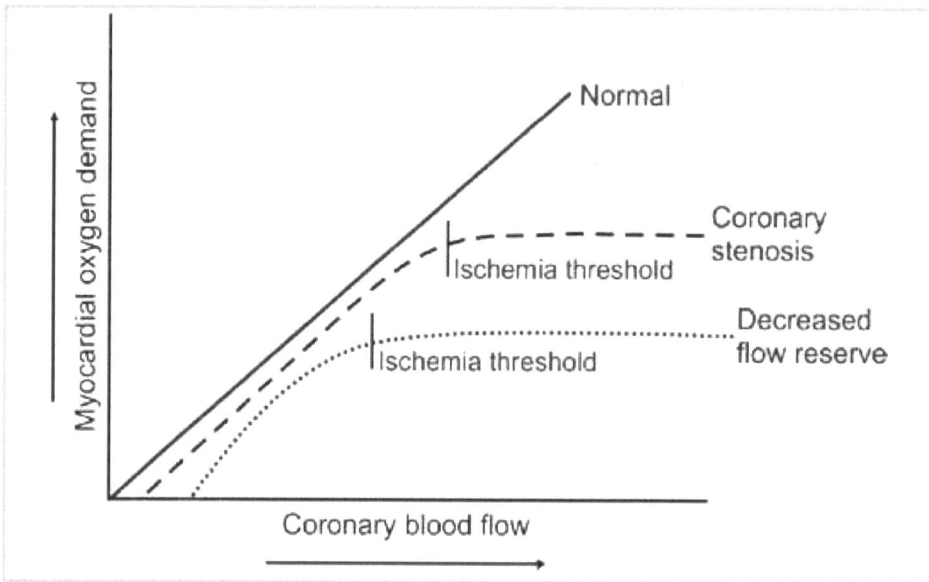

Fig. (4). Coronary blood flow occurs primarily in diastole. Aortic diastolic pressure is the perfusion pressure and is the most important determinant of coronary blood flow and left ventricular myocardial perfusion.

Laboratory Markers of ACS

ECG

Patients with symptoms suggestive of AMI/ACS, known as CP or its equivalent, should have 12-lead ECGs taken within 10 minutes and interpreted by an emergency medicine specialist or cardiologist.

In the initial ECGs of more than half of the ACS cases, the findings sought for ACS – *i.e.*, new ST segment elevation> 1 mm or new ST depression or T inversion in two adjacent leads - can be seen. Anyway, approximately one-fifth of a case may have an ECG with close to normal or barely noticeable findings.

It is thought that ECGs are frequently evaluated incorrectly or incompletely in the emergency setting, which leads to mismanagement and lawsuits. When examining why ECG is misjudged, the following points come to the fore:

- Missing the obvious changes of AMI.
- Failure to monitor/understand serial ECG changes.
- Failure to compare findings with previous ECGs.
- Ignoring non-specific ECG findings (ST-T changes).

The possibility of experiencing serious complications in the near-term future is negligible in cases whose first ECG is "normal" or similar to the old ECG and does not have clinically significant findings. However, those who have new ischemic findings in their first ECG carry a high risk in the short and long term.

In USAP cases, the sensitivity of the first ECG is even lower and should be evaluated clinically.

Pearl: The decision for AMI should not be established with a single ECG. A test with around 50% sensitivity cannot be used as a rule-out test. Serial ECGs taken within the first hours after the patient's presentation increase the sensitivity of the ECG in the diagnosis of AMI.

Figs. (**5** - **8**) give examples of different ECGs which can be encountered in patients with chest pain. The physician should keep a risk stratification in mind which should be readjusted and reborn with every specific patient, with special respect to evaluation of clinical presentation, history, signs and symptoms as a whole.

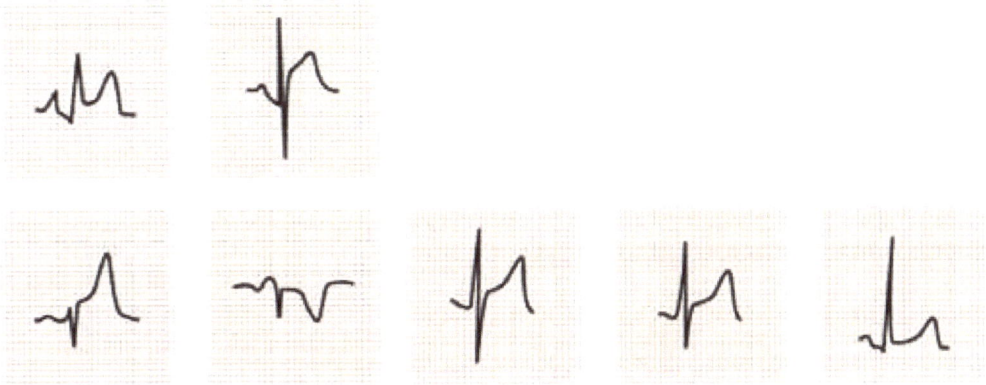

Fig. (5). Concave ST elevation with benign early repolarization. It is best seen on V4-V6.

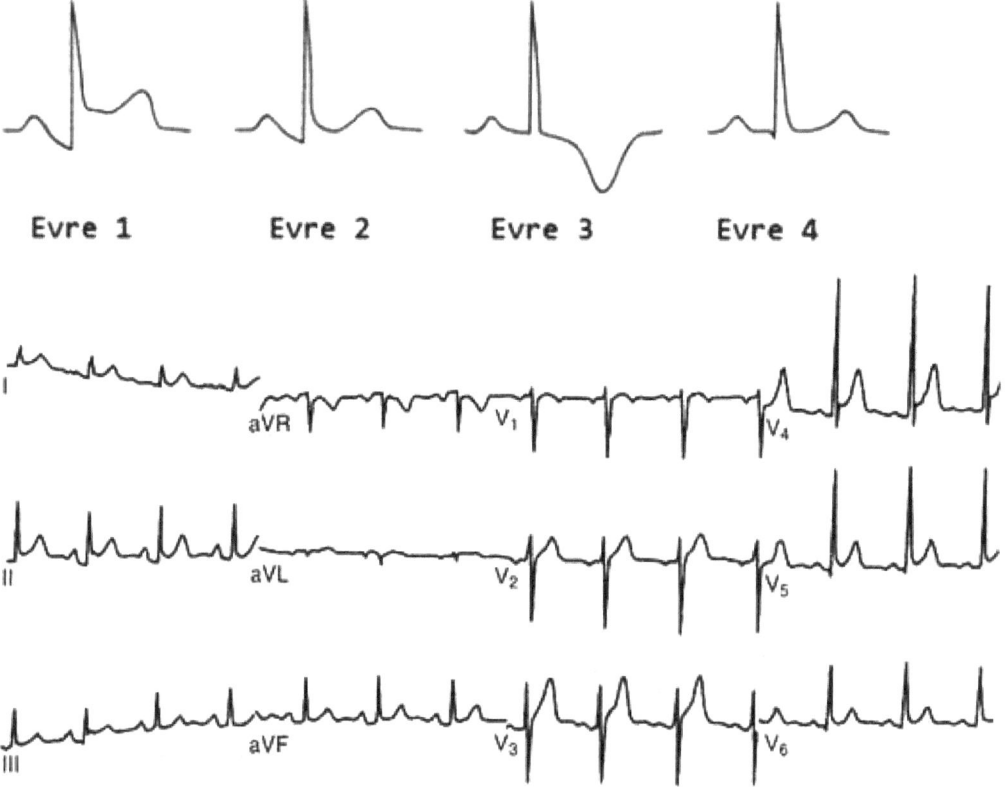

Fig. (6). ECG examples in different stages of acute pericarditis. PR depression may or may not be present with concave ST elevation.

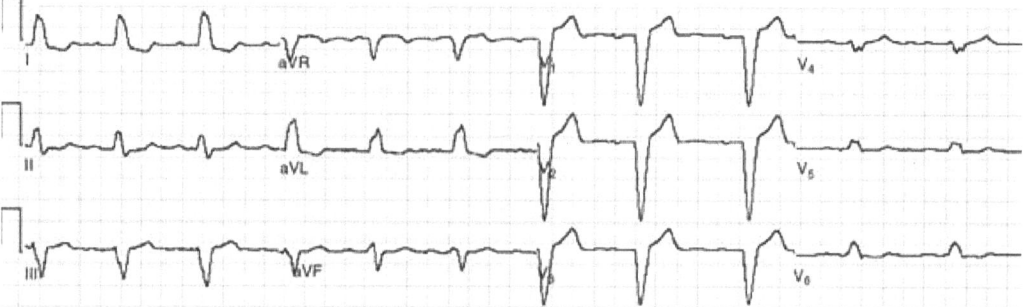

Fig. (7). Typical left bundle branch block (LBBB) appearance. Widened QRS, absence of Q wave in V6, wide monophasic R wave in lateral leads, discordant ST-T changes in anteroseptal, 1st degree AV block.

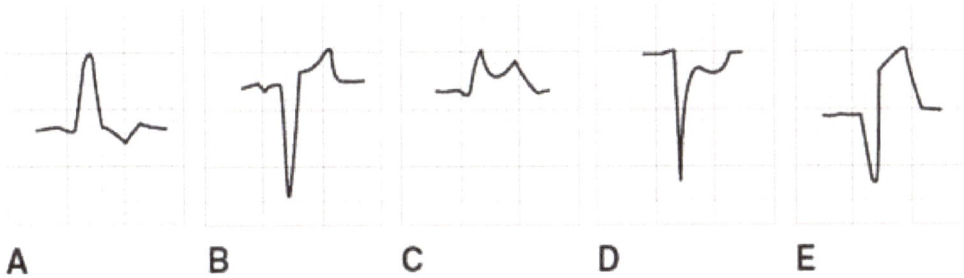

Fig. (8). In the case of LBBB, discordant and concordant ST elevation and depression. **A.** Discordant ST-segment depression (may be normal). **B.** Discordant ST-segment elevation (may be normal). **C.** concordant ST-segment elevation (suggestive of AMI). **D.** concordant ST-segment depression (suggestive of AMI). **E.** Excessive (> 5 mm) discordant ST-segment elevation (weakly suggestive of AMI).

Wellens Syndrome: It can be seen in LAD stenosis/occlusion. Although chest pain is frequently seen in patients with Wellens syndrome, it is also found in cases where chest pain is alleviated (Table **12**). Therefore, patients with Wellens syndrome or symptoms are at substantial risk for AMI (Fig. **9**).

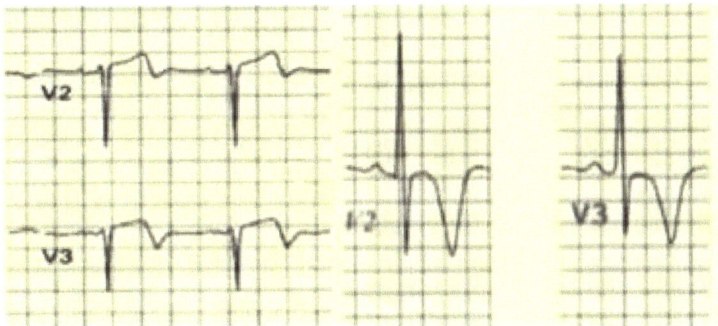

Fig. (9). Examples of Type A and B Wellens syndrome ECG. This finding is highly specific for LAD occlusion.

Table 12. Diagnostic criteria for Wellens Syndrome.

• History of CP attacks consistent with USAP
• T wave abnormalities accompanying pain +/-
• In the painless period, abnormal T waves are most prominent in V2 and V3, frequent in V1 and V4, and rarely in V5 and V6.
• Deep symmetrical T wave inversions are seen in DI and aVL in of the patients (Type B).
• Biphasic T waves are seen in 1/4 of the patients (Type A).
• No pathological Q waves or R loss
• Normal or minimal ST segment elevation
• Normal or minimal enzyme elevation

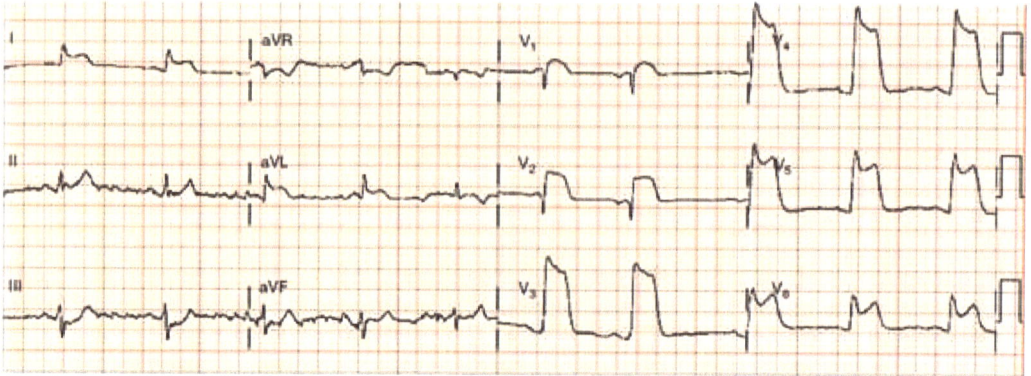

Fig. (10). Hyperacute diffuse anterior STEMI. Absence of Q waves in the anterolateral leads is of great chance for the patient. "Time is muscle" motto is intended for this patient. Immediate PCI must be performed within 120 minutes, if this cannot be done, fibrinolytics will benefit the heart muscle.

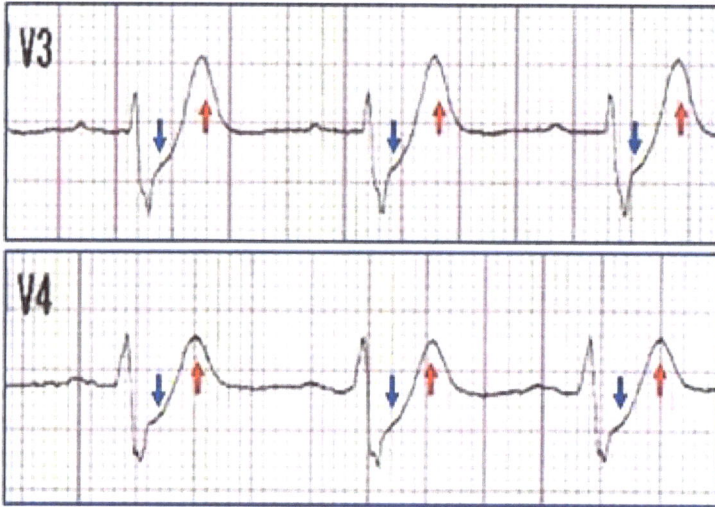

Fig. (11). De Winter waves: Evaluated as an early STEMI sign. Before ST elevation begins, sharp T waves, upslooping ST depression, ST elevation in aVR are seen.

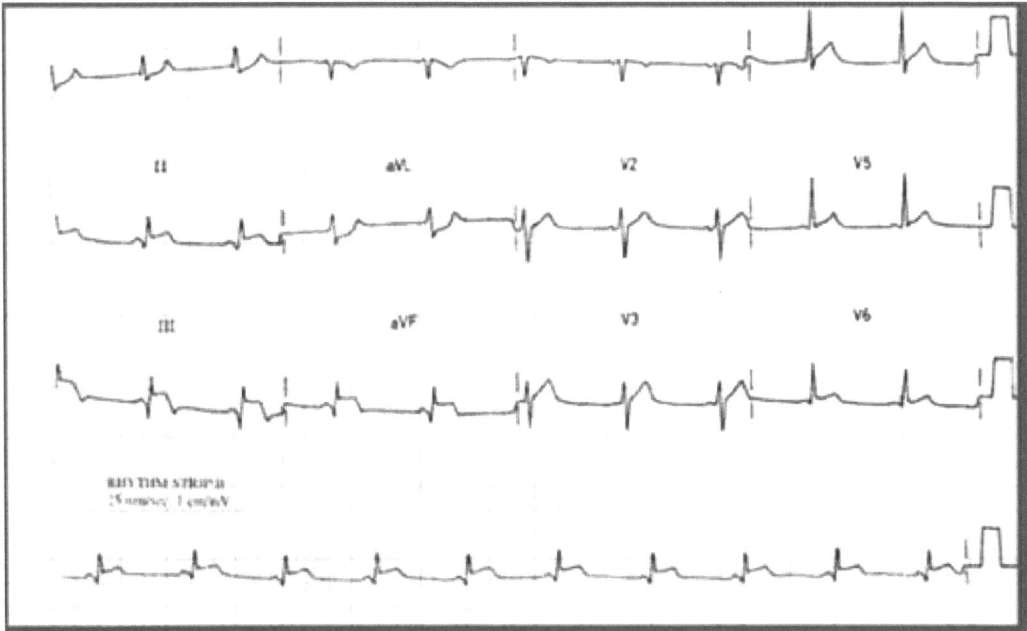

Fig. (12). The subacute period of AMI, in which the activity of the muscle cells that do not die together with the myocardial damage after passing the hyperacute phase is observed. Pathological Q waves and continuation of ST elevation are characteristic of this phase.

Left Main Coronary Artery Occlusion

ST elevation in aVR is a reliable finding indicative of ischemia involving the posterobasal face of the heart and the interventricular septum. It occurs with significant depression in DII, III, and aVF (Fig. **13**). Fig. (**14**) shows correct location of leads V7-9 on the patient's back.

Figs. (**10 - 13**) show examples of ECGs indicative of myocardial ischemia and/or infarction.

Exercise Test and Risk Assessment

The treadmill test is a valuable test performed for decades in the noninvasive work up of the presence of coronary artery disease, performed with the Bruce protocol. There are also examples of chest pain monitoring units in advanced centers and EDs that are operated in cooperation with emergency medicine and cardiology clinics.

The main principle of the test is to reduce the perfusion of the subendocardium with excessive blood flow to the striated muscles, thereby revealing the suboptimal blood flow and searching for its reflection on the ECG or clinical signs and symptoms.

The most important indication is to exclude the presence of CAD in stable patients with suspicious findings in the ECG or history.

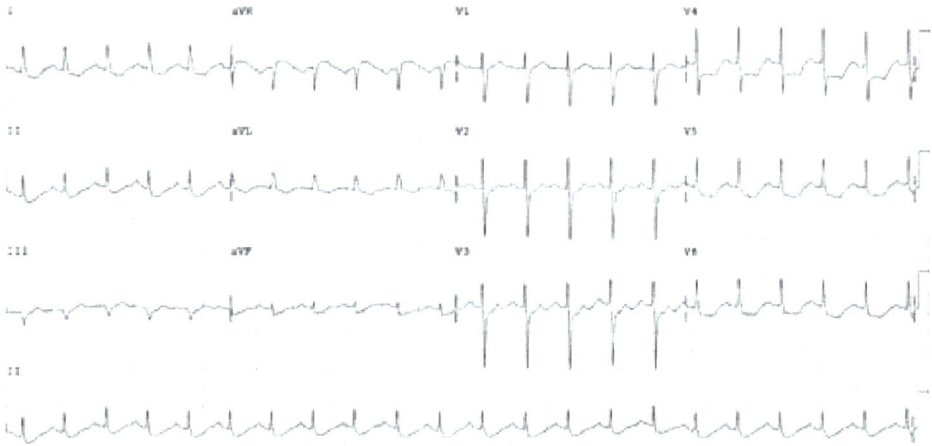

Fig. (13). ST elevation in aVR in a patient with myocardial ischemia.

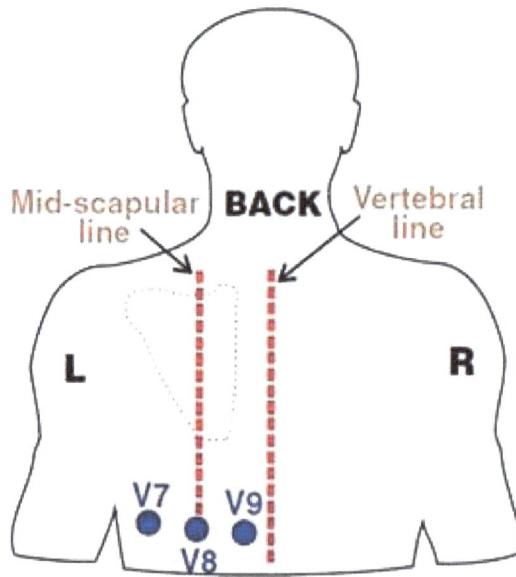

Fig. (14). Posterior leads (V7-9).

Interpretation

Almost all significant ECG changes occur in DI, V3-6. Typical ischemic response is downsloping ST depression greater than 1 mm. Such a response is sought in all leads except aVR. Slow upsloping depressions> = 1.5 mm) are also considered abnormal (Fig. **15**). The occurrence of left or right bundle branch block in treadmill exercise is often nonspecific.

Besides ECG findings, clinical conditions such as syncope, typical chest pain, shortness of breath, and extreme weakness precipitated by the exercise are considered positive.

False Positives

False positives are frequently recorded in those on digoxin therapy, those with previous LBBB or left ventricular hypertrophy.

Cardiac Enzymes

Cardiac enzymes are muscle enzymes released from damaged myocardial cells. Although the elevated cardiac enzyme level does not prove an ongoing AMI, it is suggestive of ACS. The enzymes that are usually worked up are troponins, creatine phosphokinase (CK-MB), Alanine aminotransferase (ALT or SGPT) and aspartate aminotransferase (AST or SGOT), and lactate dehydrogenase (LDH). However, since the specificities of LDH, AST and ALT are very low, their use has gradually decreased in recent decades. In recent years, it is known that levels of Brain Natriuretic Peptide (BNP), which is a substance released from ventricular myocytes in response to increased wall tension, rise in cardiovascular emergencies such as AMI, pulmonary embolism, and acute pulmonary edema. It appears to be a valuable marker in distinguishing heart failure and pulmonary disorders in routine clinical practice.

No intramuscular medication should be administered to the patient with suspected AMI because this can render muscle enzymes such as CK-MB to be released into the blood and rise the blood levels. This will hamper the diagnostic pathways.

Cardiac Troponins

Both troponin I and troponin T can be found in serum 2-4 hours following AMI. They reach peak levels in 12 hours and remains high for 7 - 10 days, so troponin is particularly useful for late presenters. Since troponin (I or T) is more cardiac specific than CK-MB, it is preferred in differentiating from striated muscle damage, recent surgery, trauma, muscle disease, or cocaine use.

Troponin elevation means a boost in complications and mortality compared to other patients, regardless of other criteria. Troponin elevation can also be detected in entities such as tachyarrhythmias, renal failure, pulmonary edema, ventricular hypertrophy, myopericarditis, APE, and sepsis/septic shock.

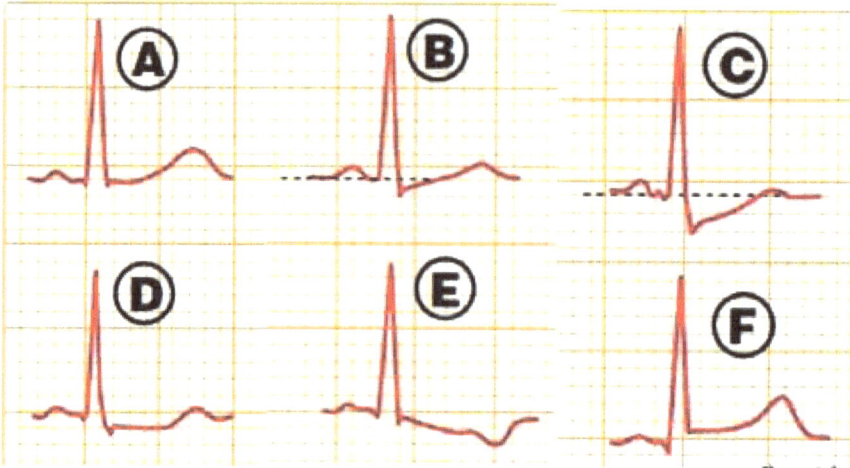

Fig. (15). Different ECGs and ST segment patterns occurring in exercise testing. **(A)** Normal **(B)** J point depression normalizes within 80 ms. **(C)** J point depression does not return to normal within 80 ms. **(D)** Horizontal ST depression **(E)** downsloping ST depression; **(F)** ST elevation.

The presumptive diagnosis of AMI should not be based solely on troponin elevation. Diagnosis is made if at least one of the following is present: ischemic complaints, *de novo* changes in ST and T waves, left bundle branch block, Q waves or signs of myocardial dysfunction, or newly emerged regional wall motion disorder.

There are important differences between Troponin I and troponin T tests. The proportion of those with high troponin T levels in patients with advanced renal failure is much higher than troponin I. Troponin values are interpreted in accord with the patient's clinical condition.

High-sensitive Cardiac Troponin T (hs-cTnT)

Its normal level is 14 ng/L. The pre-diagnosis of AMI is made when the values are above the 99th percentile of the reference population, along with supportive clinical situation and ECG findings. AMI is safely ruled out when values between 3 to 5 ng/L are obtained in a low-risk individual.

False positive results can be seen in chronic skeletal muscle disease. Hemolysis and antibodies against troponins cause a decrease in values.

Pearl Time Zero

hs-cTnT > 100 ng/L necessitates urgent cardiac evaluation and indicates high risk.

Delta TnT Value

Although some centers consider 1-hour changes, it is more appropriate to look at the 2-hour changes in a given patient. Delta> 10 ng/L makes the diagnosis more likely, while delta <4 ng/L in low risk patients may rule it out.

Rapid exclusion of AMI (Algorithm **3**, Fig. **16**) When hs-cTnT is used, AMI can be ruled out by:

- Gender-specific values below the 99th percentile (10 ng/L for women and 15 ng/L for men) (to be evaluated according to the kit and the local protocols)

- "Delta" value of 4 ng/L or less (patient's ECG should be integrated with history and risk scores).

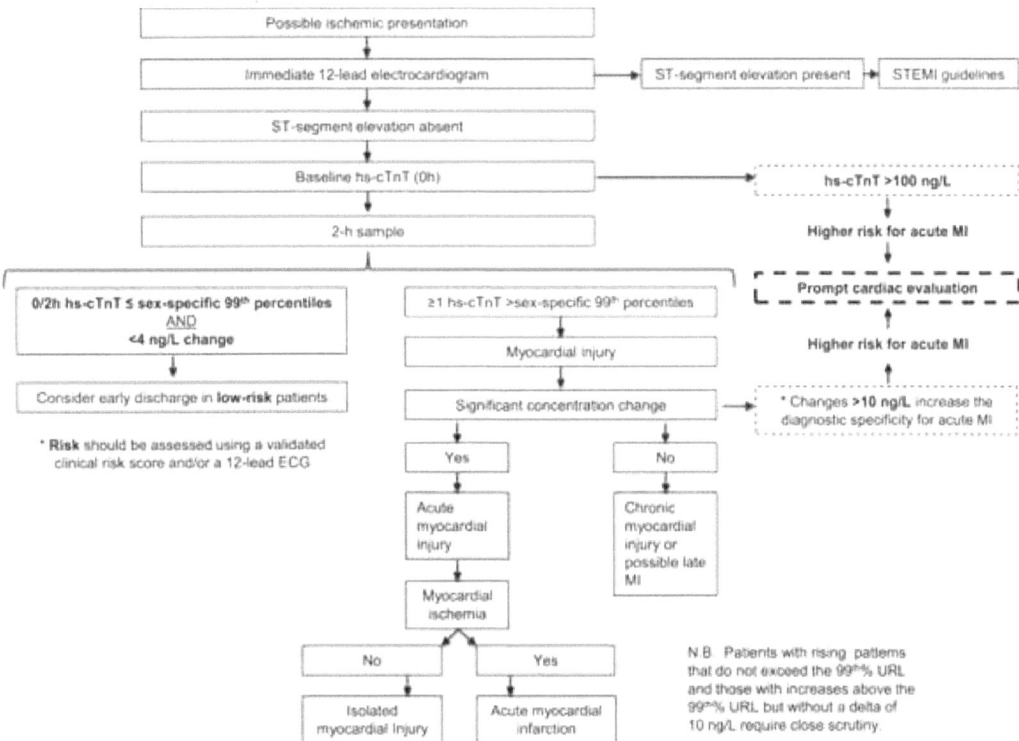

Algorithm 3. Based on ECG and hs-cTnT values in a patient with possible ischemia.

CK-MB is found more in the heart muscle. CK levels rise within 4-8 hours after the event triggering ACS, reach peak values within 16-24 hours and decrease in 4 days.

Serum myoglobin levels increase within 2-3 hours after AMI and remain high for 6-8 hours in most of the patients, peaking within 5-10 hours. Within a day, it drops back to its normal levels. It has a substantially high number of false positives, therefore, as a standard test, it is considered necessary in reinfarction research only in patients who are hospitalized with AMI diagnosis.

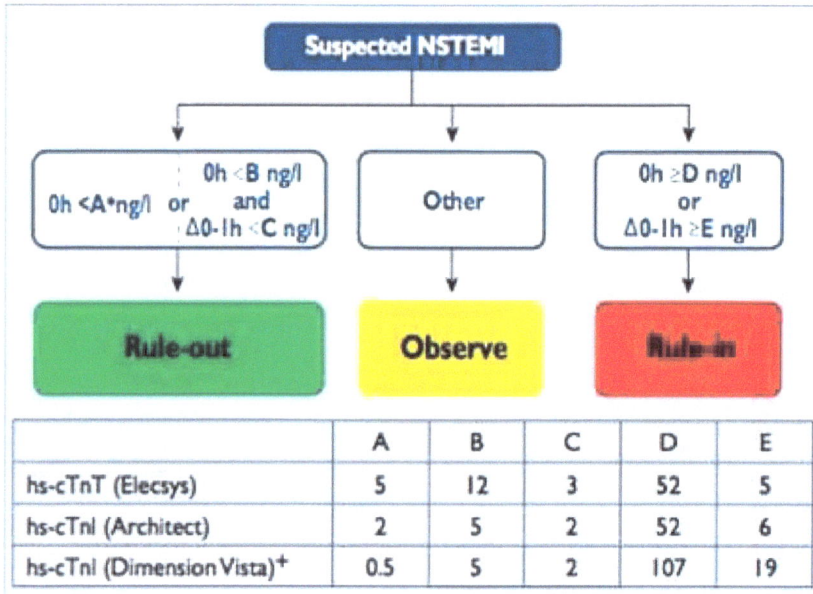

	A	B	C	D	E
hs-cTnT (Elecsys)	5	12	3	52	5
hs-cTnI (Architect)	2	5	2	52	6
hs-cTnI (Dimension Vista)+	0.5	5	2	107	19

Fig. (16). 0-1 hour rule in/rule out protocol.

B-type Natriuretic Peptide (BNP)

Represents the response of ventricular myocytes to increased wall tension and pressure loading and rises rapidly in the blood. Pro-BNP is secreted from ventricular myocytes. The half-life of BNP is about 20 minutes. The plasma half-life of NT-proBNP is 90 minutes and is excreted by the kidneys. BNP and NT-proBNP can be used in suspected ACS cases due to their high diagnostic and prognostic sensitivity. However, it is not a substitute for troponin in the diagnosis of ACS because its diagnostic accuracy is low.

ACS in The Elderly

ACS cases in the elderly present with more atypical presentations. In the elderly who present with symptoms such as drop attacks, nausea, vomiting, syncope and shortness of breath, cardiac problems should be sought for exclusion at first, unless other reasons can be determined.

While pain is more prominent in STEMI rather than NSTEMI in most subpopulations, it is seen that painless presentation is very common in both entities in the elderly. While chest pain was the chief complaint in only 40% of patients older than 85 years with NSTEMI and 57% of patients with STEMI, the same was true for 90% of STEMI patients under 65 years of age. The non-diagnostic ECG rate increases significantly with age and approaches 50%. Again, left bundle branch block accompanying STEMI can be encountered in one in every three patients of advanced age (Table **13**).

Table 13. Symptoms and ECG findings in patients with acute coronary syndrome according to age groups.

-	Pain		Nondiagnostic ECG	LBBB
	NSTEMI	STEMI	NSTEMI	STEMI
≤65	%77	%90	%23	%5
≥85	%40	%57	%43	%34

It is important to obtain the patient's previous ECG findings. In this way, the findings of the patient in the emergency setting are compared with the past situation and the management plan is highlighted.

Patients aged 80 and over receive less drug treatment than the 60-year-old patient group with ACS. Magid *et al.* reported that aspirin was not administered even if necessary in 1/5 of the elderly and 2/5 of them did not receive beta-blockers.

Pearl: Although the benefit of the invasive strategy decreases with advancing age, it is a superior approach to the conservative strategy in mitigating adverse outcomes in patients with NSTEMI aged 80 years and over.

Is Imaging Performed for AMI?

Both yes and no. Yes, bedside USG/POCUS and bedside X-ray in selected cases are valuable in excluding differential diagnoses of vital importance, such as aortic dissection and acute pulmonary embolism. In this way, for example, considering the case of DAA as STEMI and wrongly administering fibrinolytic can be prevented.

No, time should not be wasted for anything in unstable patients, who have impaired hemodynamics and planned to undergo emergency PCI and other feasible emergent procedures.

Coronary CT-angiography (CCTA)

CCTA is the tomographic imaging of coronary arteries after infusion of iodinated contrast material. 3D images can also be obtained by reformatting CT with 3D. Caution should be exercised in case of kidney failure and pregnancy. In rare cases, the contrast agent can cause kidney damage. Besides, there are risks of radiation. Invasive vascular treatment can be performed at the same time in coronary angiography (CAG), but not in CCTA. Therefore, patients with emergent and typical findings and high suspicion for ACS are suitable for CAG, instead of CCTA. Evaluation of images can be difficult in patients with multiple calcific atherosclerotic plaques.

Accuracy Rate

The sensitivity of CCTA was 85% to 99% and specificity 64% to 90% when CAG was taken as the gold standard. Since its NPV is quite high (83% to 99%), it is used as an exclusion test (Ajlan, 2013). It is performed as part of the exercise test in those with moderate risk findings (Fig. **17**).

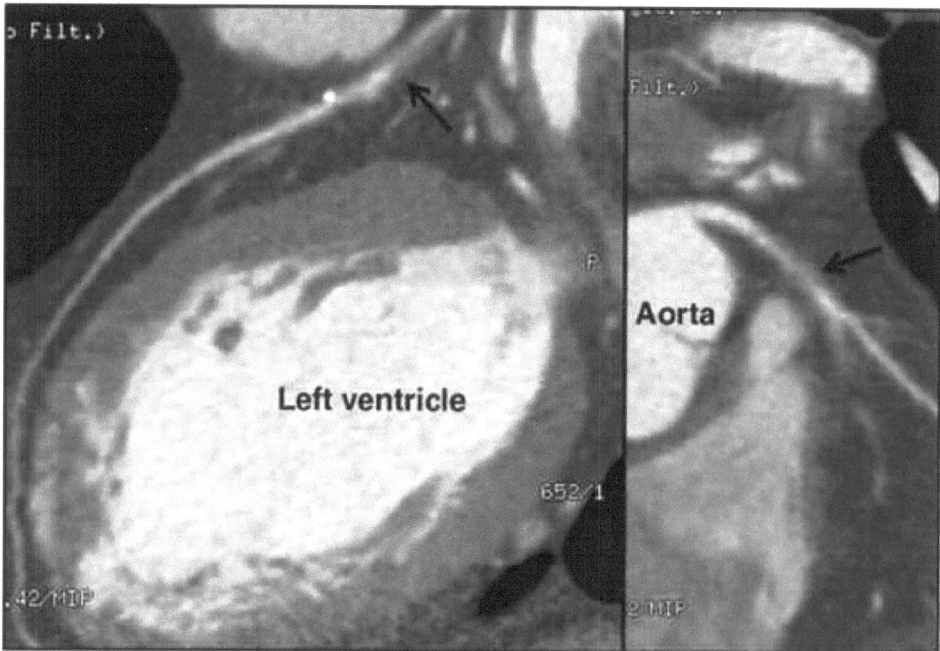

Fig. (17). CCTA images showing 70% to 99% stenosis in the proximal LAD (arrows).

Heart rate can be decreased below 65 bpm by administering beta blocker before the procedure and coronary vasodilation can be achieved with nitrates.

CCTA Advantages

• It is noninvasive.

• Fast completion, simple application.

• It is less sensitive to patient movement than MRI.

• Displays bone, soft tissue and vessels together.

• It has the advantage of simultaneously excluding pathologies related to the aortic or pulmonary tree.

• Routine CAG focuses on the lumen and plaque, while CCTA also conveys plaque characterization.

• With new technologies, hemodynamic modeling can also be demonstrated by studying fluid dynamics in CCTA.

The situations where CCTA is mostly ordered:

• Low to moderate risk atypical chest pain.
• Non-acute chest pain.
• Coronary anatomical disorder suspected.
• Suspicious findings in stress tests.
• Exacerbation of symptoms despite normal stress tests.
• In patients with suspected CABG.
• Although the risk of ACS is low to moderate, the emergence of heart failure symptoms.

"Coronary calcium" view is important in CCTA. A lesion with a density above 130 Hounsfield Units (HU) and occupying a volume larger than 1 mm^3 (2 pixels) is called calcified focus. If this focus matches the anatomical region of the coronary artery, it indicates calcified coronary artery plaque. The high calcium score indicates the excess of atherosclerotic plaque load (Figs. **18** and **19**).

How is AMI diagnosed?

Published in 2018, "3rd Universal AMI diagnosis report"

AMI is defined as a clinical condition consistent with myocardial damage +

myocardial ischemia (accompanied by at least one of the following).

- Ischemia symptoms.
- New ischemic ECG findings.
- Pathological Q waves on ECG.
- Loss of viable myocardial tissue or regional wall motion disorder.
- Intracoronary thrombus at angiography or autopsy.

In this definition, "Myocardial Damage"; It is defined as the upper reference limit of at least one of the cardiac troponin (cTn) values higher than the 99th percentile. From another point of view, AMI can also be classified by etiology (Table **14**).

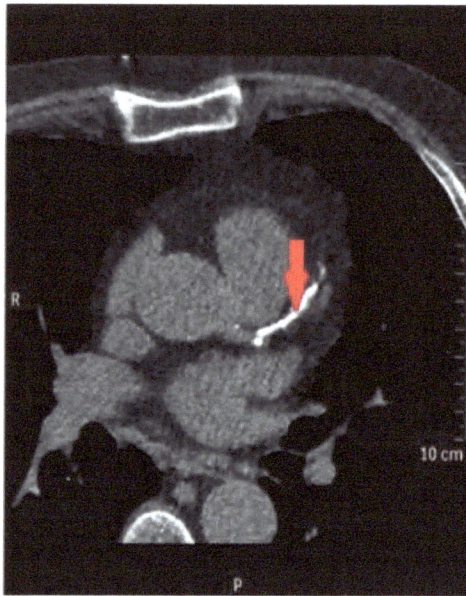

Fig. (18). "Coronary calcium" finding in LAD (arrow).

Table 14. AMI types by etiology.

• Type 1: Ruptured atherosclerotic plaque and coronary occlusion with thrombus.
• Type 2: Imbalance between oxygen supply and demand (Vasospasm, GI bleeding, coronary dissection, *etc.*).
• Type 3: sudden cardiac death with new ischemic ECG findings, in a patient with ischemic symptoms and with MI detected before enzyme elevation or autopsy.
• Type 4: AMI associated with percutaneous coronary intervention.
• Type 5: CABG-related AMI.

Unstable Angina Pectoris (USAP)

There is no clear template for USAP. In addition to the absence of typical ECG and enzymatic changes of STEMI, USAP is considered when any of the following features:

1. CP that starts at rest and exceeds 20 minutes.
2. Newly-initiated (less than 2 months of history) CP and reached at least Grade III in regard to the Canadian Cardiovascular Society (CCS) rating in severity.
3. CP exacerbated by changing characters and reached at least Grade III in the last 2 months, in accord with CCS classification in severity.

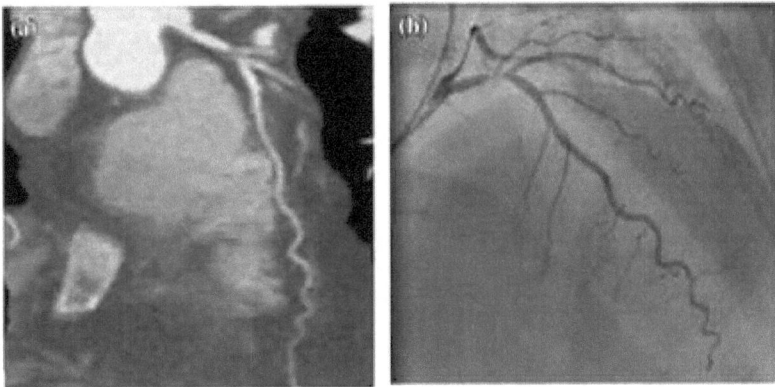

Fig. (19). Difference between CCTA and CAG. CCTA image of the proximal LAD lesion shows that there is no calcium in the lesion.

General Management Principles

Pearl: It should be noted that in some cases, ischemic attacks can also be triggered by causes such as fever, tachycardia, anemia, thyrotoxicosis, hypertension, and arrhythmia (secondary USAP). These reasons should also be investigated in a patient presenting with CP.

Low Risk Patients

Patients with CP, whose newly ensued exertional angina, which increases slightly with exercise and immediately resolves with nitroglycerine, can be treated without hospitalization with close monitoring on an outpatient basis. Patients with long-lasting pain should be hospitalized for differentiation from AMI. The risk-stratification and management principles in USAP are given in Table **10-12** and Fig. (**20**).

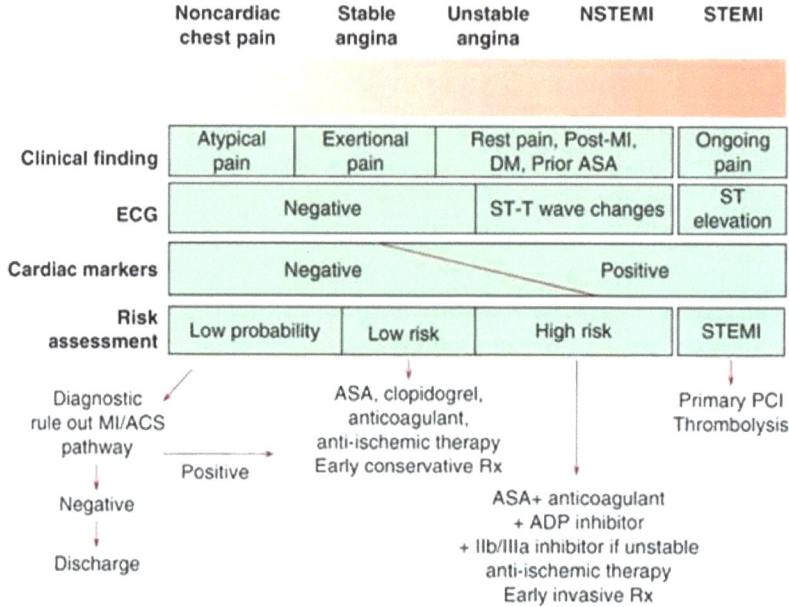

Fig. (20). Algorithm for risk stratification and treatment of patients with suspected coronary artery disease (Adapted from Harrison's Manual of Medicine, 18th Ed. Unstable Angina and Non-ST-Elevation Myocardial Infarction).

Table 15. The HEART score has been reported to predict the 30-day major adverse cardiac event (MACE) development more accurately than the TIMI and GRACE scores.

History (Characteristics of CP)	Point
Mild suspicion	+0
Moderate suspicion	+1
High suspicion	+2
ECG	
Normal ECG	+0
Nonspecific changes in repolarization (in absence of ST segment depression)	+1
Significant ST segment deviation	+2
Age	
≤45 years	+0
45-65 years	+1
≥65 years	+2
Risk Factors	
No risk factors and atherosclerotic disease	+0
1 to 2 risk factors, no atherosclerotic disease	+1
≥3 risk factors or atherosclerotic disease	+2

(Table 15) cont.....

History (Characteristics of CP)	Point
Troponin	
≤Normal limit	+0
1-3 X normal limit	+1
3 X normal limit	+2
Risk factors and atherosclerotic disease Hypertension, Hypercholesterolemia, DM, obesity, smoking, family history of CVD History of AMI, coronary revascularization (PCI, CABG), CVA/TIA, peripheral artery disease	

TIMI Risk Score

• > 65 years old

• Coronary Artery Disease ≥ 3 risk factors

• A history of ≥50% coronary stenosis

• ST segment deviation in the admission ECG

• Two or more angina attacks in the last 24 hours

• ASA use in the last 7 days

• Elevated cardiac markers

Killip Classification

Killip I: No Heart Failure (50%)

Killip II: S3 gallop rhythm + rales in lungs (30%)

Killip III: Acute Pulmonary Edema (10-15%)

Killip IV: Cardiogenic Shock (5-10%)

Treatment Goals in ACS Management

1) coronary reperfusion: (to be explained later).

a. Percutaneous coronary intervention (PCI)

b. Fibrinolytics (to be explained later).

2) Drugs that prevent re-occlusion:

a. Antithrombocyte agents-DAPT (prasugrel or ticagrelor or clopidogrel)

b. Anticoagulant agents (heparin or DOAC)

3) Agents limiting the infarct site: (will be explained later).

a. Nitrates

b. Morphine

c. β Blockers

d. Other agents

4) Management of complications: Monitoring of vital signs. Providing basic and advanced life support when necessary (Fig. **21**).

Table 16. Criteria used in CP/USAP Risk assessments.

High Risk	Intermediate Risk	Low Risk
Any of the following features must be present:	No high-risk features but must have any of the following:	No high- or intermediate-risk features but may have any of the following:
Prolonged ongoing (>20 min) rest pain	Rest angina now resolved but not low likelihood of CAD	Increased angina frequency, severity, or duration
Pulmonary edema	Rest pain (<20 min or relieved with rest or nitroglycerin therapy)	Angina provoked at a lower threshold
Angina with new or worsening mitral regurgitation murmurs	Angina with dynamic T wave changes	New-onset angina within 2 wks to 2 mos
Angina with S₃ or rales	Nocturnal angina	Normal or unchanged ECG findings
Angina with hypotension	New-onset CCSC III or IV angina in past 2 wk but not low likelihood of CAD	
	Q wave or ST depression ≥1 mm in multiple leads	
	Age >65 y	

There are 2 main goals in the treatment of USAP/NSTEMI:

- - immediate relief of ischemia,

- - Prevention of adverse consequences (death, myocardial (re) infarction)

Emergency Management of USAP

Patients with symptoms consistent with the above-mentioned USAP criteria should be given ASA, evaluated in terms of dual antiplatelet therapy (DAPT) and followed up. If any of the risk factors (symptom, rise in enzymes, ECG change) did not occur during the follow-up of the patient, the patient can be discharged from the ED to be referred to the outpatient clinic. In an ideal system, the emergency physician should be able to make the outpatient clinic appointment that such a patient will be seen the next day.

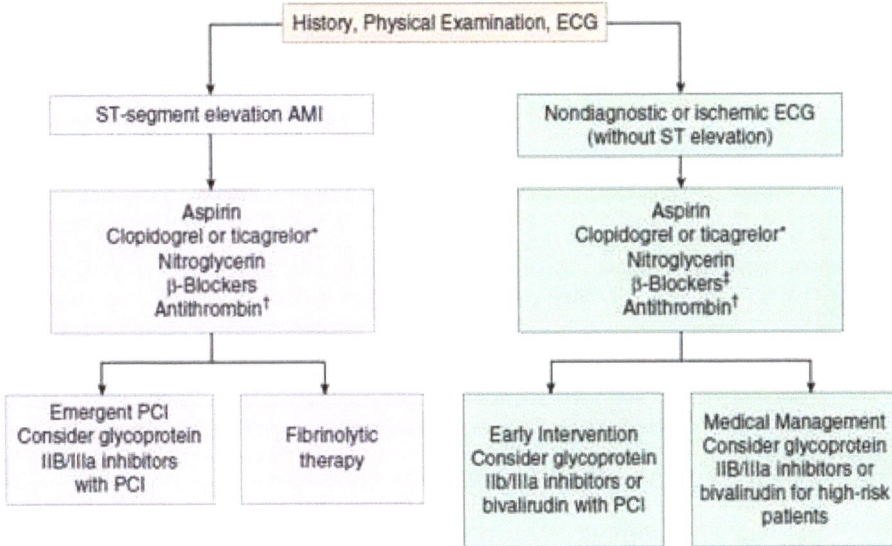

Fig. (21). Evaluation and management of the patient with suspected acute ischemia.

Case example. A 52-year-old male patient presented with new onset chest pain (Fig. **22**).

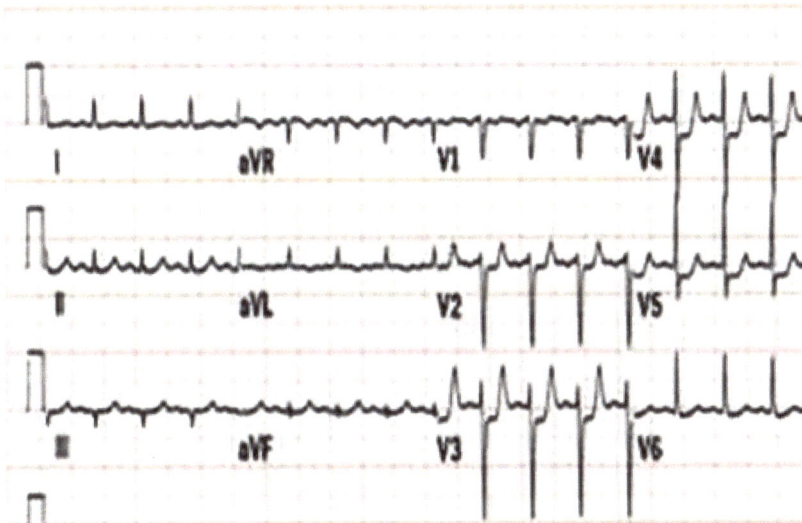

Fig. (22). ECG of a 52-year-old male patient with new onset anginal pain. Significant ST depression is observed in the anterolateral leads. IV nitrate treatment and metoprolol (beta blockade) did not relieve the patient, who was taken to catheter lab with the diagnosis of USAP.

Emergency CAG or PCI is not required in patients who are relieved by the first treatment in the ED and whose ischemia does not recur. A decision for CAG can be made with noninvasive examinations before leaving the hospital. A negative exercise test can rule out a severe coronary stenosis. These patients can be discharged by starting DAPT. Patients with persistent ischemic pain despite medical treatment and those with USAP after MI are at risk and angiography should be performed. Critical lesion (s) in these patients are opened primarily by percutaneous methods, otherwise by surgery. Intraaortic balloon pump (IABP) is recommended for patients who do not benefit from emergency treatment. IABP should be administered to patients with left ventricular dysfunction and hypotension who require urgent intervention.

How is the ACS management changed in the COVID-19 era?

Many associations and scientific bodies issued recommendations and algorithmic approaches for ACS. Recently, A position statement was published in collaboration of the Society for Cardiovascular Angiography and Interventions (SCAI), the American College of Cardiology (ACC), and the American College of Emergency Physicians (ACEP) (Mahmud, 2020) (Fig. **23**).

It can never be underemphasized that primary PCI should be performed with the strict use of personal protection equipment (PPE) for aerosolized and droplet precautions.

Another issue of vital importance is the harmonious workflow of the EDs, EMS and the CCL to improve the system-based care of these patients. First medical contact to reperfusion time (door-to-needle for EDs) is of utmost importance and should not delay primary PCI for STEMI patients.

Patients with COVID-19 concurrent with STEMI at an advanced center with PCI capabilities should be evaluated prior to transfer to a PCI center. Pre-PCI fibrinolysis (within 30 min of diagnosis), immediately followed by transfer to CCL for a rescue PCI is preferable for all STEMI patients with COVID-19.

Table 17. Likelihood classification that signs and symptoms represent an ACS secondary to CVD.

History	Known history of CAD, including MI	Age greater than 70 years Male sex Diabetes mellitus	Recent cocaine use
Examination	Transient mitral regurgitation murmur, hypotension, diaphoresis, pulmonary edema, or rales	Extracardiac vascular disease	Chest discomfort reproduced by palpation

(Table 17) cont.....

ECG	New, or presumably new, transient ST segment deviation (1 mm or greater) or T wave inversion in multiple precordial leads	Fixed Q waves ST depression 0.5 to 1 mm or T wave inversion greater than 1 mm	T wave flattening or inversion less than 1 mm in leads with dominant R waves Normal ECG
Cardiac markers	Elevated cardiac TnI, TnT, or CK-MB	Normal	Normal

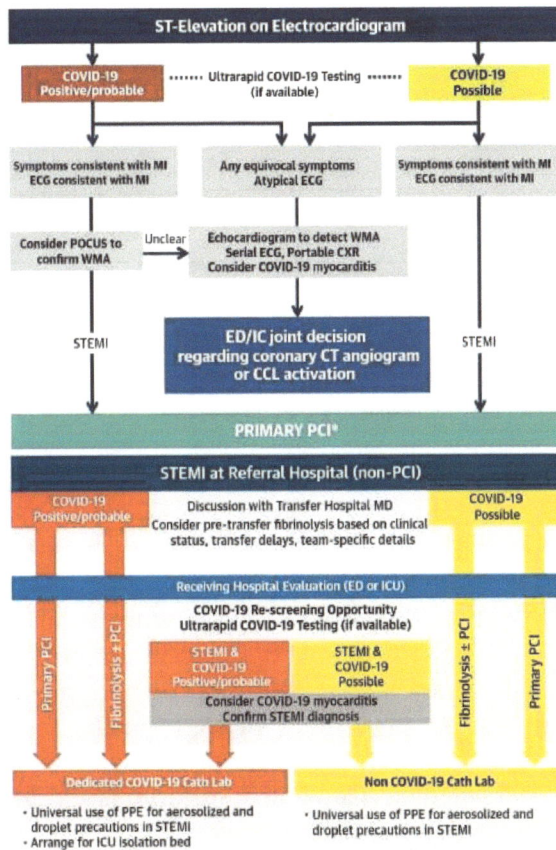

Fig. (23). The algorithm emphasizes usage of bedside ultrasound in patients with a verified diagnosis or a suspicion of COVID-19 together with clinical symptoms and ECG findings suggestive of coronary syndromes, to assess cardiac function (*i.e.*, regional wall motion abnormality, aneurysm, vave dysfunction *etc*). Patients who are considered to have a STEMI in conjunction with COVID-19 need to be transferred to cardiac cath lab (CCL) for a primary PCI. To expedite this approach, an ultrarapid COVID-19 testing can be useful to rule out the disease and warrant the use of a dedicated CCL and other resources. B. Initial fibrinolysis is also an alternative to direct transfer to CCL, especially in circumstnces where it can be difficult to summon the entire team, equipments and everything in unison. Pandemic conditions can also hamper the situation and fibrinolytics can be a more viable option for the given patient's benefit. STEMI patients with shock states and/or ROSC after arrest situation should still be prioritized for a primary PCI.

NSTEMI Treatment

PCI within 24 to 48 hours in NSTEMI cases reduces the incidence of death and recurrence by 19 to 34%. Early invasive intervention is not emphasized in NSTEMI cases as much as STEMI, but it is recommended in cases with persistent-treatment-resistant angina or hemodynamically unstable patients at high risk (Table **18**).

Table 18. Invasive evaluation and revascularization recommendations in non-ST elevation coronary artery disease (ESC-EACTS, 2018-19).

Recommendations	Sınıf	Düzey
Emergency CAG (<2 hours) is recommended in patients with high risk of ischemia.	I	C
An early invasive strategy (<24 h) is recommended in patients with at least one high risk criterion.	I	A
In patients with at least one intermediate risk criterion or recurrent symptoms, the invasive strategy (<72 hours) is recommended.	I	A
Plan the revascularization strategy (culprit lesion PCI/multi-vessel PCI/CABG) based on the clinical situation and comorbidities, disease severity (*i.e.*, according to the distribution and severity of the lesions in CAG, *e.g.*, SYNTAX score).	I	B
Routine revascularization of non-IRA lesions during PPCI is not recommended in cardiogenic shock.	III	B

IRA: infarct-related artery.

Early invasive intervention is recommended within the first 24 hours by AHA/ACC in USAP and NSTEMI cases, those with persistent angina, enzyme elevation, new ST depression, high risk findings in noninvasive stress tests, left ventricular dysfunction, ventricular arrhythmia, hemodynamic instability, those who have undergone CABG (any time) or PCI (in the last six months). The invasive strategy is recommended within 2 hours for patients with USAP/NSTEMI who are hemodynamically unstable (Fig. **24**).

Anti-ischemic Treatment in ACS

The problem in ACS is the disruption of the balance between the metabolic requirements of tissues and oxygen and nutrients brought to the myocardium.

The primary target focused on all treatment titles in ACS is reperfusion therapy.

Reperfusion therapy in ACS is the recanalization of the occluded vessel with thrombolytic therapy or percutaneous coronary intervention (PCI)/primary angioplasty in the contemporary world. In the ACCESS study conducted in 19 countries, it was reported that only 20% of STEMI cases in developing countries were intervened with PCI at the desired timeframe (ACCESS).

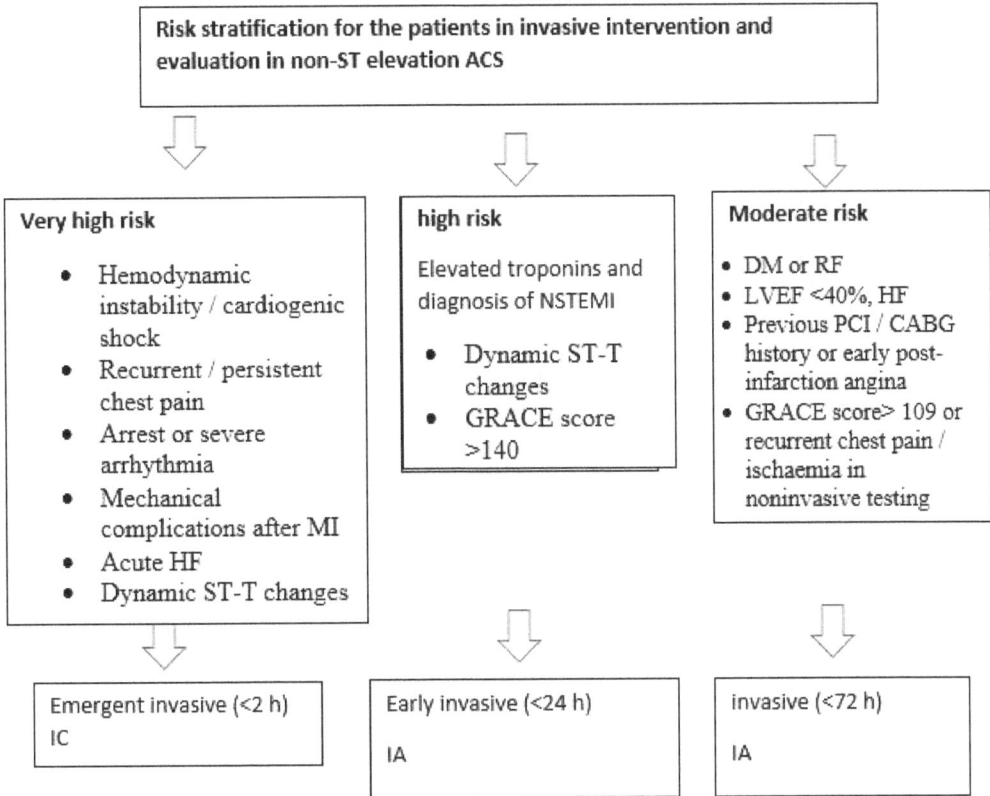

Fig. (24). Criteria used to classify the patients' risks for invasive intervention and evaluation in non-ST elevation ACS (ESC, 2018).

Significant differences in both fibrinolytic application and PCI procedure technique, equipment and timing make it difficult to compare the results of the two treatments, devoid of bias.

The preferred method primarily in STEMI is opening the occluded vessel with PCI. The physician who sees the patient first should work for transfer to the nearest center where PCI can be performed as soon as possible. Intervention without fibrinolytic administration is called primary PCI. If there is a center where primary PCI can be performed within 90 minutes from the moment the patient is first seen (door-to-balloon time <90 minutes), the patient should be transferred immediately.

Pearl: Rescue PCI should be performed immediately for STEMI patient whose fibrinolytic therapy is started against the risk of unsuccessful revascularization. Therefore, if it cannot be performed in the center where the patient is admitted, he or she should be transferred to the nearest center where PCI can be conducted. Even if revascularization is successful, patients should definitely be transferred to the appropriate center as angiography will be required.

Clinical uses of antiplatelet agents on different platelet receptors are summarized in Fig. (25).

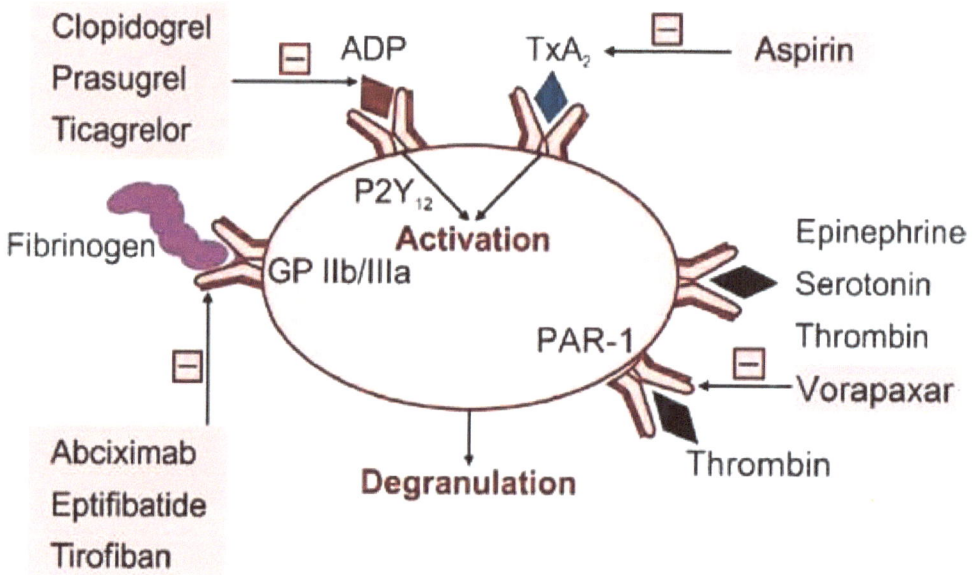

Fig. (25). Platelet activation and degranulation works through ADP, TxA2, and GP IIb/IIIa receptors. Each of these receptors is a potential target for drugs in the treatment of ACS. ADP, adenosine diphosphate; TxA2, thromboxane A2; GP, glycoprotein; PAR-1, protease activated receptor-1.

Dual Antiplatelet Therapy (DAPT)

It is started at the first contact with the patient, and if possible, in an emergency. DAPT treatment in AMI cases leads to a 25% to 50% reduction in mortality within 3 years. ASA and an ADP receptor blocker are used together. Among the P2Y12 inhibitors with ASA, prasugrel, clopidogrel or ticagrelor may be preferred. Elderly patients with ACS are at increased risk of both ischemic and hemorrhagic complications. Therefore, Savonitto *et al.* compared the effect of low dose (5 mg) prasugrel and standard 75 mg clopidogrel in the elderly who have been scheduled to have PCI in a multicenter study (Savonitto 2018). In the study in which 1443 patients (mean age = 80) were included, the stent thrombosis rate was 0.7% and 1.9% (OR 0.36, C.I. 0.13-1.00, p = 0.06), respectively. 'According to the Bleeding Academic Research Consortium, type> 2 bleeding occurred at a rate of 4.1% and

2.7, respectively (OR 1.52, C.I. 0.85-3.16, P = 0.18). In brief, it has been reported that low dose (5 mg) prasugrel and standard clopidogrel can be used equally effectively in terms of bleeding and thrombosis. Zhou *et al.* highlighted that among medically managed patients, dual antiplatelet therapy (DAPT) use at discharge was greater in NSTEMI than in UA patients (82% *vs* 65%), and was significantly associated with male sex, positive cardiac markers, and prior cardiovascular medications (p < 0.0001) (Zhou *et al.* 2020).

Prasugrel

It is a molecule from the 3rd generation thienopyridine class. In 2019, more than 4,000 patients were randomized in a new multicenter randomized study (ISAR-REACT 5). It has been demonstrated that Prasugrel has a higher success in reducing the risk of recurrent STEMI and CVA in cases of STEMI and NSTEMI than ticagrelor (Schupke S, *et al.*, 2019, ISAR-REACT 5 Trial Investigators). Bleeding frequency was similar between the two groups. In the 2017 ESC guidelines, prasugrel or ticagrelor was mentioned as a strong recommendation-Class I for STEMI cases, and clopidogrel were recommended should these be unavailable.

Attention should be paid to CVA history, age and body weight restrictions.

In the Prague-18 study published in Circulation in 2018, an equal effect in terms of ischemia and bleeding was found as a result of ticagrelor and prasugrel given in patients undergoing PCI in the acute phase of AMI (Motovska., 2018).

Most recently, a post hoc analysis combining the pre-specified subgroups of UA and NSTEMI of the randomized ISAR-REACT 5 trial was published (Valina, 2020). The safety endpoint was Bleeding Academic Research Consortium class 3-5. In accord with the findings of this study, prasugrel was superior to ticagrelor in reducing the combined 1-year risk of death, MI, and stroke without increasing the risk of bleeding in patients with NSTE-ACS.

There are other well-designed studies reporting no significant difference in the primary endpoint between prasugrel and ticagrelor in patients with STEMI undergoing primary PCI (Aytekin, 2020). However, in this study, ticagrelor was associated with a significant increase in the risk for recurrent myocardial infarction. Furthermore, Menichelli *et al.* reported that in elderly or low-weight patients with ACS, a reduced dose of prasugrel compared with the standard dose of ticagrelor is associated with maintained anti-ischemic efficacy while protecting these patients against the excess risk for bleeding (Menichelli, 2020).

Clopidogrel

clopidogrel is one of the agents preferred in the emergency department with its rapid onset of action. Maximal effect occurs within 3 to 5 days with 75 mg maintenance daily after 300 - 600 mg loading. The net benefit of loading clopidogrel 300 mg 6 hours before PCI in STEMI has been demonstrated.

Is Antiplatelet Therapy Effective on Respiratory Failure in COVID-19?

Yes, Maybe. Viecca *et al.* investigated the effects of antiplatelet therapy on arterial oxygenation and clinical outcomes in COVID-19 patients with severe respiratory failure requiring CPAP, bilateral pulmonary infiltration, and a D-dimer level higher than 3 times the upper limit of the normal reference range (Viecca *et al.*, 2020) (Fig. **26**). The study group received 250 mg ASA and 300 mg clopidogrel, followed by 25 µg/kg tirofiban IV bolus, followed by a continuous infusion of 0.15 µg/kg/min for 48 hours, in addition to standard therapy. Then, clopidogrel was given to both groups for 30 days (75 mg/day). In addition, Fondaparinux SC was administered 2.5 mg/day during the hospital stay. All control group patients were given prophylactic or therapeutic doses of heparin in addition to standard treatment, in accord with their clinical status. Treated patients had a mean (SD) reduction in A-a O_2 gradient of -32.6 mmHg (61.9, P= 0.154), -52.4 mmHg (59.4, P = 0.016) and -151.1 mmHg (56.6, P = 0.011; P = 0.047 *vs.* controls) at 24, 48 hours and 7 days after treatment. PaO_2/FiO_2 ratio increased by 52 mmHg (50, P = 0.172), 64 mmHg (47, P=0.040) and 112 mmHg (51, P = 0.036) after 24, 48 hours and 7 days, respectively. All patients but one were successfully weaned from CPAP after 3 days, while this was not the case for the control group. No major adverse events were observed.

The authors concluded that antiplatelet therapy can be effective in improving the V/Q ratio in COVID-19 patients with respiratory failure. The effects might be sustained by the prevention and interference on forming clots in lung capillary vessels. Randomized clinicaltrials are urgently needed to confirm these results.

In conclusion, thienopyridines can be alternative antithrombotic agents in the management of COVID-19, but this should be further supported by studies with robust evidence from large well-designed studies.

Ticagrelor

In patients with AMI, it is continued with 90 mg twice a day (180 mg) after 180 mg loading at time zero. The risk of bleeding decreases after the first year. There is important information indicating that intracranial and vital bleeding does not increase (Bansilal 2018). In the PEGASUS-TIMI 54 study, 21,162 patients were enrolled, resulting in a significant and significant reduction in coronary death, stent thrombosis, and AMI rates. Especially the 46% decrease in coronary deaths is striking (Bansilal 2018).

Before DAPT starts, cases with high risk of bleeding can be identified using scoring known as PRECISE-DAPT or CRUSADE. This approach will also help in agent selection (Choi, 2018) (Tables **19** and **20**).

Cangrelor is also promising for the future with its administration in IV active form, rapid effect and better prognostic expectations.

Anticoagulant Treatment

Heparin or low molecular weight heparin (LMWH) should be administered. They prevent the formation of new clots. It is not effective on thrombus that has already formed. Anticoagulants are recommended for patients scheduled for PCI or given fibrinolytics.

Table 19. Anti-thrombotic treatment recommendations in AMI according to the 2018 ESC-EACTS guideline published in 2019: (ESC/EACTS Guidelines on myocardial revascularization, European Heart Journal (2019) 40, 87--165).

Recommendations	Class	Level of Evidence
Antithrombotic Treatment Regimen in Patients with STEMI Undergoing PCI		
Aspirin should be given to all patients without contraindications: oral loading dose 150–300 mg or 75–250 mg IV), maintenance dose 75–100 mg/day.	I	A
Potent P2Y12 inhibitors (prasugrel or ticagrelor) should be administered prior to PCI, or clopidogrel if these are absent/contraindicated and continued for 12 months. (risk of excessive bleeding is a contraindication).	I	A
Antithrombotic Treatment Regimen in Patients with NSTEMI-ACS Undergoing PCI.		
Aspirin should be given to all patients without contraindications: oral loading dose 150–300 mg or 75–250 mg IV), maintenance dose 75–100 mg/day.	I	A
P2Y12 inhibitors should be administered prior to PCI, or clopidogrel if these are absent/contraindicated and continued for 12 months. (risk of excessive bleeding is a contraindication).	I	A
Prasugrel: In P2Y12-naive patients who will undergo PCI (60 mg loading dose and 10 mg/day for maintenance).	I	B
Ticagrelor: (180 mg loading dose, 90 mgX2/day) regardless of previous P2Y12-use and revascularization strategy.	I	B
Clopidogrel: (600 mg loading dose and 75 mg/day), (unless prasugrel or ticagrelor is available/if contraindicated).	I	B

(Table 19) cont.....

Recommendations	Class	Level of Evidence
GP IIb/IIIa antagonists are not recommended in patients with unknown coronary anatomy.	III	A
In patients with unknown coronary anatomy, prasugrel is not recommended.	III	B
Anticoagulation is recommended in addition to antiplatelet therapy in all patients during intervention.	I	A
UFH ve LMWH: Crossings are not recommended.	III	B
DAPT (P2Y12 inhibitor + aspirin) should be initiated and continued for 12 months in those who undergo coronary stent implantation for ACS. (risk of excessive bleeding creates contraindication) (*e.g.* PRECISE-DAPT score> = 25).	I	A

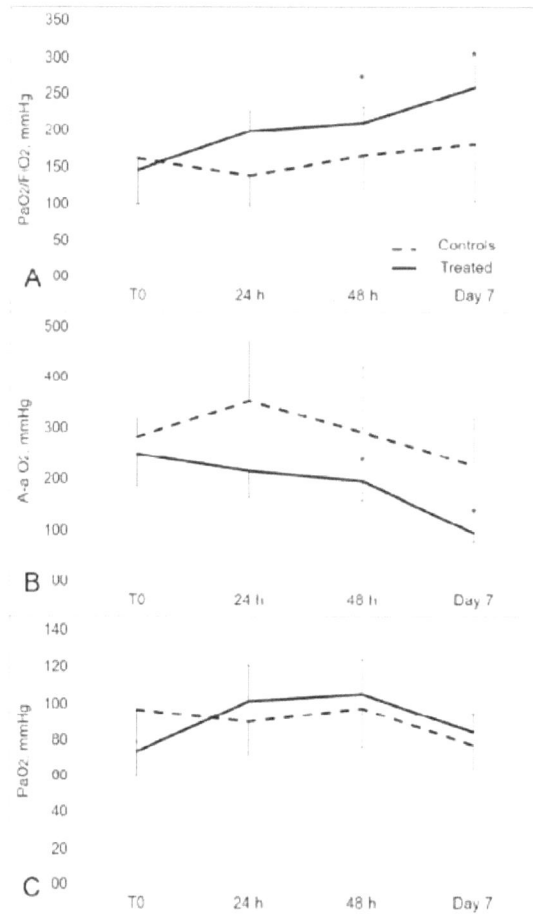

Fig. (26). Changes in PaO_2/FiO_2 ratio **(A)** , A-a O_2 gradient **(B)** and PaO_2 level **(C)** within 7 days in antiplatelet treated and controls (Adapted from Viecca *et al.*, 2020).

Table 20. Changes in 2018 guidelines for revascularization strategies: According to the 2018 ESC/EACTS Guidelines published in Eur Heart J in 2019, current recommendations are classified as follows:(ESC/EACTS Guidelines on myocardial revascularization, European Heart Journal (2019) 40, 87--165).

Class I Recommendations	Class IIa Recommendations	Class IIb Recommendations
Calculate the Syntax Score if left main coronary or multivessel disease and revascularization is contemplated.	PCI as an alternative to CABG	Routine noninvasive imaging screening of high-risk patients 6 months after revascularization
Radial intervention as standard for CAG and PCI	When considering CABG against PCI, the completion of revascularization is a priority.	The double-kissing crush technique is preferred to T-stenting in the left main bifurcations.
DES for each PCI	NOAC is preferred to VKA in nonvalvular AF patients.	Use of Cangrelor kullanımı: In patients not using P2Y12-inhibitor, who will undergo PCI.
Systematic reassessment after revascularization	"No-touch vein technique" in vein harvesting for CABG	GP IIb/IIIa inhibitors for PCI in patients with ACS who do not use P2Y12-inhibitors
Stabilized NSTE-ACS patients: Revascularization strategy is performed according to SCAD principles.	Operator should have performed left main PCI at least 25 patients a year	Dabigatran 150-mg dose is preferred to 110 mg for single APT after PCI.
Myocardial revascularization in patients with CAD, HF, and LVEF ≤35%: CABG is preferred	In patients with mild or severe CRF, if the estimated contrast volume is> 100 mL, hydration should be provided with isotonic saline before and after the procedure	Reduction of P2Y12 inhibitor by platelet function test in ACS cases

Heparin Dosage

If Primary PCI will be Performed

- UFH: 100U/kg UFH IV bolus initial dose (60 U/kg if the patient is on GP IIb/IIIa inhibitor). (ACT should be 250-350) Infusion is interrupted after the sheath is removed.

- Bivalirudin: 0.75 mg/min bolus followed by 1.75 mg/kg/hour infusion.

- Enoxaparin 0.5 mg/kg iv bolus.

If Fibrinolytic Treatment will be Ordered

Enoxaparin

30 mg IV bolus in patients under 75 years of age and creatinine <2.5 mg/ml (female 2.2), 1 mg/kg SC every 12 hours after 15 minutes. The bolus dose should not be administered to patients over 75 years of age, and the first SC dose should be reduced (0.75 mg/kg).

- UF Heparin: 30 mg/kg IV bolus (max 4000 U) and 12 U/kg/hour infusion for 24-48 hours.

Fondaparinux: 2.5 mg IV bolus, then 2.5 mg sc/day.

Fibrinolytic Therapy

Fibrinolytic therapy should be considered should the door-to-balloon time of the STEMI patient be over 90 minutes. Fibrinolytic treatment should be considered in patients presenting within the first 12 hours after the onset of symptoms. Contraindications should always be taken into account. Fibrinolytic therapy should be initiated within 30 minutes (door-to-needle time <30 minutes) after first medical contact, including the ambulance call. If there is an indication, it should be started at the prehospital stage.

Studies have shown that the combination of "accelerated" t-PA and heparin given in 90 minutes leads to better clinical results. Despite more hemorrhagic complications, still better mortality rates have been demonstrated.

Results similar to the accelerated t-PA regimen have been reported with the ease of bolus administration in the tenecteplase regimen in STEMI. 30-50 mg is given according to body weight. There is a positive change in 30-day mortality with TNK treatment in cases presenting later than 4 hours. It stands out with its easier use in pre-hospital and ED procedures.

Fibrinolytic therapy is not recommended in patients with cardiogenic shock.

In the last decade, the pharmaco-invasive approach has attracted attention at the regions where transportation to the hospital will be delayed. It can be performed in patients *via* giving "early fibrinolytic" and taken into the catheter laboratory upon admission to the hospital. Half-dose alteplase and PCI as soon as possible provided better epicardial and myocardial reperfusion when compared to insisting (and waiting) for primary PCI in patients who were admitted with STEMI in less than 6 hours but would be delayed to the laboratory (Pu *et al.*, 2017) (Table **21**).

In fibrinolytic therapy, a drug that can dissolve the blood clot inciting the infarction process is administered. This prevents death of substantial myocardial tissue. Commonly used thrombolytic agents are fibrin-specific agents, also known as tissue plasminogen activator (tPA), reteplase or tenecteplase. These agents are either administered intravenously or can be given directly into the occluded vein. When the treatment is successful, the vascular blood flow is restored and in some cases an ongoing infarction process is halted.

In 2017, a large meta-analysis comparing the efficacy of fibrinolytic agents was published in The Lancet (Jinatongthai *et al*). In the analysis involving 128,000 patients, alteplase infusion was definitely recommended to be accelerated. It was noted that tenecteplase had a significantly lower risk of bleeding (RR = 0.79). The addition of glycoprotein IIb-IIIa inhibitors to fibrinolytic agents significantly and significantly (1.3 to 8.8-fold) the risk of bleeding. It has been recommended that glycoprotein IIb-IIIa inhibitors should not be given in patients undergoing fibrinolytic. It has been reported that the administration of fibrinolytics with anticoagulants are associated with the best results. Contraindications of fibrinolytic treatment in STEMI should definitely be taken into account in the process of emergency decision making (Table **22**).

Table 21. A comparison of fibrinolytic administration and percutaneous coronary intervention in the management of AMI.

Variable	Fibrinolytic administration (fibrin-specific lytic; alteplase, tenecteplase, reteplase)	Percutaneous coronary intervention (PCI)/primary angioplasty
Cost	Cheaper	Expensive
Timing/ indication	It is indicated in AMI cases diagnosed within the first 24 hours if catheterization will not be performed in the first 120 minutes.	It is the first choice in those with diffuse anterior AMI, hypotension, heart failure, ROSC provided by CPR, and in whom intracranial hemorrhage or DAA are not ruled out.
Outcome effect	++	+++

(Table 21) cont.....

Variable		Fibrinolytic administration (fibrin-specific lytic; alteplase, tenecteplase, reteplase)	Percutaneous coronary intervention (PCI)/primary angioplasty
Cost		Cheaper	Expensive
Timing/ indication		It is indicated in AMI cases diagnosed within the first 24 hours if catheterization will not be performed in the first 120 minutes.	It is the first choice in those with diffuse anterior AMI, hypotension, heart failure, ROSC provided by CPR, and in whom intracranial hemorrhage or DAA are not ruled out.
Outcome effect		++	+++
Case scenarios	Hypotensive patient/cardiogenic shock	Not indicated	Indicated
	AMI case presented with VF arrest and ROSC provided with CPR	Not indicated	Indicated
	Prearrest patient in whom pulmonary embolism cannot be ruled out	indicated	Indicated (provided with rapid access to cath lab from ED)
	High Killip class patient with suspected pulmonary edema	Not indicated	Indicated
	Patient with difficult access to health, but accessible by ambulance	Feasible	Not indicated (inaccessible)

Table 22. Contraindications of fibrinolytic treatment in STEMI.

Absolute Contraindications
Known intracranial bleeding (at any time)
Known cerebral vascular lesion
Known intracranial mass
Ischemic stroke within last 3 months
Suspected aortic dissection or pericarditis
Active bleeding (gastrointestinal or other systems)
Relative Contraindications
Blood pressure> 180/100 mmHg
A history of chronic uncontrolled hypertension
Anticoagulant use (INR> 2)
Stroke longer than 3 months before presentation

Absolute Contraindications
Internal bleeding within the last 1 month
Other intracranial pathologies
Major surgery in the past 3 weeks
Known bleeding diathesis
CPR for longer than 30 minutes
Active peptic ulcer
Vascular interventions in places where pressure cannot be applied
Other potentially bleeding conditions such as diabetic retinopathy

Other Antiischemic Therapy

Oxygen

Although it is thought to be indicated in all cases where hypoxia and ischemia are in question, research in recent years reveals that administration of excessive oxygen is harmful. If SpO_2 is above 94% and there are no signs of shock or HF, supplemental oxygen administration should be delayed.

Nitroglycerin

Reduces myocardial workload by expanding peripheral arteries and veins. It is used in ACS and AMI, but symptoms in AMI are generally not relieved with nitroglycerin. It is also useful in pulmonary edema accompanying ACS or hypertension due to its vasodilator effect. It is administered sublingually, in gel form (ointment) and intravenously. It should not be administered in men with a history of sildenafil. It should be avoided in the case of bradycardia (pulse <60 bpm) and hypotension (systolic BP <90/60 mmHg). After large studies and meta-analyzes such as GISSI 3 and ISIS 4, it has been shown that nitrates can produce marginal benefit, if any. Nevertheless, it is currently used widely, as its usefulness is evident in cases of hypertension, pulmonary edema, and refractory ischemia, which are frequently associated with ACS cases. In recent years, some important studies have shown that administration of high dose bolus (*e.g.* 2 mg) instead of continuous infusion provides more favorable results in the treatment of hypertensive acute pulmonary edema (Wang *et al.*, 2019, Hsieh *et al.*, 2018).

Morphine Sulfate

It is a narcotic (opioid) and powerful analgesic. Besides its mild sedative effect, it also causes peripheral vasodilation. It is used in AMI, pulmonary edema and other cardiovascular emergencies. In these conditions, it should be administered IV as much as possible. Due to its histamine releasing effect, caution should be exercised against effects such as flushing. Serious or vital side effects (such as hypotension and respiratory depression) are very rare in the usual doses (0.05-0.1 mg/kg). The dose should be titrated in accord with the patient's clinical responses which are easily assessed bedside.

Beta Blockers

Used in the treatment of tachyarrhythmia, hypertension and angina pectoris. Some are non-selective (such as propranolol), while metoprolol is selective for beta-1 receptors, so the latter is more advantageous in the case of ACS/AMI. It has been proven to limit infarct size, reduce pain and reduce mortality. Beta blockers can trigger congestive heart failure, heart blocks and asthma in susceptible individuals. In the TIMI-II study, recurrent ischemia, reinfarction and death were less common in patients who underwent thrombolysis in the group receiving early (first 2 hours) beta blockade. A cohort study with the GRACE database in NSTEMI cases also revealed that those who received early metoprolol had lower mortality. This effect can be seen in Killip classes I, II and III. It is started with 2-5 mg IV slow infusion; it can be increased up to 15 mg in approximately 25-30 minutes (Table **23**).

Table 23. B-blockers used in current ACS treatment (Park, 2014).

Agent	Selectivity	β-agonist Efficacy	Dose
Acebutolol	β1	+	200–600 mg bid
Atenolol	β1	-	50–200 mg/g
Betaxolol	β1	-	10–20 mg/g
Bisoprolol	β1	-	10 mg/g
Carvedilol	-	+	6.25–25 mg bid
Esmolol	β1	-	50–300 µg/kg/min
Labetalol	-	+	200–600 mg bid
Metoprolol	β1	-	50–200 mg bid
Nadolol	-	-	40–80 mg/g
Pindolol	-	+	2.5–7.5 mg tid
Propronalol	-	-	20–80 mg bid
Timolol	-	-	10 mg bid

Drug Selectivity Agonist Activity Dose.

Esmolol

It is a fast-acting beta blocker. It is indicated in the emergency treatment of ventricular tachyarrhythmias and to prevent relapse of VF in patients who have undergone CPR/ACLS due to ventricular fibrillation and provided ROSC.

Calcium Channel Blockers

Verapamil, diltiazem and nifedipine are from this group. The dihydropyridine group (nifedipine and the like) is not used in patients with or suspected of having ACS. Nondihydropyridine agents are more cardioselective CCBs and thus are increasingly used in supraventricular tachycardia, hypertension and some other cardiovascular problems. It is used in supraventricular tachyarrhythmias accompanying ACS, especially when tachycardia reduces cardiac output. More favorable side effect profile has promoted the use of diltiazem. In patients with chest pain and ACS (except vasospastic angina), this group of agents is administered very carefully and should generally be avoided.

Benzodiazepines (Diazepam, Midazolam)

These agents with prominent anxiolytic effects can be given to distressed and agitated patients with ACS/AMI and to conscious patients undergoing cardioversion. A slow IV bolus is administered. Diazepam is not administered intramuscularly. In case of sedation in patients who are administered morphine, diazepam may not be needed in general. Although the dose is titrated according to the patient's responses, initially, midazolam 0.05 mg/kg and diazepam 0.15 mg/kg can be given initially.

Epinephrine (adrenaline)

It is indicated in resuscitation of sudden cardiac death; arrest and prearrest situations, which are considered to be in the ACS group. It is used in the case of cardiovascular collapse and life-threatening dysrhythmias such as ventricular fibrillation and asystole. It has no place in other ACS.

Dopamine

Although it is one of the amines similar to epinephrine, it is effective especially in bradycardia associated with hypotension.

Ivabradine

Can be used to treat persistent sinus tachycardia. It selectively inhibits primary stimulation in the sinus node and can be used in people for whom B-blockers are contraindicated.

Other treatments considered in the hospital are placement of cardiac pacemakers, enlargement of blocked arteries by balloon angioplasty method, emergency bypass surgery and placement of aortic counterpulsation balloon pump in cardiogenic shock cases.

Cardiogenic Shock

It is the most important and fatal complication of ACS/AMI except arrhythmias. Dyspnea due to heart failure, and shocky state plus hypotension due to circulatory failure are noted together. It is the most severe form of cardiac pump failure. Left ventricular functions cannot meet the body's metabolic requirements; In addition, corrective mechanisms have also failed to restore the physiology to convey the cellular substrates. Cardiogenic shock can be resistant even if existing dysrhythmias, hypovolemia and impaired vascular tone are corrected. It often develops after extensive AMI involving more than 40% of the left ventricle.

Signs and Symptoms

Since cardiogenic shock mostly follows AMI, signs and symptoms are like AMI. However, as the corrective mechanism fails in cardiogenic shock, hypotension is also seen. Systolic blood pressure is often below 80 mmHg. The mental status can range from anxiety to confusion and coma. Usually there is sinus tachycardia while dysrhythmias may also ocur. It will be difficult to distinguish whether this is a cause or a consequence of hypotension. Therefore, dysrhythmias should be treated. The skin is usually pale, cold, and sweaty. Since pulmonary edema is the rule, tachypnea is almost always seen.

Treatment

Mortality rate is high; it can go up to 4 out of 5 cases. If the patient is in the field or at home, he/she should be transported to hospital immediately. Give high flow oxygen by maintaining the airway patent. Keep the patient in a supine (supine) position. Establish a vascular access so that little fluid is removed. Stick the ECG electrodes. If the patient is sweaty, apply the gel first. Take the baseline ECG, do not rule out anything with this. Pay special attention to blood pressure, JVD and breathing sounds on physical examination. The rhythm and heart rate should be treated first.

Medicines to be Used

Dopamine

Dopamine increases cardiac output and stimulates both alpha and beta receptors. Its advantage over other drugs is that it can preserve renal perfusion by dose adjustment. Care should be taken in ischemic myocardium, namely ACS, because it may increase the oxygen and blood requirement of the myocardium.

Norepinephrine

It is considered the first vasopressor of choice in some cases of cardiogenic shock. After the availability of dopamine, norepinephrine is used selectively, because it impairs renal perfusion and lacks beta effects.

If there is left HF and pulmonary edema, they should be treated simultaneously. The first choice of treatment agents are morphine, furosemide and oxygen administration with positive pressure ventilation. Some authors have suggested the application of PASG (pneumatic anti-shock pants) in cardiogenic shock. This tool can be used if pulmonary edema has not developed. It is recommended that you follow your institution's protocols as it is a controversial subject.

CONCLUSION

Timely recognition of ACS is critical to save lives and improve cardiac functions of the involved individuals with these CV emergencies. System-based interventions need to be organized and coordinated in a multidisciplinary approach. An important point is the harmonious workflow of the EDs, EMS and the CCL to improve the general systematic care of these patients. First medical contact to reperfusion time (door-to-needle for EDs) is of utmost importance and should not delay primary PCI for STEMI patients.

Patients with COVID-19 concurrent with STEMI at an advanced center with PCI capabilities should be evaluated prior to transfer to a PCI center. Pre-PCI fibrinolysis (within 30 min of diagnosis), immediately followed by transfer to CCL for a rescue PCI is preferable for all STEMI patients with COVID-19.

REFERENCES

ACCESS Investigators. (2011). Management of acute coronary syndromes in developing countries: acute coronary events-a multinational survey of current management strategies. *Am. Heart J., 162*(5), 852-859.e22. [http://dx.doi.org/10.1016/j.ahj.2011.07.029] [PMID: 22093201]

Adabag, A.S., Luepker, R.V., Roger, V.L., Gersh, B.J. (2010). Sudden cardiac death: epidemiology and risk factors. *Nat. Rev. Cardiol., 7*(4), 216-225. [http://dx.doi.org/10.1038/nrcardio.2010.3] [PMID: 20142817]

Alexander, K.P., Newby, L.K., Cannon, C.P., Armstrong, P.W., Gibler, W.B., Rich, M.W., Van de Werf, F., White, H.D., Weaver, W.D., Naylor, M.D., Gore, J.M., Krumholz, H.M., Ohman, E.M. (2007). Acute coronary care in the elderly, part I: Non-ST-segment-elevation acute coronary syndromes: a scientific statement for healthcare professionals from the American Heart Association Council on Clinical Cardiology: in collaboration with the Society of Geriatric Cardiology. *Circulation, 115*(19), 2549-2569.
[http://dx.doi.org/10.1161/CIRCULATIONAHA.107.182615] [PMID: 17502590]

Al-Khatib, S.M., Stevenson, W.G., Ackerman, M.J., Bryant, W.J., Callans, D.J., Curtis, A.B., Deal, B.J., Dickfeld, T., Field, M.E., Fonarow, G.C., Gillis, A.M., Granger, C.B., Hammill, S.C., Hlatky, M.A., Joglar, J.A., Kay, G.N., Matlock, D.D., Myerburg, R.J., Page, R.L. (2018). 2017 AHA/ACC/HRS guideline for management of patients with ventricular arrhythmias and the prevention of sudden cardiac death: Executive summary: A Report of the American College of Cardiology/American Heart Association Task Force on Clinical Practice Guidelines and the Heart Rhythm Society. *Heart Rhythm, 15*(10), e190-e252.
[http://dx.doi.org/10.1016/j.hrthm.2017.10.035] [PMID: 29097320]

Altenberger, J., Gustafsson, F., Harjola, V.P., Karason, K., Kindgen-Milles, D., Kivikko, M., Malfatto, G., Papp, Z., Parissis, J., Pollesello, P., Pölzl, G., Tschöpe, C. (2018). Levosimendan in acute and advanced heart failure: an appraisal of the clinical database and evaluation of its therapeutic applications. *J. Cardiovasc. Pharmacol., 71*(3), 129-136.
[http://dx.doi.org/10.1097/FJC.0000000000000533] [PMID: 28817484]

Aytekin, A., Ndrepepa, G., Neumann, F.J., Menichelli, M., Mayer, K., Wöhrle, J., Bernlochner, I., Lahu, S., Richardt, G., Witzenbichler, B., Sibbing, D., Cassese, S., Angiolillo, D.J., Valina, C., Kufner, S., Liebetrau, C., Hamm, C.W., Xhepa, E., Hapfelmeier, A., Sager, H.B., Wustrow, I., Joner, M., Trenk, D., Fusaro, M., Laugwitz, K.L., Schunkert, H., Schüpke, S., Kastrati, A. (2020). Ticagrelor or prasugrel in patients with st-segment-elevation myocardial infarction undergoing primary percutaneous coronary intervention. *Circulation, 142*(24), 2329-2337.
[http://dx.doi.org/10.1161/CIRCULATIONAHA.120.050244] [PMID: 33115278]

Bansilal, S., Bonaca, M.P., Cornel, J.H., Storey, R.F., Bhatt, D.L., Steg, P.G., Im, K., Murphy, S.A., Angiolillo, D.J., Kiss, R.G., Parkhomenko, A.N., Lopez-Sendon, J., Isaza, D., Goudev, A., Kontny, F., Held, P., Jensen, E.C., Braunwald, E., Sabatine, M.S., Oude Ophuis, A.J. (2018). Ticagrelor for secondary prevention of atherothrombotic events in patients with multivessel coronary disease. *J. Am. Coll. Cardiol., 71*(5), 489-496.
[http://dx.doi.org/10.1016/j.jacc.2017.11.050] [PMID: 29406853]

Belletti, A., Castro, M.L., Silvetti, S., Greco, T., Biondi-Zoccai, G., Pasin, L., Zangrillo, A., Landoni, G. (2015). The effect of inotropes and vasopressors on mortality: a meta-analysis of randomized clinical trials. *Br. J. Anaesth., 115*(5), 656-675.
[http://dx.doi.org/10.1093/bja/aev284] [PMID: 26475799]

Carugo, S., Ferlini, M., Castini, D., Andreassi, A., Guagliumi, G., Metra, M., Lombardi, C., Cuccia, C., Savonitto, S., Piatti, L., D'Urbano, M., Lettieri, C., Vandoni, P., Lettino, M., Marenzi, G., Montorfano, M., Zangrillo, A., Castiglioni, B., De Ponti, R., Oltrona Visconti, L. (2020). Management of acute coronary syndromes during the COVID-19 outbreak in Lombardy: The "macro-hub" experience. *Int. J. Cardiol. Heart Vasc., 31*, 100662.
[http://dx.doi.org/10.1016/j.ijcha.2020.100662] [PMID: 33173807]

Chobanian, A.V., Bakris, G.L., Black, H.R., Cushman, W.C., Green, L.A., Izzo, J.L., Jr, Jones, D.W., Materson, B.J., Oparil, S., Wright, J.T., Jr, Roccella, E.J. National Heart, Lung, and Blood Institute Joint National Committee on Prevention, Detection, Evaluation, and Treatment of High Blood Pressure; (2003). National High Blood Pressure Education Program Coordinating Committee. (2003). The Seventh Report of the Joint National Committee on Prevention, Detection, Evaluation, and Treatment of High Blood Pressure: the JNC 7 report. *JAMA, 289*(19), 2560-2572.
[http://dx.doi.org/10.1001/jama.289.19.2560] [PMID: 12748199]

Choi, S.Y., Kim, M.H., Cho, Y.R., Sung Park, J., Min Lee, K., Park, T.H., Yun, S.C. (2018). Performance of precise-dapt score for predicting bleeding complication during dual antiplatelet therapy. *Circ. Cardiovasc. Interv., 11*(12), e006837.

[http://dx.doi.org/10.1161/CIRCINTERVENTIONS.118.006837] [PMID: 30545256]

Gruppo Italiano per lo Studio della Sopravvivenza nell'infarto Miocardico. (1994). GISSI-3: effects of lisinopril and transdermal glyceryl trinitrate singly and together on 6-week mortality and ventricular function after acute myocardial infarction. *Lancet, 343*, 1115-1122.

Harrison's Manual of Medicine. (2016). Chapter 122. Unstable Angina and Non-ST-Elevation Myocardial Infarction. URL: https://accessmedicine.mhmedical.com/content.aspx?bookid=2738&sectionid=227558042 Accessed: 08. June, 2021

Hsieh, Y.T., Lee, T.Y., Kao, J.S., Hsu, H.L., Chong, C.F. (2018). Treating acute hypertensive cardiogenic pulmonary edema with high-dose nitroglycerin. *Turk. J. Emerg. Med., 18*(1), 34-36.
[http://dx.doi.org/10.1016/j.tjem.2018.01.004] [PMID: 29942881]

ISIS-4: a randomised factorial trial assessing early oral captopril, oral mononitrate, and intravenous magnesium sulphate in 58,050 patients with suspected acute myocardial infarction. *ISIS-4 (Fourth International Study of Infarct Survival) Collaborative Group. Lancet, 18; 345*(8951), 669-685.
[http://dx.doi.org/10.1016/S0140-6736(95)90865-X] [PMID: 7661937]

Jinatongthai, P., Kongwatcharapong, J., Foo, C.Y., Phrommintikul, A., Nathisuwan, S., Thakkinstian, A., Reid, C.M., Chaiyakunapruk, N. (2017). Comparative efficacy and safety of reperfusion therapy with fibrinolytic agents in patients with ST-segment elevation myocardial infarction: a systematic review and network meta-analysis. *Lancet, 390*(10096), 747-759.
[http://dx.doi.org/10.1016/S0140-6736(17)31441-1] [PMID: 28831992]

Magid, D.J., Masoudi, F.A., Vinson, D.R., van der Vlugt, T.M., Padgett, T.G., Tricomi, A.J., Lyons, E.E., Crounse, L., Brand, D.W., Go, A.S., Ho, P.M., Rumsfeld, J.S. (2005). Older emergency department patients with acute myocardial infarction receive lower quality of care than younger patients. *Ann. Emerg. Med., 46*(1), 14-21.
[http://dx.doi.org/10.1016/j.annemergmed.2004.12.012] [PMID: 15988420]

Mahmud, E., Dauerman, H.L., Welt, F.G.P., Messenger, J.C., Rao, S.V., Grines, C., Mattu, A., Kirtane, A.J., Jauhar, R., Meraj, P., Rokos, I.C., Rumsfeld, J.S., Henry, T.D. (2020). Management of acute myocardial infarction during the COVID-19 pandemic: a position statement from the society for cardiovascular angiography and interventions (SCAI), the American college of cardiology (ACC), and the American college of emergency physicians (ACEP). *J. Am. Coll. Cardiol., 76*(11), 1375-1384.
[http://dx.doi.org/10.1016/j.jacc.2020.04.039] [PMID: 32330544]

Masip, J., Roque, M., Sánchez, B., Fernández, R., Subirana, M., Expósito, J.A. (2005). Noninvasive ventilation in acute cardiogenic pulmonary edema: systematic review and meta-analysis. *JAMA, 294*(24), 3124-3130.
[http://dx.doi.org/10.1001/jama.294.24.3124] [PMID: 16380593]

Menichelli, M., Neumann, F.J., Ndrepepa, G., Mayer, K., Wöhrle, J., Bernlochner, I., Richardt, G., Witzenbichler, B., Sibbing, D., Gewalt, S., Angiolillo, D.J., Lahu, S., Hamm, C.W., Hapfelmeier, A., Trenk, D., Laugwitz, K.L., Schunkert, H., Schüpke, S., Kastrati, A. (2020). Age and weight-adapted dose of prasugrel *Versus* standard dose of ticagrelor in patients with acute coronary syndromes : results from a randomized trial. *Ann. Intern. Med., 173*(6), 436-444.
[http://dx.doi.org/10.7326/M20-1806] [PMID: 32687741]

Miró, Ò., Martínez, G., Masip, J., Gil, V., Martín-Sánchez, F.J., Llorens, P., Herrero-Puente, P., Sánchez, C., Richard, F., Lucas-Invernón, J., Garrido, J.M., Mebazaa, A., Ríos, J., Peacock, W.F., Hollander, J.E., Jacob, J. ICA-SEMES Research Group Researchers. (2018). Effects on short term outcome of non-invasive ventilation use in the emergency department to treat patients with acute heart failure: A propensity score-based analysis of the EAHFE Registry. *Eur. J. Intern. Med., 53*, 45-51.
[http://dx.doi.org/10.1016/j.ejim.2018.03.008] [PMID: 29572091]

National Clinical Guideline Centre. (2014). Acute heart failure. diagnosing and managing acute heart failure in adults. *NICE Clinical Guidelines* (Vol. 187). London: National Institute for Health and Care Excellence (UK).

Neumann, F.J., Sousa-Uva, M., Ahlsson, A., Alfonso, F., Banning, A.P., Benedetto, U., Byrne, R.A., Collet, J.P., Falk, V., Head, S.J., Jüni, P., Kastrati, A., Koller, A., Kristensen, S.D., Niebauer, J., Richter, D.J., Seferovic, P.M., Sibbing, D., Stefanini, G.G., Windecker, S., Yadav, R., Zembala, M.O. (2019). 2018 ESC/EACTS Guidelines on myocardial revascularization. *Eur. Heart J., 40*(2), 87-165. [published correction appears in Eur Heart J. 2019 Oct 1;40(37):3096].
[http://dx.doi.org/10.1093/eurheartj/ehy394] [PMID: 30165437]

Pollesello, P., Parissis, J., Kivikko, M., Harjola, V.P. (2016). Levosimendan meta-analyses: Is there a pattern in the effect on mortality? *Int. J. Cardiol., 209*, 77-83.
[http://dx.doi.org/10.1016/j.ijcard.2016.02.014] [PMID: 26882190]

Ponikowski, P., Voors, A.A., Anker, S.D., Bueno, H., Cleland, J.G.F., Coats, A.J.S., Falk, V., González-Juanatey, J.R., Harjola, V.P., Jankowska, E.A., Jessup, M., Linde, C., Nihoyannopoulos, P., Parissis, J.T., Pieske, B., Riley, J.P., Rosano, G.M.C., Ruilope, L.M., Ruschitzka, F., Rutten, F.H., van der Meer, P. (2016). 2016 ESC Guidelines for the diagnosis and treatment of acute and chronic heart failure: The Task Force for the diagnosis and treatment of acute and chronic heart failure of the European Society of Cardiology (ESC)Developed with the special contribution of the Heart Failure Association (HFA) of the ESC. *Eur. Heart J., 37*(27), 2129-2200.
[http://dx.doi.org/10.1093/eurheartj/ehw128] [PMID: 27206819]

Pu, J., Ding, S., Ge, H., Han, Y., Guo, J., Lin, R., Su, X., Zhang, H., Chen, L., He, B. EARLY-MYO Investigators. (2017). Efficacy and safety of a pharmaco-invasive strategy with half-dose alteplase *Versus* primary angioplasty in st-segment-elevation myocardial infarction: early-myo trial (early routine catheterization after alteplase fibrinolysis *versus* primary PCI in acute ST-segment-elevation myocardial infarction). *Circulation, 136*(16), 1462-1473.
[http://dx.doi.org/10.1161/CIRCULATIONAHA.117.030582] [PMID: 28844990]

Roberts, R. (1991). Immediate *versus* deferred beta-blockade following thrombolytic therapy in patients with acute myocardial infarction (TIMI) IIB study. *Circulation, 83*, 422-437.
[http://dx.doi.org/10.1161/01.CIR.83.2.422] [PMID: 1671346]

Schüpke, S., Neumann, F.J., Menichelli, M., Mayer, K., Bernlochner, I., Wöhrle, J., Richardt, G., Liebetrau, C., Witzenbichler, B., Antoniucci, D., Akin, I., Bott-Flügel, L., Fischer, M., Landmesser, U., Katus, H.A., Sibbing, D., Seyfarth, M., Janisch, M., Boncompagni, D., Hilz, R., Rottbauer, W., Okrojek, R., Möllmann, H., Hochholzer, W., Migliorini, A., Cassese, S., Mollo, P., Xhepa, E., Kufner, S., Strehle, A., Leggewie, S., Allali, A., Ndrepepa, G., Schühlen, H., Angiolillo, D.J., Hamm, C.W., Hapfelmeier, A., Tölg, R., Trenk, D., Schunkert, H., Laugwitz, K.L., Kastrati, A. ISAR-REACT 5 trial investigators. (2019). Ticagrelor or prasugrel in patients with acute coronary syndromes. *N. Engl. J. Med., 381*(16), 1524-1534.
[http://dx.doi.org/10.1056/NEJMoa1908973] [PMID: 31475799]

Valina, C., Neumann, F.J., Menichelli, M., Mayer, K., Wöhrle, J., Bernlochner, I., Aytekin, A., Richardt, G., Witzenbichler, B., Sibbing, D., Cassese, S., Angiolillo, D.J., Kufner, S., Liebetrau, C., Hamm, C.W., Xhepa, E., Hapfelmeier, A., Sager, H.B., Wustrow, I., Joner, M., Trenk, D., Laugwitz, K.L., Schunkert, H., Schüpke, S., Kastrati, A. (2020). Ticagrelor or prasugrel in patients with non-st-segment elevation acute coronary syndromes. *J. Am. Coll. Cardiol., 76*(21), 2436-2446.
[http://dx.doi.org/10.1016/j.jacc.2020.09.584] [PMID: 33213722]

Viecca, M., Radovanovic, D., Forleo, G.B., Santus, P. (2020). Enhanced platelet inhibition treatment improves hypoxemia in patients with severe Covid-19 and hypercoagulability. A case control, proof of concept study. *Pharmacol. Res., 158*, 104950.
[http://dx.doi.org/10.1016/j.phrs.2020.104950] [PMID: 32450344]

Wang, K., Samai, K. (2020). Role of high-dose intravenous nitrates in hypertensive acute heart failure. *Am. J. Emerg. Med., 38*(1), 132-137.
[http://dx.doi.org/10.1016/j.ajem.2019.06.046] [PMID: 31327485]

Yancy, C.W., Jessup, M., Bozkurt, B., Butler, J., Casey, D.E., Jr, Colvin, M.M., Drazner, M.H., Filippatos, G., Fonarow, G.C., Givertz, M.M., Hollenberg, S.M., Lindenfeld, J., Masoudi, F.A., McBride, P.E., Peterson, P.N., Stevenson, L.W., Westlake, C. (2016). 2016 ACC/AHA/HFSA focused update on new pharmacological therapy for heart failure: an update of the 2013 ACCF/AHA guideline for the management of heart failure: a report of the american college of cardiology/American heart association task Force on clinical practice guidelines and the heart failure society of America. *J. Am. Coll. Cardiol., 68*(13), 1476-1488. [http://dx.doi.org/10.1016/j.jacc.2016.05.011] [PMID: 27216111]

Zhou, J, Chin, CT, Huang, X (2020). Long-term antiplatelet therapy in medically managed non-ST-segment elevation acute coronary syndromes: The EPICOR Asia study. *Int. J. Cardiol., S0167-5273*(20), 34089-4.

CHAPTER 6

Heart Failure and Acute Pulmonary Edema (APEd)

Abstract: Heart failure (HF) is a complex syndrome in which the cardiac output cannot meet the demand, *i.e.*, metabolic needs of the tissues and reflect the impairment of the heart's pump function. This condition is also referred to as congestive heart failure (CHF) as it is mostly associated with fluid retention.

The four main factors that determine the pump function of the left ventricle, which are contractility (contractility), preload, afterload and heart rate.

Accepted guidelines divided patients with HF into three groups according to their left ventricular ejection fraction (EF). The group with a EF below 40% continues to be known as a "low/reduced EF" (HF-REF), and a group of 50% and above remains "preserved EF" (HF-PEF), while a group of 40–49% is at the border (mid-range), thus it was named mildly reduced EF" (HF-MREF). The incidence of HF-PEF increases with age. The majority of cases in the elderly is due to HF-PEF. Acute decompensated HF is a deadly cause of cardiac dysfunction that can present with acute respiratory distress. There are many different causes of APEd, though cardiogenic pulmonary edema is usually a result of acutely elevated cardiac filling pressures. Clinical findings develop as a result of impaired perfusion and/or venous distension, with resultant surge in pressure. The patient mostly present with progressive symptoms of HF or acutely appeared signs of left-sided decompensation.

Patients who are diagnosed with HF for the first time and who is admitted with APEd should be hospitalized and treated accordingly. HF develops in 10 to 20% of AMI cases. Since this group has a high mortality, it must be identified and treated.

The main objective of the treatment in the Acute Left HF is to provide the respiratory and cardiovascular stability as soon as possible. The main goal is to "dry" the lungs, not just throwing off water.

COVID-19 pneumonia and respiratory distress can masquerade APEd in the pandemic period. Most "typical" radiological findings including ground-glass opacities are common in both entities. It is very frequent that a clinician mixes up the two entities, especially misinterpret APEd as COVID-19, because the outbreak affects so many people that every physician is conditioned to see the viral pneumonia. Therefore, educational resources should stress on how to implement correct differential diagnosis of cardiopulmonary entities including AHF/APEd in the pandemics in both hospital and outpatient conditions. This chapter provides a general overview of the diagnosis and management of HF and APEd with a special emphasis on the acute presentation in the pandemic era.

Keywords: Acute pulmonary edema, Congestive heart failure, COVID-19, Dyspnea, Heart failure, Left ventricular dysfunction.

INTRODUCTION

Heart failure (HF) is a complex syndrome in which the cardiac output cannot meet the demand, *i.e.*, metabolic needs of the tissues and reflect the impairment of the heart's pump function. This condition is also referred to as congestive heart failure (CHF) as it is mostly associated with fluid retention. Between 90% and 95% of patients with HF are considered congestive patients.

ETIOLOGY FRANK-STARLING LAW

The mechanisms underlying the "Frank-Starling Law of the heart" states that the stroke volume of the left ventricle will increase as the left ventricular volume increases due to the myocyte stretch causing a more forceful systolic contraction. This assumes that other factors remain constant. The functional importance of the Frank-Starling mechanism lies mainly in adapting left to right ventricular output. In a clinical situation, when increased volumes of blood flow into the heart (increasing preload), the walls of the heart stretch (Seres, 2011). The myocytes contract with increased force and, within limits, empties the expanded chambers with increasing stroke volume. Lengths of myocytes and sarcomere eventually become supranormal and therefore contraction forces are reduced below normal.

Types and Clinical Presentation

Patients with HF mostly present to the ED or call an ambulance with left ventricular dysfunction, briefly "left HF" and resultant respiratory signs and complaints (such as dyspnea/APEd, shortness of breath, paroxysmal nocturnal dyspnea, *etc.*).

The basic mechanism of "right HF" is that excess water is sequestered in the body (venous system) due to pump failure. Complaints occur with pretibial edema, fluid accumulation in third cavities, hepatomegaly, hepatojugular reflux, and jugular venous distinction. However, life-threatening or critical condition due to right HF is very rare.

European and American Cardiology associations have published new consensus reports on the diagnosis and treatment of HF. For example, in the 2016 ESC HF guidelines, patients with HF were divided into three groups according to their left ventricular ejection fraction (EF). The group with a EF below 40% continues to be known as a "low/reduced EF" (HF-REF), and a group of 50% and above remains "preserved EF" (HF-PEF), while a group of 40% to 49% is at the border (mid-range), thus it was named mildly reduced EF" (HF-MREF) (Ponikowski *et al.*; Yancy *et al.*, Nadar S).

Characteristics of patients with HF

The EAHFE registry has prospectively collected 13,971 consecutive AHF patients diagnosed in 41 Spanish EDs (Llorens, ICA-SEMES Research Group, 2018). Compared to other large registries, patients in the EAHFE registry were older (80 years), more frequently women (55.5%), and had a higher prevalence of hypertension (83.5%) and a lower prevalence of ischaemic cardiomyopathy (29.4%). *De novo* AHF was observed in 39.6%. More than half of the sample (56.1%) had HF-PEF. 56.8% of the patients arrived at the ED by ambulance, 4.5% arrived hypotensive, and 21.3% hypertensive. Direct discharge from the ED was noted in one-fourth of the patients. The length of hospitalisation was 9.3 (8.6) days, and in-hospital, 30-day, and 1-year all-cause mortality were 7.8, 10.2 and 30.3%, respectively; and 30-day re-hospitalisation and ED revisit rates due to AHF were 16.9 and 24.8%, respectively.

The incidence of HFpEF increases with age. The majority of cases in the elderly is due to HFpEF. Acute decompensated HF is a deadly cause of cardiac dysfunction that can present with acute respiratory distress. In decompensated cases, pulmonary edema and the rapid accumulation of fluid within the interstitial and alveolar spaces leads to significant dyspnea and respiratory distress. There are many different causes of APEd, though cardiogenic pulmonary edema is usually a result of acutely elevated cardiac filling pressures (King, 2020) (Table 1).

Table 1. HF types (from severe to mild) and associated clinical and laboratory variables.

HF-LEF (low EF)	HF-MEF (medium EF)	HF-PEF (protected EF)
Symptoms + signs		
LVEF<40%	LVEF=40%-49%	LVEF>50%
BNP can rise (not a rule)	BNP rises	
Systolic dysfunction	Structural heart disease and/or diastolic dysfunction	

Pathogenesis

Four main factors determine the pump function of the left ventricle: Contractility, preload, afterload and heart rate. CHF occurs because of a marked decrease in myocardial contractility, tissue loss in the myocardium, or increased volume or pressure load of the myocardium. Examples of pressure loading include hypertension and aortic stenosis, volume loading, aortic or mitral insufficiency and left-to-right shunt, decreased contractility, and cardiomyopathy.

Low-flow failure results from inadequate myocardial contraction. In high-flow failure, the myocardium is intact, but there is excessive functional demand (such as anemia, thyrotoxicosis, beriberi, large A-V shunts). CHF is either due to dysfunction of the heart or insufficient peripheral compensatory response despite decreased heart rate.

Diastolic Dysfunction (DD)

DD is the result of normal left ventricular EF in a patient with signs and symptoms of CHF, and failure of left ventricular compliance and relaxation as the main pathomechanism. A history of hypertension is common in these patients. In USG/Echo, left ventricular concentric hypertrophy is viewed as a rule. In histology, increase fibrillar collagen is detected in myocytes. The diagnosis is mostly established by ruling other dyspnea etiologies out. Treatment is initiated with preventing tachycardia, and alleviating blood pressure. Beta blockers, nitrates and diuretics have beneficial effects in addition to lifestyle modification.

HF Accompanying ACS

One of the most important and vital complications of ACS is the development of HF. Patients who are diagnosed with HF for the first time and who is admitted with APEd should be hospitalized and treated accordingly. HF develops in 10% to 20% of AMI cases. Since this group has a high mortality, it must be identified and treated. Killip-Kimball classification is used in the classification of patients who present with HF signs and symptoms accompanying AMI (Table 2).

Patients with HF can be divided into 4 different subgroups regarding clinical appearance, signs and symptoms. Main characteristics are given in the Table.

Table 2. Killip-Kimball classification.

Class I: No clinical signs of HF
Class II: Rales and S3 gallop rhythm
Class III: APEd
Class IV: Hypoperfusion complicating dyspnea: Cardiogenic shock, SBP <90 mmHg, peripheral vasoconstriction (cyanosis, oliguria, diaphoresis)

According to ICA-SEMES Research Group, the AHF phenotypes were categorized as: warm/wet 82.0%, warm/dry 6.2%, cold/wet 11.1%, and cold/dry 0.7% (Llorens, 2018) (Table **3**).

Table **3**. **Assessment of hemodynamic status and findings on auscultation of the lungs, patient classification and relevant treatment options in patients admitted with HF signs and symptoms.**

Group Definition	Hot-Wet	Hot-Dry	Cold-Wet (Most Common)	Cold-Dry
Summary of Presentation	well perfused and congested	poorly perfused-no--congested	poorly perfused-congested	poorly perfused-no--congested
Blood Pressure, Rales and Dyspnea	hypertensive or normotensive + rales + dyspnea	often normotensive + no rales + no dyspnea	often hypotensive + rales + dyspnea	often hypotensive + no rales + no dyspnea
General Treatment: Fluids, Diuretics, Drugs	It may benefit from diuretics, give calcium channel blocker, unless ACS.	Search for the differential diagnoses, it may be purely right-HF. Careful monitoring may suffice	Examine IVC and caval index with USG, if needed, fluid can be given carefully.	Examine IVC and caval index with USG, if needed, fluid can be given carefully.
Treatment: Fluids, Diuretics, Drugs	Furosemide + nicardipine + -Ultrafiltration	Follow-up, rule out ACS, discharge if there are no other serious diagnoses	Inotropes (dopamine/noradrenaline) is mostly required. CVP monitoring may be performed. Furosemide can be given with caution. Mechanical circulatory support may be needed.	An inotrope may be needed, unless recovered quickly.
Admission/discharge	Admit to wards or ICU in accord with clinical status and comorbid/associated factors	Oral treatment, admit to wards or discharge	ICU admission.	ICU admission, unless recovered quickly.

Diagnosis, Physical Examination and Findings

Clinical findings develop as a result of impaired perfusion and/or venous distension, with resultant surge in pressure. The patients mostly present with progressive symptoms of HF or acutely appeared signs of left-sided decompensation. Insufficient perfusion leads to fatigue and weakness, especially when the metabolic needs of the musculoskeletal system are not adequately met. Activation of the renin-angiotensin-aldosterone system (RAS) causes retention of water and sodium (volume loading and edema) and a boost in systemic vascular resistance. In addition, impaired perfusion triggers tachycardia through the sympathetic nervous system (Table **4**).

Increased Venous Pressure, *i.e.*, Signs of Retrograde Circulatory Failure

In parallel with the increase in left ventricular end-diastolic pressure, the left atrium faces with an increase in pressure in the pulmonary veins and capillaries. As a result of this process, the development of interstitial edema followed by alveolar edema appears in the early phase. The main complaint, dyspnea, ensues with heavy exertion at first, then with moderate exertion, while doing daily routine, and finally at rest (orthopnea). Paroxysmal nocturnal dyspnea (PND), and coughing attacks are very typical.

Table 4. The most common etiologies of acute HF and APEd.

Precipitating Cause in *de novo* Acute HF	Precipitating Causes in Acute HF on Previously Diagnosed HF
Myocardial ischemia: Acute or chronic Valve dysfunction: Aortic valve diseases: Aortic stenosis, aortic insufficiency (dissection, infective endocarditis) Mitral valve diseases: Mitral stenosis, mitral regurgitation (rupture of chordae tendinea in papillary muscle) Other causes of left ventricular outflow obstruction: Aortic stenosis, membranous subvalvular aortic stenosis Idiopathic cardiomyopathy (CMP): Hypertrophic, dilated, restrictive Acquired CMP: Toxic (alcohol, cocaine), Metabolic (thyrotoxicosis) Myocarditis: Radiation, infection Constrictive Pericarditis Cardiac dysrhythmias Cardiac Tamponade Systemic Hypertension Anemia	Infections (infective endocarditis, bronchitis *etc.*) Pulmonary embolism Tachyarrhythmias (Atrial tachycardia/fibrillation, ventricular tachycardia) Bradyarrhythmias (sinus, nodal, AV block) Myocardial ischemia or infarction Systemic hypertension Anemia Thyroid diseases (Hyper/hypothyroidism) Treatment incompatibility/drug cessation Excessive salt intake Agents resulting in sodium retention Negative inotropic drugs Physical/emotional stress Pregnancy

The clinical picture of HF depends on which ventricle is affected primarily. The main symptoms and physical examination findings in accord with the involved ventricle are shown in Table **5**.

Table 5. Significant symptoms and signs regarding ventricular involvement in patients with heart failure.

Symptom	Physical examination findings
Left HF	

(Table 5) cont....

Fatigue	Tachycardia, tachypnea
Shortness of breath (effort dyspnea), angina	S3 gallop, sometimes S4
Orthopnea	Diaphoresis
Bendopnea (dyspnea increasing bending forward)	Cyanosis
	Rales in lung areas
Paroxysmal nocturnal dyspnea	Pulsus alternans (in severe cases)
Oliguria	Hypotension (in severe cases)
Nocturia	Altered mental status, syncope
	Pink frothy sputum-hemoptysis
Right HF	
Edema and swelling, weight gain,	Jugular venous distension
Pain/tenderness on the right upper quadrant	Edema of the periphery; i.e., pretibial, scrotal and abdominal skin, ascites
Anorexia	Hepatomegaly
Nausea	Hepatojugular reflux
Jaundice	Palmar erythema, spider angioma, gynecomastia
	CVP increase

RADIOLOGICAL AND LABORATORY FINDINGS

Telecardiogram

The main findings are cardiomegaly and pulmonary effusion. If pulmonary venous pressure (PVP)> 15 mm Hg, vascular redistribution occurs, if above 20 mmHg; interstitial and interlobular edema is triggered and "Reindeer Horn" and "Kerley-B Lines" can be seen; if PVP is above 25 mmHg, alveolar pulmonary edema; "Discarded Cotton view" and "Butterfly Image" can be noted (Table **6**). If pleural effusion can be monitored, the capillary wedge pressure is at least 18 to 25 mm Hg in these patients. In this case, they are typically on the right or bilateral.

Table 6. The relationship between pulmonary venous pressure (PVP) and radiological findings.

PVP	Pathophysiology	What is it Called?
> 15 mm Hg	vascular redistribution	-
>20 mm Hg	interstitial and interlobular edema	"Reindeer Horn" and "Kerley-B Lines"
>25 mm Hg	alveolar edema	"Discarded Cotton view" and "Butterfly Image"

Conventional Chest X-Ray (CXR)

The main findings are cardiomegaly and pulmonary effusion, and as the PVP exceeds 15 mmHg, the pressure levels are parallel to radiological findings. Table shows the relationship between PVP and radiological findings. Fig. (**1A**) shows a CXR of a patient who is newly symptomatic for the interstitial edema phase. In

Fig. (**1**), the radiological imaging of the patient in whom alveolar congestion is evident and the clinical course is expected to be more severe.

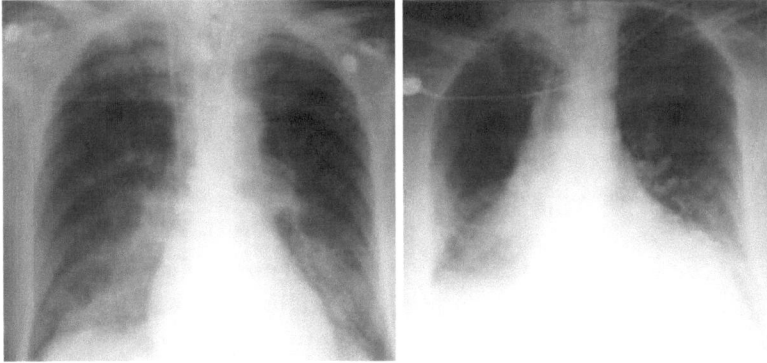

Fig. (1). CXR depicting interstitial edema. (**1A**). No abnormality can be noted other than the Kerley-B lines. (**1B**). CXR findings of alveolar pulmonary edema.

On the other hand, neurogenic pulmonary edema can be manifested with non-occupied costodiaphragmatic sinuses, absence of cardiomegaly and Kerley-B lines as distinguishing features (Fig. **2**).

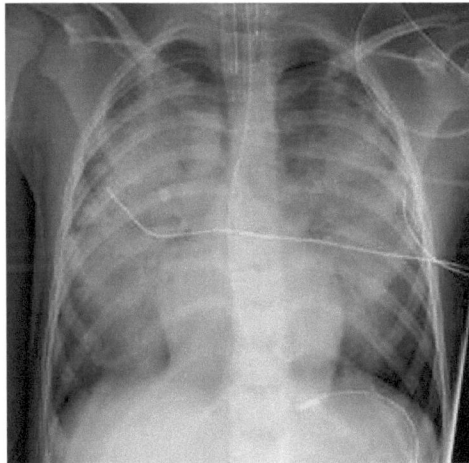

Fig. (2). Neurogenic pulmonary edema.

Can COVID-19 Masquerade for APEd?

Yes. Ground-glass opacities (GGO) are somehow a common finding in both entities. In the pandemic era, it is very frequent that a clinician mixes up the two entities, especially misinterpret APEd as COVID-19, because the outbreak affects so many people that every physician is conditioned to see the viral pneumonia in every patient in both outpatient and inpatient circumstances.

Ultrasonography (USG)/POCUS

Bedside USG has 97% sensitivity and 95% specificity in the diagnosis of APEd. Apart from B-lines, USG findings indicative of APEd include pleural fluid, loss of respiratory collapse and enlargement in the inferior vena cava, a decrease in heart contraction (Fig. **3**).

Bedside USG/POCUS: Modified LuCUS Protocol

Detection of 3 or more diffuse B lines in bilateral anterosuperior lung regions with POCUS is predictive for acute decompensated HF, pulmonary edema. In addition, the fact that EF <45% is diagnostic. The specificity of this protocol is 100%, that is, when found, it ensures acute lung edema, excluding other diagnoses.

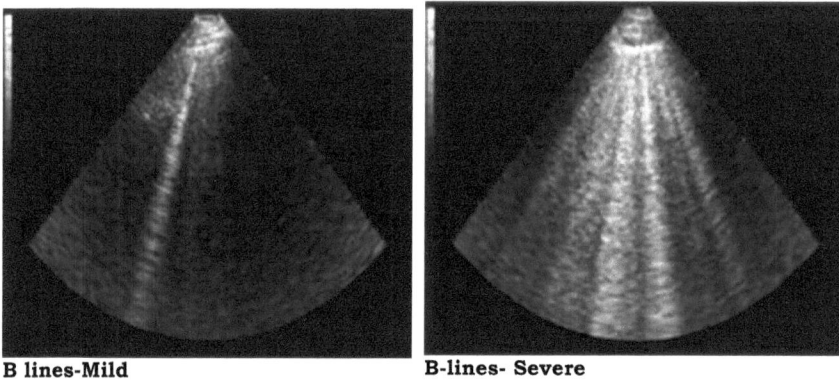

B lines-Mild   **B-lines- Severe**

Fig. **(3).** B-lines compatible with mild and severe pulmonary edema and cardiogenic shock.

CT

In a case with a diagnosis of HF, the CT indication is in the 'rule rule out' phenomenon. Pulmonary embolism, aortic aneurysm/dissection, ACS are tried to be excluded in CT with a single contrast injection (Fig. **4**). If nephrotoxicity and allergic events are excluded, no reservations have been reported. CT can also be used for characterization of the myocardium, such as the stunning phenomenon following ACS/AMI.

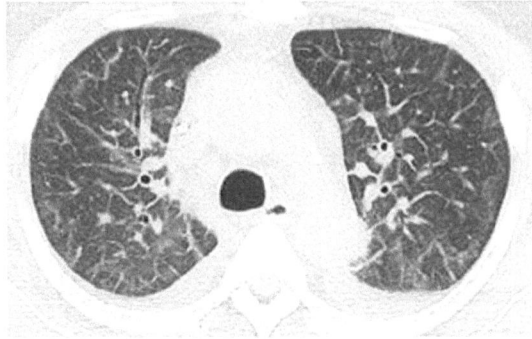

Fig. (4). CT Findings compatible with pleural effusion in a patient with moderate APEd. It is noted that fluid accumulations are more remarkable in dependent areas.

Case example: Chest X-ray and ECG of a 67-year-old woman admitted to hospital due to respiratory symptoms and was diagnosed with COVID-19 (Adapted from Dabbagh, 2020) (Fig. **5**).

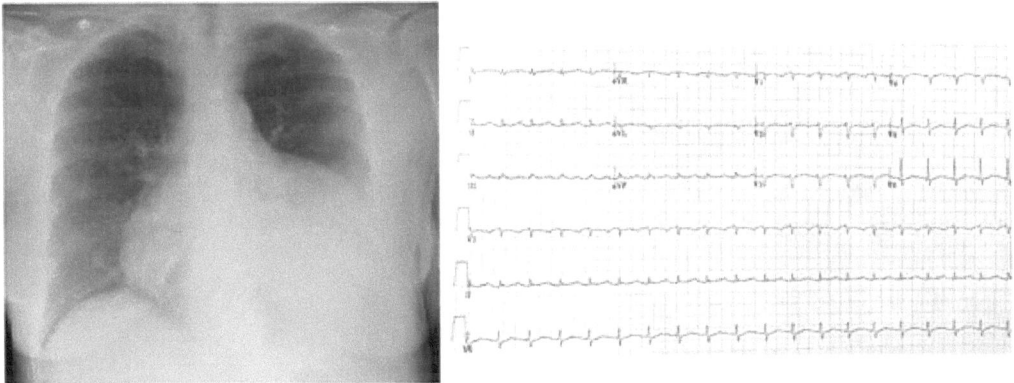

Fig. (5). CXR demonstrates markedly enlarged cardiac silhouette, while ECG shows sinus tachycardia with low-voltage QRS complex in limb leads and nonspecific STsegment changes in precordial leads. She was found to have a large hemorrhagic pericardial effusion with echocardiographic signs of tamponade and mild left ventricular impairment which was also complicated by Takotsubo cardiomyopathy in a few days. She was treated with pericardiocentesis, colchicine, corticosteroids, and hydroxychloroquine, with improvement in symptoms.

Case example. CT scan with IV contrast obtained with "triple rule out" procedure in a patient presenting with dyspnea (Fig. **6**).

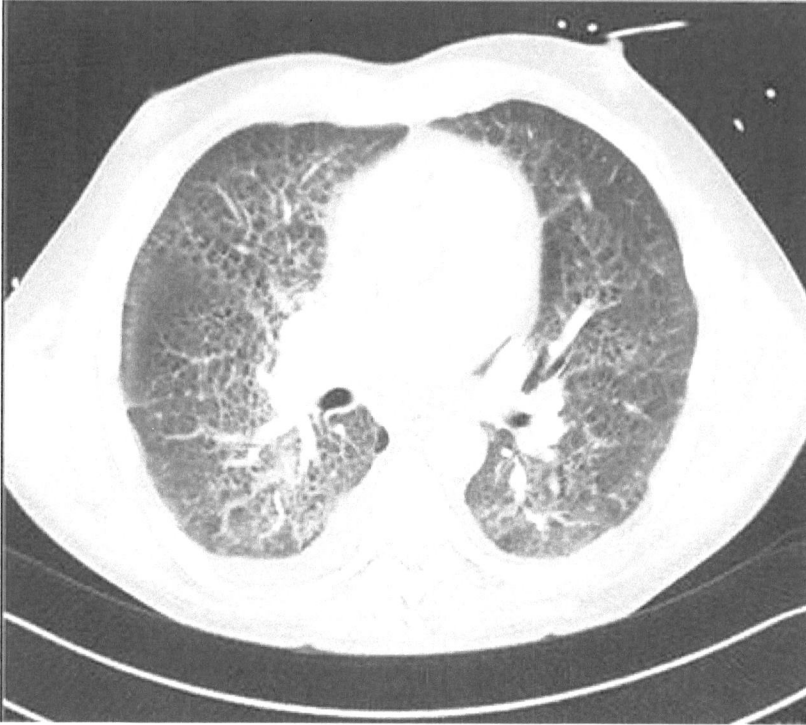

Fig. (6). Pulmonary embolism was not identified in the CT scan, but suboptimal opacification of the distal subsegmental arteries is remarkable. Diffuse "crazy paving type pattern" is seen in both lung areas. Apart from pulmonary edema, pulmonary hemorrhage, pulmonary alveolar proteinosis, acute interstitial pneumonitis and diffuse alveolar damage should be considered and distinguished in emergency situations. The patient was diagnosed with APEd.

Gadolinium-enhanced Cardiac MRI

Gadolinium-enhanced Cardiac MRI is useful for revealing viable myocardium and recording the percentage of viable portion after PCI, displaying sections that are in hibernation or stunning phenomenon.

ECG

There is no typical ECG sign for heart failure. The most important reason for taking an ECG in a case with a left HF is to rule out ACS, especially myocardial infarction. In addition, acute, subacute or chronic rhythm disturbances such as acute atrial fibrillation, ventricular dysrhythmias, assist in recognizing the etiology by disclosing conduction problems. "P mitrale" appears in valve failure (*e.g.*, mitral stenosis) and "p pulmonale" in pulmonary hypertension.

P has an amplitude of > 2.5 mm in inferior leads in p pulmonale, and> 1.5 mm in V1 and V2 (Fig. **7**).

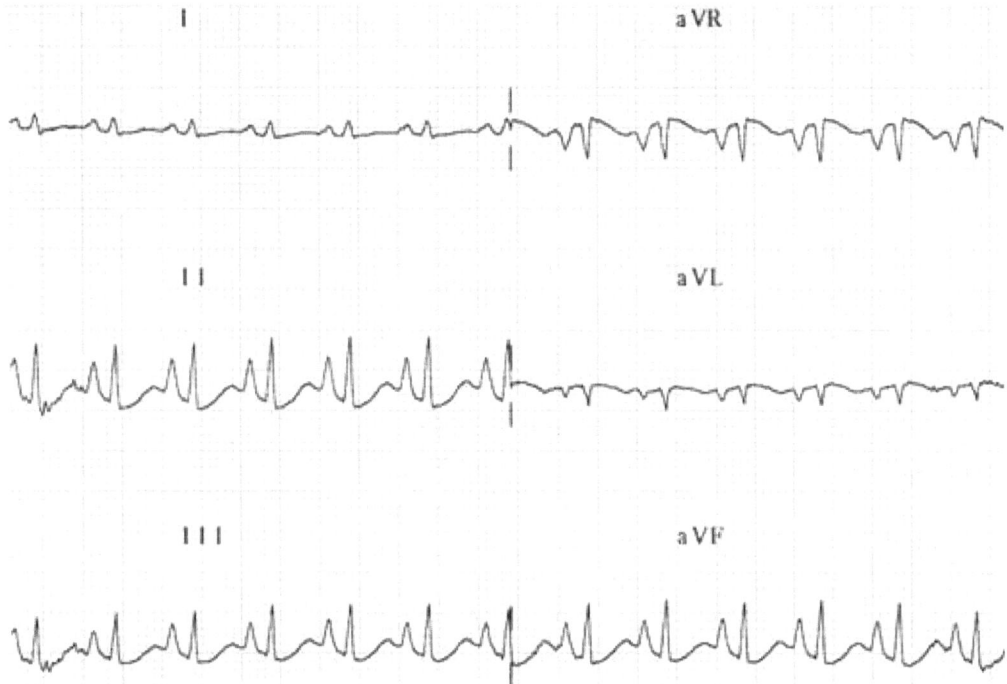

Fig. (7). P pulmonale view in limb lead DII.

P mitrale is a double-crested or "notched" P wave view in DII (Fig. **8**). This is due to delayed left atrium activation. P wave amplitude is> 120 ms.

It should be known that the S1 Q3 T3 finding sought in PE is detected only in a small percentage (3% to 10%) of all embolism cases, that is, it cannot be used as an exclusion (rule out) test.

USG/Echocardiography

It is an indispensable diagnostic tool in the verification of HF because it provides invaluable information about the anatomical and functional status (condition of the ventricles and ejection fraction), which enables rapid and bedside peformance and noninvasive evaluation. It provides information about wall motion disorders, valves and the state of the pericardium. Diastolic HF can also be diagnosed. It allows measuring pulmonary artery pressure (PAP) with the Doppler function. The widespread use of USG will make wedge pressure measurement largely unnecessary, possibly, which was used previously through pulmonary artery catheterization. CVP measurement, which is a more common procedure, will also have an increasingly rare indication. Fluid excess can be largely recognized with caval index or IVC measurements, and fluid loading test can be done simply with passive leg raising.

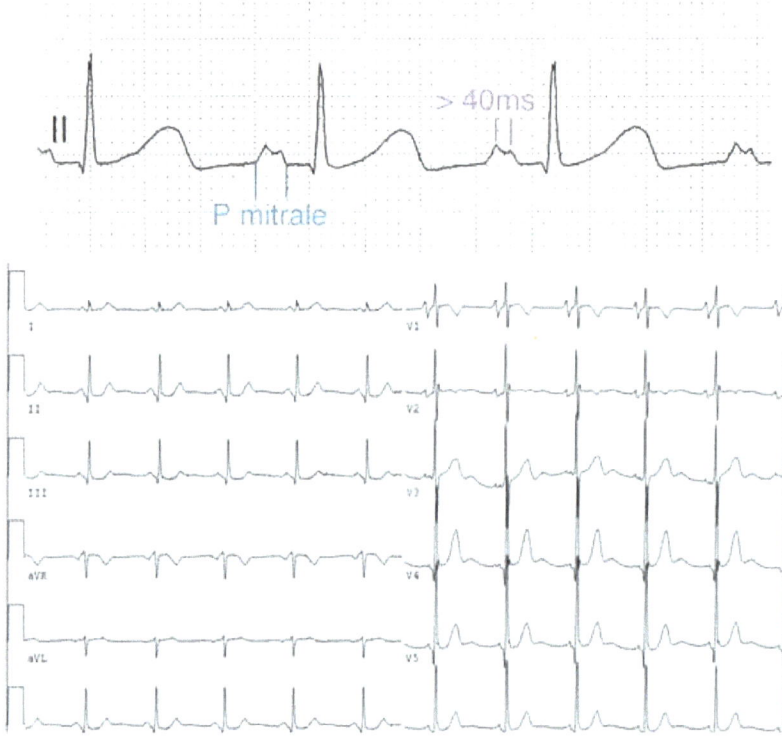

Fig. (8). P mitrale view.

Pulse Oximeter

Its widespread use has reduced the need for arterial blood gases. It should be drawn as soon as the patient with dyspnea presents into the ED. Acutely subnormal values (*i.e.*, below 90%) should suggest ventilatory support and tracheal intubation if necessary. While interpreting the values, it should be kept in mind that there is a +/- 3% margin of error, and the value of 92% can actually be 89%. Values between 90 and 95% are evaluated according to the patient, it can be interpreted in favor of intubation, and other measures such as CPAP, increasing the supplemental O_2 dose can be considered as well. It is comforting if values above 95% are also compatible with the clinical status. In a patient whose clinical status is not stable, measurements below 90% persistently require urgent endotracheal intubation unless otherwise proven. It should be noted that in some important clinical entities such as pulmonary embolism, carbon monoxide intoxication, pulse oximetry measurement may appear misleadingly normal. Again, it should be known that misleading results zcan be obtained when the ambient temperature is very low, in African/black patients and in the interference of additional substances such as nail polish and in newborns.

Arterial Blood Gases (ABG)

It gives information about the acid-base balance and the level of respiratory effort. It can provide information about hypoxia, hypercarbia and acidosis. It is the preliminary finding of respiratory failure. Lactic acid and base deficits can clearly demonstrate the inability to meet the body's metabolic needs, the transition to anaerobic metabolism. It is not necessary to take ABG in all cases where CHF or lung edema is considered. Pulmonary edema triggered especially by hypertension is rapidly treated if COPD is not present in the history. ABG does not provide any additional diagnostic value in these cases. In cases of COPD exacerbation and between CHF-AMS, ABG may be useful, in addition to clinical findings, BNP and bedside USG have adequate diagnostic power for CHF.

Biochemistry

Liver function tests and kidney function tests, may help detection of oliguria-related kidney dysfunction. As prerenal failure will be seen in cases where CHF is prolonged, firstly BUN/urea value and then creatinine levels will increase. Electrolyte and other blood chemistry abnormalities related to paraneoplastic syndromes may be encountered. For example, hypercalcemia is seen in primary lung non-small cell carcinomas in addition to bone metastases. In mesenchymal cancers, persistent hypoglycaemia may occur.

Complete Blood Count

It may be of help in the demonstration of etiology rather than definite diagnosis. It may indicate anemia or infection. It should be noted that leukocytosis is not directly related to infections. In many subgroups such as elderly, immunosuppressed, and debilitated, leukocytosis may not be expected and may cause the infection to be overlooked. Chronic disease anemia can be seen in patients with cancer, renal failure and hypothyroidism. Shortness of breath can also be noted in acute anemia. Acute blood loss should be sought for and ruled out primarily in case of anemia, especially if MCV and MCHC is normal, and reticulocyte count is higher than normal.

B-Type Natriuretic Peptide (Brain natriuretic Peptide, BNP) and N-Terminal ProBNP (NT-ProBNP)

It is a pressure-induced marker released from ventricular myocytes in response to ventricular wall tension, and in recent years this test has been increasingly used for the diagnosis of CHF/APEd and to monitor the effectiveness of treatment. While BNP is better at reflecting acute hemodynamic changes, NT-ProBNP is more effective at demonstrating chronic disease. Therefore, BNP is very useful in discerning HF in dyspnea patients in EDs.

Natriuretic peptide level will take different values in different biochemical forms as pmol/mL. For example, normal values are NP <100 pg/mL, NT-proBNP <300 pg/mL, MR-proANP <120 pmol/mL.

Clinical interpretation with BNP should be undertaken in accord with the whole clinical picture.

It can be attributed to HF following ruling out other possible causes. For example, a patient with STEMI or PTE can also have high BNP levels (Table 7).

Table 7. Threshold values of BNP and NT-ProBNP to help diagnose or rule out acute and chronic HF (Adapted from Ponikowski 2016, Januzzi 2018, Maisel 2002, Murphy, 2020).

To rule in acute HF	NT-proBNP	>450 pg/mL (<50 y); >900 pg/mL (50-75 y); >1800 pg/mL (>75 y)
	BNP	>100 pg/mL (values >400 pg/mL have higher specificity)
To rule out acute HF	NT-proBNP	<300 pg/mL
	BNP	<50 pg/mL
To rule out chronic HF	NT-proBNP	<125 pg/mL
	BNP	<35 pg/mL

Other Blood Tests

Thyroid function tests may show HF caused or precipitated by a thyroid disorder. Cardiac enzyme levels can indicate acute cardiac ischemia resulting in myocardial cellular injury or AMI.

DIFFERENTIAL DIAGNOSIS

COPD Exacerbations

The patient's history, smoking history, the list of medications used, posture, cyanosis, clubbing of the fingers generally give an idea for inclusion of COPD in the differential diagnosis.

Right Ventricular AMI

A history of chest pain, clear lung areas, jugular venous distension, and hypotension are noted in these patients. Typical V4R sign on ECG (in addition to inferior AMI with majority, 1 mm and more ST elevation when V4 lead is placed on the right border of the sternum) are mostly recorded in patients with right ventricular AMI.

Cardiac Tamponade

There are one or more of the findings that include the Beck triad (jugular venous distention, hypotension, pulsus paradoxus, deep heart sounds). As a rule, it is easily recognized by USG. There are no rales on auscultation of the lungs. Unlike APEd, shortness of breath is subtle or absent.

Pulmonary Embolism

Presence of certain risk factors, positive Homans'test indicative of DVT, a history of immobilization lasting longer than 12-24 hours can help in differential diagnosis. It is reasonable to exclude it by Wells' criteria or PERC. In low-risk cases, a negative d-dimer rules out the diagnosis in almost 100% of cases. Echo/POCUS can also be of invaluable help in presumptive diagnosis if acute right ventricular strain could be demonstrated. On the other hand, definitive diagnosis can be made with CTPA in high-risk patients thought to have high pretest probability.

Pneumonia

High fever, flank pain and progressive cough in the patient's history together with leukocytosis and left shift are suggestive of pneumonia which should be investigated further *via* laboratory and radiological adjuncts. Since the signs and symptoms such as fever, pain, and leukocytosis will be more subtle in elderly, the rate of false negative diagnoses can rise in patients with moribund status. In this case, it will be necessary to refer to radiological investigations. There is a risk of missing the diagnosis because the 3rd dimension cannot be visualized in one-way shots on the CXRs. Plain radiographs should be shot in at least two directions. Finally, it should not be forgotten that pneumonia may have triggered APEd, that is, both pathologies may coexist in a given patient (Fig. **9**).

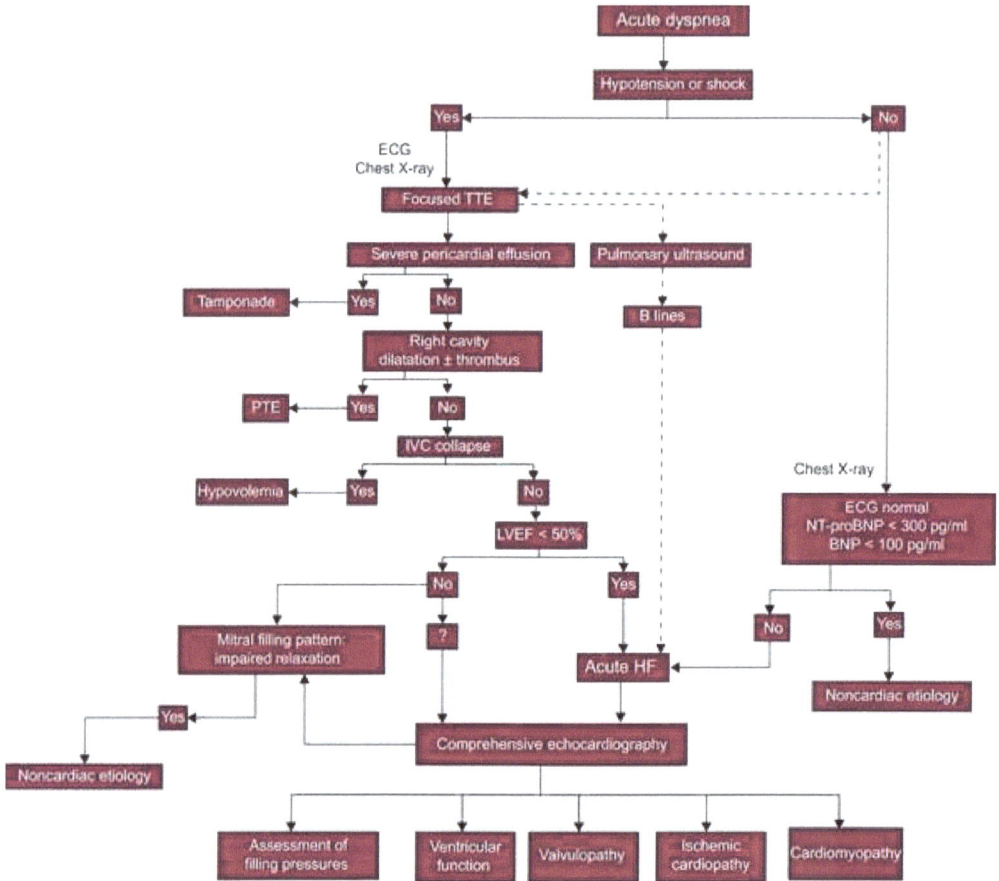

Fig. (9). Proposed algorithm for the diagnostic and therapeutic management of the patient with acute dyspnea. Apart from clinical examination, ECG, chest X-ray, ultrasonography and echocardiography play pivotal roles in this decision-making process.

ACUTE PULMONARY EDEMA (APED)

Heart-induced APEd is an advanced and fatal form of acute left ventricular failure, which must be recognized and treated immediately. While it is generally encountered with the presence of precipitating factor(s) in those with chronic HF, it can rarely be seen in people who have not been diagnosed with HF.

APEd almost always occurs with a triggering event which should be identified and treated in the management of the patient. Since it is common for hypertension to be precipitating event, it is also called "hypertensive acute pulmonary edema".

Etiology includes left HF, hypertensive attack, ischemic heart disease, water-salt loading, kidney failure, acute atrial fibrillation, and other arrhythmias (Table **8**).

Table 8. Triggering causes of APEd.

exacerbation of the underlying HF
ischemic heart disease
dysrhythmia
incompatibility between drugs and/or diet
valve failure
hyperthyroidism

Signs and Symptoms

Dyspnea on exertion, paroxysmal nocturnal dyspnea, orthopnea, chest pain, abdominal pain, syncope or altered mental status are the leading signs and symptoms. The patient has either severe acute shortness of breath or a sudden increase in pre-existing shortness of breath. Air hunger, anxiety/agitation, pink frothy sputum, weakness and fatigue, and feeling of fainting can be seen. Auxiliary muscles of respiration can participate in breathing. The patient can feel better by holding his legs below the edge of the bed in a sitting position to perform phlebotomy. The skin is pale and sweaty. In physical examination, breathing sounds are rough and noisy with rales, starting from the dependent areas-lung bases and spreading to higher zones. Tachycardia, S3 and sometimes S4 can be taken in cardiac auscultation. Patients' pre-existing diagnosis of HF, or existing shortness of breath, orthopedic and paroxysmal nocturnal dyspnea (PND) facilitates diagnosis and differential diagnosis.

Left HF Findings

Basilar/bibasilar rales, infrequently silent lung, hypo- or hypertension, parasternal lift, pulsus alternans, decreased urine output, cold and moist skin, supraclavicular/intercostal muscular retractions, atrial and ventricular arrhythmias, marked dyspnea, impaired consciousness. In some cases, right HF findings (JVD; hepatojugular reflux; pretibial edema, ascites, abdominal pain) may accompany but are not a prerequisite.

TREATMENT OF LEFT HF/APED

The main objective of the treatment in the Acute Left HF is to provide the respiratory and cardiovascular stability as soon as possible. The main goal is to "dry" the lungs, not throwing off water.

In a recent article in JAMA cited that treatment strategies should include diuretics to relieve symptoms and application of an expanding armamentarium of disease-modifying drug and device therapies (Murphy, 2020). Unless there are specific contraindications, patients with HF-REF should be treated with β-blockers (BB) and an angiotensin receptor-neprilysin inhibitor, angiotensin-converting enzyme inhibitor (ACEI), or angiotensin receptor blocker (ARB) at the beginning. Mineralocorticoid receptor antagonist can be added in patients with symptoms unrelieved with these measures. Ivabradine and hydralazine/isosorbide dinitrate can also be administered to selected patients with HF-REF.

BB agents have beneficial effect in the management of HF. These compounds occupy cellular β-receptors and mitigate the effects of catecholamines on β-adrenergic receptors. Some BBs are "partial agonists" (*e.g.*, acebutolol, pindolol, and celiprolol), which cause inhibition only in the presence of high concentrations of catecholamines. Negative inotropic (decreased stroke volume) and chronotropic effects (slowed AV conduction) of BB represent the role of adrenoceptors in the regulation of myocardial contractility and electrical activity of the sino-atrial (SA) node. An evidence-based BB agent (metoprolol succinate, carvedilol, or bisoprolol) should be prescribed in all patients with HFrEF unless contraindicated or not tolerated (eg, patients with symptomatic bradycardia despite lowest dose, patients with advanced HF and low cardiac output or on home inotropes, or patients with high-grade AV block); as these agents reduce mortality, sudden cardiac death, and hospitalizations in patients with HF-REF (Murphy, 2020).

Our goals in treatment are;

1. To recognize the underlying cardiac condition/pathology,

2. To treat congestion and excess water (in most patients),

3. Identification and management of the precipitating factor that brings the patient to the ED at the moment.

Follow-up

Continuous cardiac monitoring and 12-lead ECG monitoring are important to detect ACS and arrhythmias.

The First-line Treatment

The First-line Treatment that should be commenced in the ED can be summarized as MONA-FB. Since it is not possible to rule out ACS immediately in a typical patient presenting to the ED with shortness of breath, treatment should be arranged by presumption of ACS.

The patient should be placed in a comfortable position. Orthopneic position is the most comfortable in the majority of these patients. In the case of hypervolemia, it may also be beneficial for some patients to sit on the bedside, hanging the feet down, called 'dry' phlebotomy. 16G or wider vascular access should be opened and made sure that it is kept open. The intraosseous route is an alternative to usual IV routes. It should be remembered that the patient may have cardiac arrest at any time as a result of hypoxia or complication of ACS.

In the guidelines published in 2016, the follow-up of the patients with cardiogenic shock in intensive care units with continuous cardiac catheterization and temporary mechanical support is emphasized as Class 1 recommendation. In these updates, the primary approach to acute HF algorithm is to reveal whether it is APEd solely or whether it is complicated by circulatory failure (cardiogenic shock). In the presence of cardiogenic shock, the focus of the treatment is shifted radically.

Fluid Therapy

For centuries, hypervolemia has been associated with congestion, thus a belief has been established in physicians that no additional fluid should be administered to any patient with CHF. However, the truth is not so simple. Fluid administration in patients was deemed a Class 1 recommendation and included in the 2016 NICE guidelines. Patients with marked hypervolemic fluid loading were excluded and the rest were recommended the infusion of normal saline or lactated Ringer's to be> 200 ml/15–30 min as an initial treatment. Naturally, in patients with low EF with hypervolemia accompanied by pulmonary edema, IV administration of fluids carries the risk of disrupting oxygenation even further. For this, bedside USG should be used as a guide, if hypervolemia can be excluded with evaluation of IVC diameter and caval index, crystalloids should be given, starting at 100 mL/kg.

Ensuring Oxygenation

Ensuring Oxygenation is a priority in the emergent management. In cases where cyanotic, and/or hypoxic (SpO_2 below 90%), time should not be wasted with other measures and oxygenation of vital organs should be ensured immediately. All patients should be evaluated rapidly and aggressive treatments including endotracheal intubation, should be initiated expediently in patients who do not respond immediately to supplemental O_2 administration and nitrate therapy and deterioration is noted. In selected cases, Venturi mask and CPAP treatments can be time-saving methods that delay intubation and can sometimes eliminate the need for it.

Oxygenation with High Flow Nasal Cannula (HFNCO)

It has been demonstrated in many studies in the last decade that oxygenation with HFNC can be an effective option before permanent airway control (intubation) in patients with respiratory failure. The humidified and heated air/oxygen mixture is delivered to the nostrils through the nasal cannula. High current up to 60 L/min can be given with this method. Although the data obtained from the studies are quite heterogeneous, it has been clarified that with HFNCO treatment, respiratory work and the respiratory rate (bpm) are diminished and the need for ventilatory support occurs more rarely. We are sure that it is apparently more advantageous compared to standard O2 in patients with HF, especially after NIV application. HFNCO strategy was reported to be associated with more favorable findings in a study in which NYHA Class III cases were examined ultrasonographically for vena caval collapse in inspiration. With this method, it has been a generally accepted rule that patients who do not have sufficient oxygenation within 24 hours will go to intubation somehow.

Non-invasive Ventilation (NIV)

It has become an important option in the treatment of acute HF, especially in the management of APEd. In 2005, a meta-analysis revealed that NIV application reduced intubation rate and mortality in these patients (Masip *et al*. 2005). It is reported that this result is valid for both "continuous positive airway pressure" (CPAP) and "bi-level positive airway pressure" (BIPAP). CPAP and BIPAP are noninvasive methods of respiratory support to treat respiratory insufficiency secondary to pulmonary vascular congestion and APEd. The use of CPAP and BIBAP has reduced the need for intubation and MV in HF with respiratory decompensation (Bello, 2018). In situations where CPAP and BIPAP are ineffective in improving the patient's respiratory status, one should consider early intubation and MV to prevent further decompensation (King, 2020).

Avoiding complications of intubation is its most important advantage. In the EAHFE study involving more than 11,000 patients, it was suggested that the practice of BIPAP in the ED did not reduce the mortality rates, and more attention should be paid to the patients with accompanying ACS and the elderly, especially if hypotensive (Miro, 2018). Longer hospital stay was also noted in those who received NIV.

The common topic is that initiating NIV in pre-hospital conditions and ED often leads to an improvement in the first minutes and hours, but this is not so clear in long-term results, it may be better to avoid in high-risk patient groups (hypotensive, elderly, with ACS).

Coronary Revascularization

This approach can also reduce mortality and morbidity by improving diastolic and systolic dysfunction in selected circumstances. It is accepted as an intervention for HF patients with angina, LV dysfunction, and CAD. Interventional cardiology should be consulted early for patients according to AHA recommendations (Yancy, 2013, King, 2020).

MONA-FB TREATMENT

M: Morphine Sulfate

It should be given by titrating 0.05-0.1 mg/kg in complicated cases with anxiety and agitation. The emergency team should be prepared for the need for endotracheal intubation in such a patient. Another drawback of the agent is histamine-releasing effect, which can even masquerade as anaphylaxis. It can also cause hypotension and respiratory depression. Nonetheless, it is very rare to encounter a need for acute decompensation just because of using opiates in patients with acute HF or APEd. Although there are beneficial effects of opiates in APEd, some researchers cited that it can be associated with an increase in 30-day mortality of patients with acute HF (Miro, 2017).

O: (Oxygen)

All patients who are admitted with signs and symptoms indicative of instability, such as respiratory distress, impaired consciousness, cyanosis, chest pain and dyspnea should be started supplemental O2 as soon as the patient arrives in the ED or ambulance, with the exception of those with SpO2 value of 95% and above in whom the general condition is completely stable. General dose of application is 10 to 15 L/min.

N: Nitrates, Glycerol Trinitrate

It is effective in direct treatment of HF because of both ACS assumption and venodilator effect. It relieves symptoms within minutes. As can be started as SL, IV treatment is advantageous in cases where the general condition is impaired and ACS is not excluded. The use of sildenafil should be inquired in the history and nitrates should not be administered in case of doubt. Since its effect is limited to minutes, it is given by infusion. If 10 mcg/min is started and sufficient effect is not seen within a few minutes, it should be titrated up quickly. It is administered by monitoring blood pressure closely and infusion should be stopped at systolic BP values below 100 mmHg. In recent studies, initial treatment with a rapid infusion of 400 mcg to 2 mg is also recommended. Wang and Samai reported that high-dose nitrates appear to be safe and may be effective, as demonstrated in the studies reviewed in their article (Wang, 2020). Administration of high-dose nitrates may be appropriate in hypertensive patients with HF presenting with severe respiratory distress and SBP ≥160 mmHg or MAP ≥120 mmHg.

A: Aspirin, Acetylsalicylic Acid (ASA)

It is the standard treatment for left HF cases, as it is indicated for the management of ACS and atrial fibrillation, which plays a role in the etiology of APEd. ASA should be given in all cases except for those with active bleeding from GI or another source, those with active bleeding diathesis even in the absence of bleeding, and those known to be allergic. 325 mg ASA should be chewed and swallowed with some water. It can also be given *via* nasogastric tube after dispersed in water, in patients with altered mental status or inability of swallowing for any reason.

F: Furosemide

In cases considered to be hypervolemic, 40-100 mg IV furosemide and subsequent infusion therapy can be commenced in addition to MONA treatment. Volume loading is not a rule in patients with left HF, although it is present in a majority of them. In other words, it should be known that there may be hypo- or normovolemic cases, and thus furosemide will not be useful in every case. Volume status and potassium level should be monitored. Its antihypertensive effect becomes evident through vascular dilatation in the first minutes and diuretic effect will emerge after 30 minutes. Both mechanisms are beneficial in patients with volume loading *via* facilitating O_2 transport through alveolocapillary membrane and draining excess water from the lungs related to increased afterload.

Update

The initial IV furosemide dose was recommended as 20–40 mg for diuretic-virgin patients, while it was emphasized that parenteral dose should be at least equal to the oral dose in those who used it before.

B: Beta-blocker

Due to its beta-1 cardioselective effect, Metoprolol 15 mg IV should be given in divided doses (*e.g.*, 3x5 mg in around 20 to 30 minutes) with slow infusion. It should be given in all patients with HF except for these with asthma, peripheral artery disease (*e.g.*, Raynaud's disease), severe hypotension, profound and resistant bradycardia and decompensated left HF. It has been shown to be effective in alleviating symptoms and signs of mild to moderate HF. Since these agents have direct therapeutic effects on hypertension and ischemic heart disease, beta blockade should be considered when these factors are considered in the etiology of HF.

A history of bronchial asthma, bradycardia and heart failure do not constitute definitive contraindications for beta-blocker therapy. Cardioselective beta-blockers can be administered with close monitoring at low doses.

ADDITIONAL TREATMENTS

ACE Inhibitors

Although it has no place in preventing life threatening events in the emergency setting, it has benefits such as controlling urgent hypertension and preventing long-term myocardial remodeling. It should not be used in patients with hereditary angioneurotic edema and anuric CKD.

Digoxin

The effect of digitalis glycoside derivatives is minimal in these patients, since APEd is often triggered by ischemic heart disease. The 2016 ESC guideline recommended that it can be used to slow the ventricular rate in patients with atrial fibrillation, in digoxin-naive patients in NYHA IV group with Class IIa level recommendation. Although it has no importance in the treatment of acute HF, if the triggering factor is AF with rapid ventricular response, it may be useful to slow the rate and thus improve cardiac output. It is indicated in these patients at a dose of 0.25-0.50 mg iv.

Vasopressors

The agents to be selected are norepinephrine and dopamine. These agents are safer in terms of side effects and mortality than epinephrine. It is necessary to avoid epinephrine especially in resistant hypotensive patients.

Dopamine

It is considered in cases where emergent positive inotropic support is required, especially if SBP is below 90 mmHg in whom there is a substantial vital risk. Therefore, the patient should be admitted to the hospital, and that referral to a center where invasive interventions can also be performed by an experienced cardiology team should be evaluated. It can be administered in the dose range of 2 to 20 mcg/kg/min. Doses smaller than 8-10 mcg/kg/min are not suitable in the hypotensive patients. It is titrated in accord with the patient's response.

Dobutamine

Unlike dopamine, it is a positive inotropic agent to be selected in normotensive cases, not in hypotensive situations. It should be used with caution, due to its proarrhythmogenic potential, It is given in a dose of 2.5-20 mcg/kg/min. It is titrated regarding the patient's response. Long-term infusions have been claimed to increase mortality.

Levosimendan

This agent has been approved as a safe inodilator agent with an increase in calcium sensitivity in cardiomyocytes and a potassium channel opening effect in vascular smooth muscle cells. In acute and advanced HF cases, IV administration leads to a dose-dependent increase in cardiac output and stroke volume. Many studies have reported that its administration is associated with a reduction in rehospitalization rates. The beneficial effect of intermittent or repetitive treatments has also been demonstrated. Although contradictory results have been obtained, there are researchers who claim that it is superior to dobutamine. In brief, it is thought to be useful as an adjunctive therapy, if not an alternative to conventional definitive therapies.

Milrinon

It has been demonstrated in the level of meta-analysis that it significantly increases left ventricular ejection fraction and cardiac output in acute HF following AMI. Its effect on mortality is not evident. It has been reported that it is more beneficial in nonischemic cardiomyopathy and may be inconvenient in HF triggered by acute ischemia. It is a safe agent. Milrinon therapy combined with beta blockers has also been shown to be a viable strategy for inotrope weaning. In 2016, it was suggested to be administered in Class IIa level in hypotensive, hypoperfused patients after beta blocker use together with levosimendan in ESC guidelines. It also has beneficial effects on amyloidosis-related HF.

Istaroxim

It stands out as a promising new treatment. Since Na-K inhibits ATPase, it has digoxin-like effects. It is a promising new agent, unique in its class with its effects that reduce the heart rate and increase systolic blood pressure, improve the cardiac index, pulmonary wedge pressure. It has no effect on the kidney and does not interfere with troponins.

Anxiolytic and Sedatives

These can be used in excited and agitated patients. Because if agitation is not intervened, it will affect many physiological variables such as blood pressure and pulse, and increase the use of oxygen and substrates of the myocardial cells. Short-acting benzodiazepines are the best option in acute situations. Administration of IM or IV midazolam is the most practical. Treatment with diazepam *via* IM route is not recommended, because of undredictable pharmacokinetics. It should also be known that its effect can last as long as 6 hours and even longer in patients with liver failure and some others.

Renal Replacement Therapy

Patients should be chosen well due to the risk of infection and other complications.

It is more accurate to try loop diuretics in hypervolemic HF. Ongoing oliguria despite treatment, severe hyperkalaemia (K> 6.5 mmol/L), severe acidosis (pH <7.2), BUN> 25 mmol/L, creatinine> 3.4 mg/dL, RRT it will be an urgent and right option.

TREATMENT IN CARDIOGENIC SHOCK

Class I Recommendations

- ECG should be taken in every patient suspected of cardiogenic shock and bedside USG (POCUS) should be evaluated.
- Any patient with cardiogenic shock should be transferred to a center with cardiac catheterization and coronary ICU.
- Angiography and revascularization should be provided within 2 hours after entering the ED for every patient with cardiogenic shock due to ACS.
- Continuous ECG and blood pressure monitoring should be done.
- Invasive arterial monitoring should be maintained.
- If there is no hypervolemia, crystalloid fluid treatment is recommended first.

Class IIb Recommendations

- IV inotropic agents may be useful for increasing cardiac output.
- If resistant hypoperfusion is available, vasopressors can be used to ensure adequate perfusion.
- If there is resistant cardiogenic shock, short-term mechanical circulation support can be used depending on age, comorbidity status and neurological status.

CONCLUSION

HF is an important diagnosis with high mortality and morbidity rate, therefore clinicians should be alerted to distinguish the entity among alternatives. Patients who are diagnosed with *de novo* HF and/or admitted with APEd should be hospitalized and treated accordingly. Although right HF is mostly a non-urgent entity, acute left HF carries a high death toll. The main objective of the treatment in the acute left HF is to provide the respiratory and cardiovascular stability as soon as possible.

Pandemic period made all these processes even more complex. COVID-19 pneumonia and respiratory distress originating from APEd can be mixed up easily. Most "typical" radiological findings are common in both entities. Therefore, educational resources should stress on how to implement correct differential diagnosis of cardiopulmonary entities including AHF/APEd in the pandemics in both hospital and outpatient conditions.

REFERENCES

Ailani, R.K., Rovakhab, K., DiGiovine, B. (1997). A new method for the rapid separation of cardiac and pulmonary dyspnea. *Chest,* 1100-1104.
[PMID: 10531178]

Bello, G., De Santis, P., Antonelli, M. (2018). Non-invasive ventilation in cardiogenic pulmonary edema. *Ann. Transl. Med., 6*(18), 355.
[http://dx.doi.org/10.21037/atm.2018.04.39] [PMID: 30370282]

Boldanova, T., Noveanu, M., Breidthardt, T., Potocki, M., Reichlin, T., Taegtmeyer, A., Christ, M., Laule, K., Stelzig, C., Mueller, C. (2010). Impact of history of heart failure on diagnostic and prognostic value of BNP: results from the B-type Natriuretic Peptide for Acute Shortness of Breath Evaluation (BASEL) study. *Int. J. Cardiol., 142*(3), 265-272.
[http://dx.doi.org/10.1016/j.ijcard.2008.12.214] [PMID: 19185372]

Braithwaite, S., Perina, D. *Marx: Rosen's Emergency Medicine: Concept and Clinical Practice* (5th ed.). Mosby.

Cabanes, L., Richaud-Thiriez, B., Fulla, Y., Heloire, F., Vuillemard, C., Weber, S., Dusser, D. (2001). Brain natriuretic peptide blood levels in the differential diagnosis of dyspnea. *Chest, 120*(6), 2047-2050.
[http://dx.doi.org/10.1378/chest.120.6.2047] [PMID: 11742939]

Cummins, R.O., Field, J.M., Hazinski, M.F. (2003). *ACLS: Principles and Practice.* American Heart Association.

Dabbagh, M.F., Aurora, L., D'Souza, P., Weinmann, A.J., Bhargava, P., Basir, M.B. (2020). Cardiac Tamponade Secondary to COVID-19. *JACC Case Rep, 2*(9), 1326-1330.
[http://dx.doi.org/10.1016/j.jaccas.2020.04.009] [PMID: 32328588]

Danzl, D.F. (2004). Tracheal intubation and mechanical ventilation. In: Tintinalli, J.E., Kelen, G.D., Stapczynski, J.S., (Eds.), *Emergency Medicine: A Comprehensive Study Guide. FACEP.* McGraw-Hill.

DePaso, W.J., Winterbauer, R.H., Lusk, J.A., Dreis, D.F., Springmeyer, S.C. (1991). Chronic dyspnea unexplained by history, physical examination, chest roentgenogram, and spirometry. Analysis of a seven-year experience. *Chest, 100*(5), 1293-1299.
[http://dx.doi.org/10.1378/chest.100.5.1293] [PMID: 1935284]

Duzgun, S.A., Durhan, G., Demirkazik, F.B., Akpinar, M.G., Ariyurek, O.M. (2020). COVID-19 pneumonia: the great radiological mimicker. *Insights Imaging, 11*(1), 118.
[http://dx.doi.org/10.1186/s13244-020-00933-z] [PMID: 33226521]

Fischer, Q., Darmon, A., Ducrocq, G., Feldman, L. (2020). Case report of anterior ST-elevation myocardial

infarction in a patient with coronavirus disease-2019. *Eur Heart J Case Rep, 4*(FI1), 1-5.
[PMID: 33089044]

Grant, H.D., Murray, R.H., Bergeron, J.D. (1994). *Respiratory Emergencies. Emergency Care.* (6th ed., pp. 369-380). New Jersey: Prentice Hall Inc.

Januzzi, J.L., Jr, Chen-Tournoux, A.A., Christenson, R.H., Doros, G., Hollander, J.E., Levy, P.D., Nagurney, J.T., Nowak, R.M., Pang, P.S., Patel, D., Peacock, W.F., Rivers, E.J., Walters, E.L., Gaggin, H.K. (2018). N-terminal pro-B-type natriuretic peptide in the emergency department: the ICON-RELOADED study. *J. Am. Coll. Cardiol., 71*(11), 1191-1200.
[http://dx.doi.org/10.1016/j.jacc.2018.01.021] [PMID: 29544601]

King, K.C., Goldstein, S. (2020). Congestive Heart Failure and Pulmonary Edema. In: StatPearls [Internet].: StatPearls Publishing.
[PMID: 32119444]

Llorens, P., Javaloyes, P., Martín-Sánchez, F.J., Jacob, J., Herrero-Puente, P., Gil, V., Garrido, J.M., Salvo, E., Fuentes, M., Alonso, H., Richard, F., Lucas, F.J., Bueno, H., Parissis, J., Müller, C.E., Miró, Ò. (2018). Time trends in characteristics, clinical course, and outcomes of 13,791 patients with acute heart failure. *Clin. Res. Cardiol., 107*(10), 897-913.
[http://dx.doi.org/10.1007/s00392-018-1261-z] [PMID: 29728831]

Maisel, A, Hollander, JE, Guss, D (2004). Primary results of the Rapid Emergency Department Heart Failure Outpatient Trial (REDHOT). A multicenter study of B-type natriuretic peptide levels, emergency department decision making, and outcomes in patients presenting with shortness of breath. *J Am Coll Cardiol, 44*(6), 1328-33.24.

Maisel, A.S., Krishnaswamy, P., Nowak, R.M., McCord, J., Hollander, J.E., Duc, P., Omland, T., Storrow, A.B., Abraham, W.T., Wu, A.H., Clopton, P., Steg, P.G., Westheim, A., Knudsen, C.W., Perez, A., Kazanegra, R., Herrmann, H.C., McCullough, P.A. (2002). Rapid measurement of B-type natriuretic peptide in the emergency diagnosis of heart failure. *N. Engl. J. Med., 347*(3), 161-167.
[http://dx.doi.org/10.1056/NEJMoa020233] [PMID: 12124404]

Miró, Ò., Gil, V., Martín-Sánchez, F.J., Herrero-Puente, P., Jacob, J., Mebazaa, A., Harjola, V.P., Ríos, J., Hollander, J.E., Peacock, W.F., Llorens, P. ICA-SEMES research group(□). (2017). Morphine use in the ed and outcomes of patients with acute heart failure: a propensity score-matching analysis based on the eahfe registry. *Chest, 152*(4), 821-832.
[http://dx.doi.org/10.1016/j.chest.2017.03.037] [PMID: 28411112]

Miró, Ò., Martínez, G., Masip, J., Gil, V., Martín-Sánchez, F.J., Llorens, P., Herrero-Puente, P., Sánchez, C., Richard, F., Lucas-Invernón, J., Garrido, J.M., Mebazaa, A., Ríos, J., Peacock, W.F., Hollander, J.E., Jacob, J. (2018). Effects on short term outcome of non-invasive ventilation use in the emergency department to treat patients with acute heart failure: A propensity score-based analysis of the EAHFE Registry. *Eur. J. Intern. Med., 53*, 45-51.
[http://dx.doi.org/10.1016/j.ejim.2018.03.008] [PMID: 29572091]

Murphy, S.P., Ibrahim, N.E., Januzzi, J.L., Jr (2020). Heart failure with reduced ejection fraction: a review. *JAMA, 324*(5), 488-504.
[http://dx.doi.org/10.1001/jama.2020.10262] [PMID: 32749493]

Nadar, S. (2017). New classification for heart failure with mildly reduced ejection fraction: greater clarity or more confusion? *Sultan Qaboos Univ. Med. J., 17*(1), e23-e26.
[http://dx.doi.org/10.18295/squmj.2016.17.01.005] [PMID: 28417024]

O'Connor, R.E., Levine, B.J. (2001). Airway management in the trauma setting. In: Ferrera, P.C., Colucciello, S.A., Marx, J.A., Verdile, V.P., Gibbs, M.A., (Eds.), *Trauma management: An emergency medicine approach.* (pp. 52-74). St. Louis, USA: Harcourt Co.

O'Connor, CM, Starling, RC, Hernandez, AF (2011). Effect of nesiritide in patients with acute decompensated heart failure. *N. Engl. J. Med., 365*(1), 32-43.

Ponikowski, P., Voors, A.A., Anker, S.D., Bueno, H., Cleland, J.G.F., Coats, A.J.S., Falk, V., González-

Juanatey, J.R., Harjola, V.P., Jankowska, E.A., Jessup, M., Linde, C., Nihoyannopoulos, P., Parissis, J.T., Pieske, B., Riley, J.P., Rosano, G.M.C., Ruilope, L.M., Ruschitzka, F., Rutten, F.H., van der Meer, P. ESC Scientific Document Group. (2016). 2016 ESC Guidelines for the diagnosis and treatment of acute and chronic heart failure: The Task Force for the diagnosis and treatment of acute and chronic heart failure of the European Society of Cardiology (ESC)Developed with the special contribution of the Heart Failure Association (HFA) of the ESC. *Eur. Heart J., 37*(27), 2129-2200.
[http://dx.doi.org/10.1093/eurheartj/ehw128] [PMID: 27206819]

Ray, P., Arthaud, M., Lefort, Y., Birolleau, S., Beigelman, C., Riou, B. EPIDASA Study Group. (2004). Usefulness of B-type natriuretic peptide in elderly patients with acute dyspnea. *Intensive Care Med., 30*(12), 2230-2236.
[http://dx.doi.org/10.1007/s00134-004-2469-0] [PMID: 15502931]

Seres, T. (2011). *Heart Failure.* Mosby. https://www.sciencedirect.com/science/article/pii/B978032 3065245000350
[http://dx.doi.org/10.1016/B978-0-323-06524-5.00035-0]

Stulbarg, M.S., Lewis, A. (2000). *Dyspnea. Murray& Nadel: Textbook of Respiratory Medicine.* W. B. Saunders.

Walls, R.M. (1998). Airway management. In: Rosen, P., Barkin, R., (Eds.), *Emergency Medicine: Concept and Clinical Practice.* (4th ed., pp. 2-24). St. Louis: Mosby-Year Book, Inc..

Wang, K., Samai, K. (2020). Role of high-dose intravenous nitrates in hypertensive acute heart failure. *Am. J. Emerg. Med., 38*(1), 132-137.
[http://dx.doi.org/10.1016/j.ajem.2019.06.046] [PMID: 31327485]

Yancy, C.W., Jessup, M., Bozkurt, B., Butler, J., Casey, D.E., Jr, Colvin, M.M., Drazner, M.H., Filippatos, G., Fonarow, G.C., Givertz, M.M., Hollenberg, S.M., Lindenfeld, J., Masoudi, F.A., McBride, P.E., Peterson, P.N., Stevenson, L.W., Westlake, C. (2016). 2016 ACC/AHA/HFSA Focused Update on New Pharmacological Therapy for Heart Failure: An Update of the 2013 ACCF/AHA Guideline for the Management of Heart Failure: A Report of the American College of Cardiology/American Heart Association Task Force on Clinical Practice Guidelines and the Heart Failure Society of America. *J. Am. Coll. Cardiol., 68*(13), 1476-1488.
[http://dx.doi.org/10.1016/j.jacc.2016.05.011] [PMID: 27216111]

CHAPTER 7

Acute Pulmonary Embolism (APE)

Abstract: Acute pulmonary embolism (APE) is one of the diseases posing immense death rates and a great burden to public health. APE defines a blood clot or other substance in the deep leg/calf vein that traverses through the right heart and blocks the pulmonary arterial bloodflow (venous thromboembolism, VTE). The severity of the signs and symptoms of APE depends on the size of the thrombus and location of the occlusion, together with the previous reserves of the individual. A presentation template that will fit all cases cannot be put forward. "Massive" or hemodynamically unstable PE has a high death rate despite contemporary management. Healthcare personnel should be alerted to recognize untreated patient with high probability for APE in the ED and primary care institutions. Treatment should be expedient and aggressive in accord with the patient's instability. Systemic or catheter-mediated thrombolysis, anticoagulation and other approaches should be contemplated immediately after general supportive measures.

This chapter delineates diagnostic dilemmas, distinctive properties and management principles of APE in the emergency setting. Also, challenges brought into scene with COVID-19 pandemics is discussed.

Keywords: Acute pulmonary embolism, Thromboembolism.

APE causes 200,000 deaths annually in the USA and is the 3rd cause of death in hospitalized patients. Most cases are recognized at autopsy, which means they die without being recognized. Less than one-tenth of fatal cases can receive specific treatment.

The reason it is difficult to recognize is that its symptoms and signs are usually among those that can be found in many other entities.

APE is a pathologically formed blood clot or other substance in the deep leg/calf or –rarely- upper extremity venous system that passes through the right heart and blocks the pulmonary arterial bloodflow. When the clot migrates (embolism), it is called venous thromboembolism (VTE) (Table **1**).

Ozgur KARCIOGLU

Table 1. Some materials reported to be embolized into the pulmonary circulation are as follows.

Material	Mechanism/Cause
air	neurosurgical interventions, central venous catheter,
amniotic fluid	labor
fat	long bone fracture
foreign bodies	injection in IV drug addicts,
parasite eggs	schistosomiasis,
septic embolism	acute bacterial endocarditis,
tumor cells	renal cell carcinoma.

Risk factors for thrombosis in the venous system are prolonged immobility (such as prolonged bed rest, post-operative period), thrombophlebitis, use of certain drugs (such as oral contraceptives), heart failure, advanced age, DVT, malignancy and some rare blood diseases (Table **2**).

Table 2. Predisposing factors for APE.

Strong (OR > 10)	Moderate (OR 2-9)	Weak (OR<2)
Lower extremity fractures	Arthroscopic knee surgery Use of agents stimulating erythropoiesis.	Bed rest >3 days
Hospitalization with heart failure or atrial fibrillation/flutter in the last 3 months		Diabetes mellitus
	Congestive heart failure/respiratory failure	Hypertension
Hip or knee replacement surgery		Prolonged journeys
Major trauma	Malignancy and/or metastases	Advanced age
ACS/AMI in the last 3 months	Infections (esp. pneumonia, UTI/HIV)	Laparoscopic surgery
Past APE/VTE	IVF procedures	Obesity
Spinal cord injury	CVA, stroke	Pregnancy
	Inflammatory bowel diseases	Varices

Thromboembolism is defined as 'provoked' if it occurs with temporary or reversible reasons within 6 to 12 weeks from diagnosis (such as surgery, trauma, immobilization, pregnancy, use of oral contraceptives).

Since pulmonary arterial bloodflow is blocked due to APE, the right heart works against a substantially increased resistance. This causes an increase in pulmonary capillary pressure (wedge pressure, PAWP). As a result of the sequestration of the area fed by the occluded vessel, the mechanics of A-a gradient, in other words gas exchange, are impaired.

The severity of the signs and symptoms of VTE and APE depends on the size of the thrombus and occlusion, which vessels are occluded, and the person's previous reserves. A presentation template that will fit all cases should not be sought.

The patient usually complains of acute onset, dyspnea unexplained by an obvious cause. This may be accompanied by chest pain and tachypnea. Immobilization history is often detected but is not the rule. Dyspnea occurs in 75% to 85% of the cases, and pain on inspiration occurs in 65% to 75%. Tachypnea is the only reliable finding found in more than half of the patients.

Pearl: If none of The Trio *i.e.*, Dyspnoea, Tachypnea, Chest Pain, Tachycardia is Present in a Given Patient, APE Can Be Safely Ruled Out.

In the PIOPED I (Prospective Investigation of Pulmonary Embolism Diagnosis) study involving patients with angiographically proven PE, at least one of the following three findings was found in 97% of the patients; dyspnea, chest pain triggered with inspiration and tachypnea (PIOPED Investigators, 1990). On physical examination, tachypnea, dyspnea and tachycardia are usually found together. In a patient with massive PE, signs of right HF/ventricular strain such as neck vein distension and sometimes hypotension are observed.

Massive or nonmassive? Massive PE was defined as featured by hypotension (systolic BP below 90 mmHg or a drop of >= 40 mmHg persisted for at least 15 min which is not caused by *de novo* arrhythmias) or apparent findings consistent with shock (Sekhri, 2012). Massive PE has a high death rate despite contemporary management. Of note, some patients with hemodynamically stable, nonmassive PE but documented to have right ventricular dysfunction *via* echocardiography is classified as "submassive PE".

CASE

In Italy, a 50-year-old man presented with acute chest pain and exertion dyspnea eventually had respiratory failure worsening with PTE, during the COVID-19 pandemics (Lorenzo, 2020). There is no thrombosis related medical history. There is a history of fever, weakness and cough two weeks before admission. The home PCR test had been found positive and the patient was isolated at home. He recovered within 10 days without any medications. On the 13th day, she presented to the ED with sudden-onset dyspnea and chest pain. Hypoxic and hypocapnic respiratory failure were noted. Hypercoagulability has been demonstrated by thrombelastometry. Hemodynamics are stable. USG revealed DVT in the left tibial vein, and CTPA demonstrated left lobar, segmental and subsegmental PTE, and bilateral interstitial pneumonia (Fig. **1**). IgM and IgG tests are also positive for mycoplasma pneumonia.

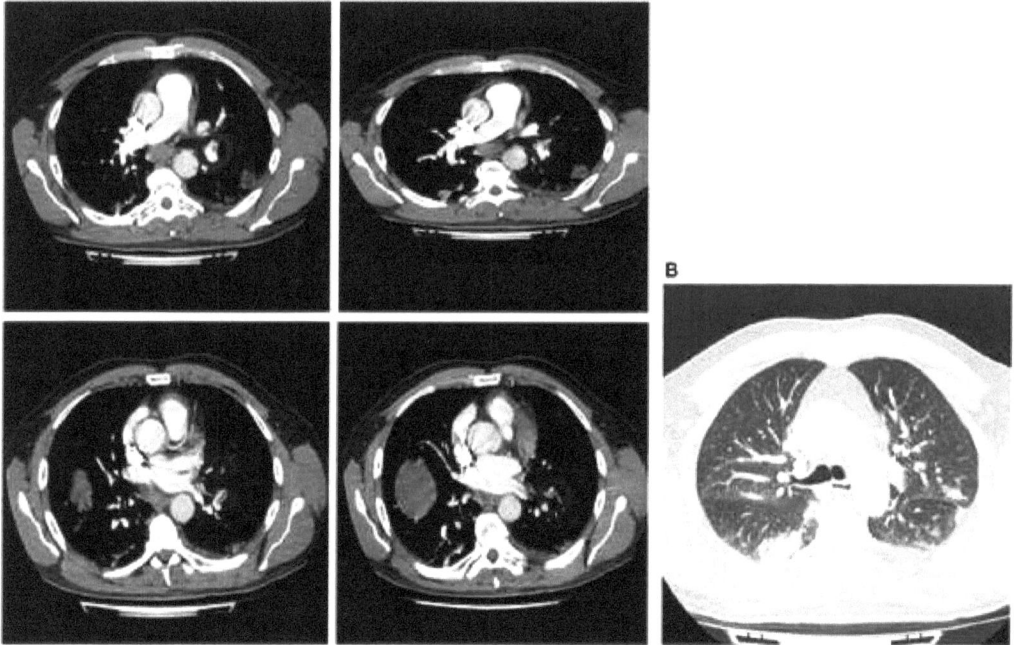

Fig. (1). Left lobar, segmental and subsegmental PTE, and bilateral interstitial pneumonia were remarkable in low-dose CTPA images.

The patient was treated with LMWH and azithromycin, hydroxychloroquine and levofloxacin. After recovery, LMWH was discontinued and apixaban was started. He was discharged healthily after 10 days of hospitalization.

DIAGNOSIS

High index of suspicion is mandatory in those with signs or symptoms of VTE or relevant risk factors. This risk status should be assessed using validated risk scoring systems, *e.g.*, the Wells and modified Wells score or the PE rule-out criteria (PERC) helpful in estimating the likelihood for PE.

"PRE-TEST PROBABILITY" (PTP) FOR APE

An assessment of PTP is a mandatory step before all diagnostic evaluations for APE. The percentages of definitively diagnosed APE cases is expected to be 10% in "PTP-low probability", 30% in "PTP-medium probability" and 65% in "PTP-high probability".

Should the PTP is high and POCUS reveals loaded right heart in an unstable patient (in shock/hypotensive), reperfusion therapy is to be commenced with the presumptive diagnosis of APE without further examination. CTPA can be obtained once the patient is stabilized.

In the hemodynamically stable patient PTP is low to moderate.

DIAGNOSTIC STRATEGY

If D-Dimer is found negative, APE is ruled out. If D-dimer is positive in this group, CT can be obtained. MR angiography should not be used to exclude PTE.

Hypoxemia is common, but two-fifths of the patients have normal SaO2 and 1/5 of them have a normal A-a oxygen gradient. Hypocapnia is also identified frequently. Pathological findings can often be encountered on chest radiography, although these are non-specific, they can be used to rule out alternative diagnoses.

ECG Findings for APE

ECG is abnormal in 2/3 of APE patients. The most frequently noted abnormalities are sinus tachycardia and nonspecific ST-T wave changes, each of which is detected in approximately half of the patients. In the PIOPED I study, 5% or less of the patients had P pulmonale, right ventricular hypertrophy, right axis deviation and right bundle branch block.

Findings showing right ventricular loading (T wave inversion in the anterior leads, QR in V1, S1Q3T3 pattern and RBBB in 12-lead ECG) are encountered in patients with severe APE (Fig. **2**).

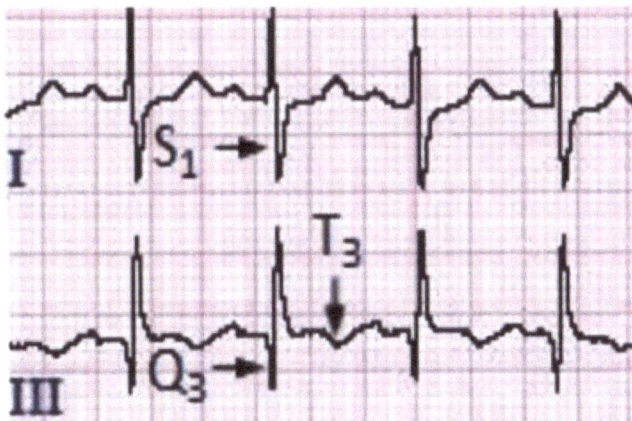

Fig. (2). The so-called "S1Q3T3 pattern" represents acute cor pulmonale. This finding is also referred to as the McGinn-White Sign and only around 10% to 15% sensitive for the diagnosis of APE.

Clinical prediction scoring: Wells (Canadian) clinical prediction scoring system is among the most commonly used scales used to assess pulmonary thromboembolism risk in a given patient (Tables **3** and **4**).

Table 3. Wells (Canadian) pulmonary thromboembolism clinical prediction scoring.

Sign/Variable	Point (Original)	Point (Simplified)
Signs and symptoms of DVT (swollen leg and pain on palpation of deep veins)	3	1
The probability of alternate diagnoses is lower than APE	3	1
Heart rate > 100 bpm	1.5	1
A history of > 3 days of immobilization or surgery in the last four weeks	1.5	1
previous DVT and/or APE	1.5	1
Hemoptysis	1	1
Malignancy (treatment or palliative care in the last 6 months)	1	1

Table 4. Wells' score can be interpreted in either ways.

Three-step (PTP) interpretation	-
High	>6
Moderate	2-6
Low	<2
Two-step (PTP) interpretation	
Strong probability for APE	>4
Weak probability for APE	<4

Hemodynamic instability is to be evaluated first in those with high-risk for having APE as the cause of the signs and symptoms.

HOW TO RULE OUT APE?

In clinical practice, exclusion is vital in the management in the ED, since the number of cases with suspected APE is high and the number of cases diagnosed is low. Without a rational exclusion strategy, unnecessary tests are performed on hundreds of patients who are exposed to radiation, the crowdedness of ED cannot be avoided. Therefore, PERC is used. In many well-designed studies, it has been reported that APE can be safely ruled out in suspicious cases with low PERC scores, that is, low clinical probability.

Lab Biomarkers

The increase in BNP and NT-proBNP in APE is associated with hemodynamic status and right ventricular dysfunction. An elevation of Troponin-I or T was found in a half of patients with APE. Troponin increase is associated with high mortality.

Table 5. Criteria for the definition of hemodynamic instability which are sought for high-risk APE.*.

Cardiac arrest[1]	Obstructive shock[2]	Persistent hypotension[3]
-	SBP <90 mmHg or vasopressor requirement despite volume replacement And Hypoperfusion-related findings (such as altered mental status, oliguria, hyperlactatemia, cold sweating)	Hypotension not due to hypovolemia, sepsis or dysrhythmia and lasting longer than 15 minutes (SBP <90 mmHg or decrease from baseline values> 40 mmHg)

* Presence of any one of 1, 2, or 3 is considered positive.

H-FABP (Heart-type fatty acid-binding protein) is an early marker of myocardial damage. It is considered to have prognostic significance. Its negative predictive power is 99%. Bedside measurements are consistent with the imaging findings with POCUS, showing right ventricular dysfunction.

An elevation of blood levels of creatinine, neutrophil gelatinase-associated lipocalin (NGAL) and cystatin C have prognostic value for APE.

D-DIMER

D-dimer rises when acutely thrombus is formed in any vessel in the body. The NPV of the D-dimer level is high and the development of APE is not expected in a patient with a normal D-dimer level. However, high D-dimer level does not make a diagnosis of APE, so its positive predictive value is low. PE is considered to be excluded when a low D-dimer level is found in a patient with low PTP in the ED.

D-dimer increases in many conditions such as cancer, GI or other bleeding, trauma, inflammation, operation, or advanced age. Therefore, a positive D-dimer does not indicate that it is APE/DVT.

This factor should also be taken into account, as the normal limits of the D-dimer test may vary with age. In this context, it is recommended to add 0.01 mg/mL for all ages in patients over 50 years of age, instead of the standard 0.5 mg/mL for everyone. This approach facilitates ruling out APE in elderly patients without causing missed diagnosis.

As the diagnostic sensitivity in D-dimer measurement with ELISA method is 95%, it is recommended to examine D-dimer with this technique. The reliability of the test measured with other methods such as latex is low.

POCUS/Bedside USG/Echocardiography

USG helps to rule out some alternative diagnoses and APE in certain situations rather than establishing the diagnosis in the etiology of acute dyspnea.

The absence of acute volume loading and/or dysfunction findings in the right ventricle in a patient with moderate or low probability of PTP excludes APE among the causes of hemodynamic instability.

APE causes significant increase in right ventricular pressure and dysfunction because of its pathophysiology. Since the negative predictive value (NPV) is not high enough (50%), a "normal" result does not indicate that our patient does not have APE.

In a hemodynamically unstable patient with high suspicion of PTP, the findings of increased right ventricular pressure are suggestive of APE and warrant a reperfusion therapy *via* administration of thrombolytics. These findings are the 60/60 sign (Figure), McConnell's sign (decreased right ventricular free wall contractility), direct visualization of the thrombus in the right atrium/ventricle. Afonso *et al*. cited that the 60/60 sign was 51% sensitive and 96% specific for massive and submassive PE (AUC, 0.74; 95% CI, 0.68-0.79) (Afonso *et al*. 2020) (Fig. 3). Likewise, McConnell's sign has been shown to have 52% sensitivity and 97% specificity in the same study.

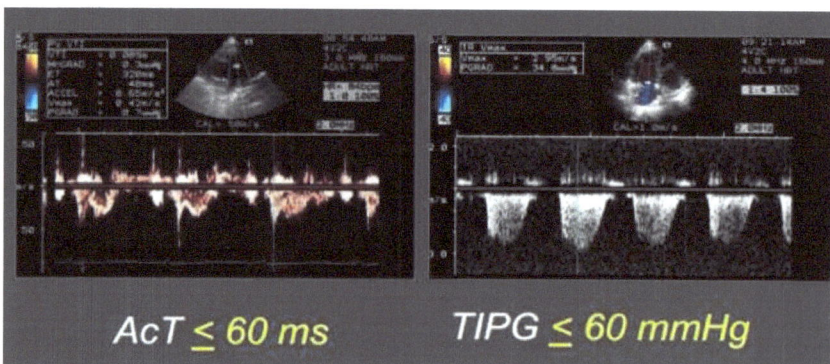

Fig. (3). Explanation of the 60/60 finding. Pulmonary ejection acceleration time (AcT) <= 60 ms and tricuspid insufficiency pressure gradient (TIPG) <= 60mmHg.

If CT angiography is available in emergency setting, this should be evaluated individually for confirmation of the diagnosis. Since the unstable case cannot be transferred to the CT unit, it is often in the patient's interest to start emergency treatment immediately, without searching for any further evidence with the available advanced technological resources. A stable patient in the gray zone, whose treatment could not be decided, should certainly be sent to CTPA.

Compression Ultrasonography (CUS)

APE is most commonly caused by lower extremity DVTs and much less frequently by arm veins. In suspected APE, DVTs can be identified *via* CUS by performing USG at four points, bilateral femoral and popliteal veins. The only diagnostic criterion for DVT is inadequate venous compression, indicating thrombus. Although the sensitivity of CUS is low (41%), it provides invaluable information as it is known that its diagnostic specificity is very high (96%) which means if the sign is positive, it rules out differential diagnoses.

Ruling out APE with USG

Normal CUS findings seems to be sufficient in a patient with stable hemodynamics and no right ventricular dysfunction with POCUS to rule out APE.

On the other hand, treatment can be initiated without further examination in patients with suspected APE and proximal DVT visualized with CUS.

CT Pulmonary Angiography (CTPA)

It is a 'gold standard' method that is diagnostic for hemodynamically stable cases, with a moderate to high suspicion in APE. CTPA sensitivity is 83% and specificity is 96%.

In cases considered low to moderate risk, the diagnosis is ruled out when CTPA is found negative. The diagnosis is established when CTPA is positive (segmental or more proximal filling defect) was found in cases considered high to moderate risk.

Further investigation is required when there is a subsegmental filling defect. CT venography is not recommended in addition to CTPA (Figs. **4** and **5**).

In order to estimate the outcome, it is recommended to first evaluate the clinical findings, then note the biomarkers and search for right ventricular overload and pursue a risk stratification by PTP. Besides shock and hypotension, Pulmonary Embolism Severity Index (PESI) or simplified PESI (sPESI) scoring systems have been proposed as predictors of poor prognosis (Table **6**).

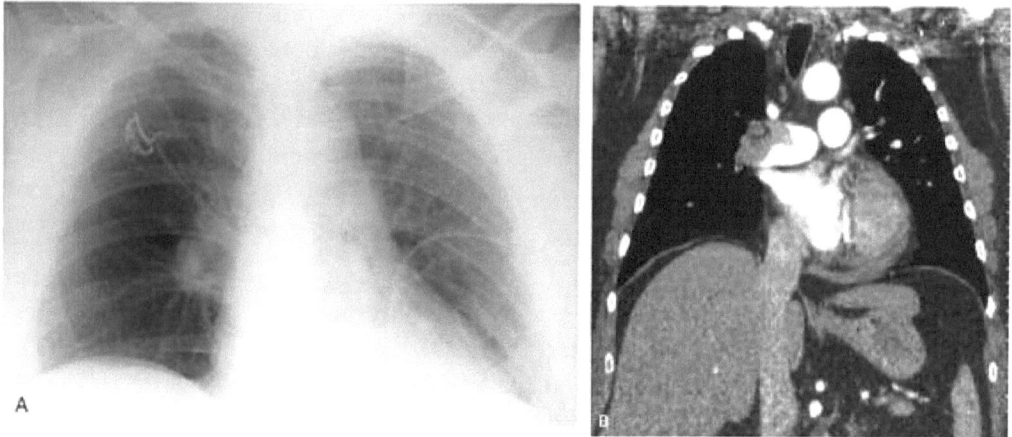

Fig. (4).   A. Hyperlucent appearance in the lower lobe of the right lung in the patient with APE (Westermark's sign). Hypovascularity is marked when normal left lung and vascular branches are compared. B. CT angiography of the same case shows a large thrombus occluding the right pulmonary artery.

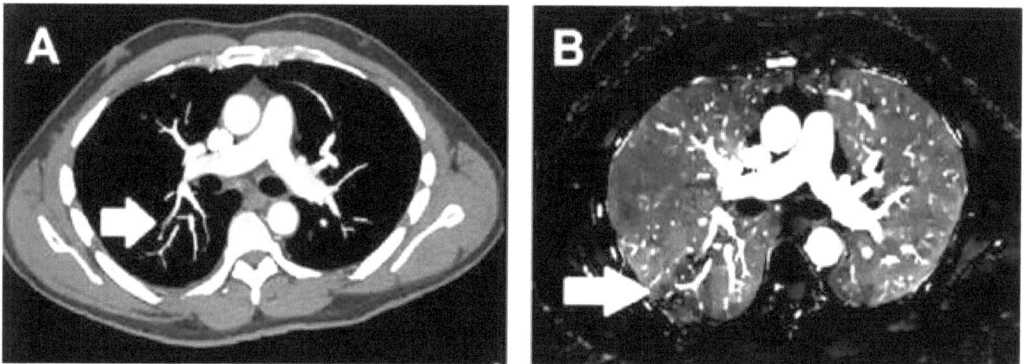

Fig. (5). (A) Axial CTPA image shows an occlusive APE in a subsegmental artery of the right lower lobe (white arrow). **(B)** Matching wedge-shaped perfusion defects are visualized on the axial iodine distribution map taken from the same level (white arrow).

Table 6. Original and Simplified Pulmonary Embolism Severity Index (PESI and sPESI).

Variable	PESI Score	sPESI Score
Age>80	Yaş (yıl)	1
Male	+10	-
Cancer in history	+30	1
Heart failure in history	10	1 (if either of these is positive)
Chronic respiratory disease in history	10	
Heart rate>110 bpm	20	1
SBP<100 mmHg	30	1
Respiratory rate >=30 bpm	20	-

Variable	PESI Score	sPESI Score
T<36C	20	-
Altered mental status	60	-
SaO$_2$<90%	20	1

General management strategies related to sPESI and PESI are

1. Those with sPESI 0 or PESI I-II, negative markers and without right ventricular dysfunction can be followed up in an outpatient setting. The 30-day mortality rate in these patients is 1%, thus the patient can be discharged regarding APE.
2. In those with sPESI ≥1, right ventricular loading findings should be worked up with lab and radiological examination.
3. Cases with sPESI ≥1 and having both high markers and right ventricular overload are in the moderate to high-risk group. These patients should be monitored closely and rescue reperfusion (thrombolytic) may be warranted.

Risk-Stratification: For those with confirmed PE, patients should be categorized and triaged according to the presence or absence of shock or hypotension.

High-risk patients are those who are hypotensive or exhibit signs and symptoms of shock. It is associated with almost 50% risk of death. These patients necessitate emergency CTA to rule out the diagnosis and administer reperfusion (Algorithm. **1**).

EMERGENCY MANAGEMENT AND TREATMENT

When the patient is considered to have APE, first priority should be the patency of the airway, and necessary support should be given to breathing. Fluid infusion should be gauged *via* assessment of deficits or congestion, if any. POCUS can be an inappreciable guide for this, with collapse found in vena cavae or in contrast, motionless fullness in the vessels. All vital signs are recorded and continuous cardiac monitoring is commenced. Give oxygen to all patients, except for the completely stable cases with SpO$_2$ of 95% and above.

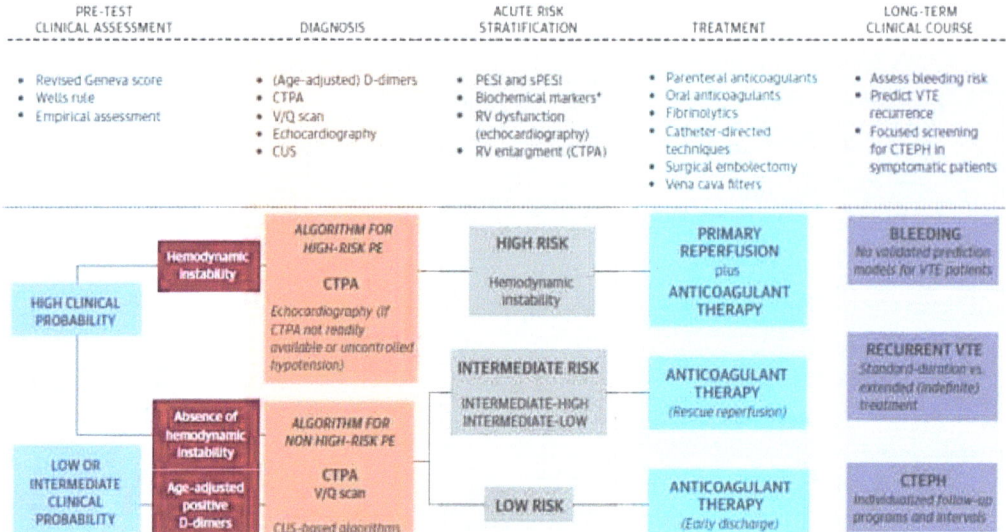

Algorithm 1. Risk management in APE in acute phase and long term.

In hemodynamically unstable patients, thrombolytic agents (streptokinase, urokinase and recombinant tissue plasminogen activator, rt-PA) are used for emergency reperfusion (Tables **7** and **8**). Thrombolytic therapy has been shown to reduce mortality and recurrence in high-risk PE patients with unstable hemodynamics.

Table 7. Anticoagulants recommended in DVT and APE.

Agent	Dosa	Half-Life	Renal Dose
Direct Factor Xa Inhibitors (NOAC/DOAC)			
Apixaban	10 mg PO BID; 7 days, then 5 mg PO BID	12 hrs	27% renal clearance
Edoxaban	Adults > 60 kg: 60 mg PO Adults = 60 kg: 30 mg PO daily parenteral anticoagulation for 5 to 10 days	10-14 hrs	50% renal clearance CrCl 15 - 50 mL/min/1.73 m^2 (0.25 to 0.83 mL/s/m^2): 30 mg PO/day Do not use if CrCl < 15 mL/min/1.73 m^2 Do not use if CrCl > 95 mL/min/1.73 m^2 (1.59 mL/s/m^2)

Agent	Dosa	Half-Life	Renal Dose
Rivaroxaban (Xarelto)	15 mg PO (with food) BID/21 days, then 20 mg PO daily	5 - 9 hrs	66% renal clearance Do not use if CrCl = 30 mL/dak/1.73 m² (0.50/s/m²)
Direct Thrombin Inhibitors			
Dabigatran (Pradaxa)	150 mg PO BID with parenteral anticoagulation, 5 to 10 days	12 –17 hrs	80% renal clearance CrCl = 30 mL/min/1.73 m²: dosage recommendations are not specified by the manufacturer. Do not use if CrCl < 50 mL/min/1.73 m² and on P-glycoprotein inhibitor treatment
Indirect Factor Xa Inhibitors			
Fondaparinux (Arixtra)	Warfarin should be started as soon as possible Adults < 50 kg: 5 mg SC daily Adults: 50 - 100 kg: 7.5 mg SC daily Adults > 100 kg: 10 mg SC daily	17 –21 hrs	100% renal clearance CrCl 30 - 50 mL/min/1.73 m²: use with caution, you can cut the dose in half Do not use if CrCl < 30 mL/min/1.73 m² 100% renal clearance
LMWH			
Dalteparin (Fragmin)	100 U/kg SC/12 hrs, or 200 U/kg SC daily	3 - 5 hrs	Its excretion is primarily renal CrCl <30 mL/min/1.73 m²: see anti-Xa levels
Enoxaparin (Lovenox)	1 mg/kg SC/12 hrs, or 1.5 mg/kg SC daily	4.5- 7 hrs	Its excretion is primarily renal CrCl <30 mL/min/1.73 m²: consider reducing the dose to 1 mg/kg/day
Fibrinolytics			
Alteplase (Activase)	100-mg IV infusion/2 hrs	30- 45 min	80% renal clearance No need for dose adjustment
Unfractionated heparin (UFH)	80 U/kg IV bolus, then 18 U/kg/s IV infusion; *or* 8,000 - 10,000 U SC/8 hrs, or 15,000 -20,000 U SC/12 hrs	1-5 hrs	Adjust the dose with aPTT
Vitamin K Antagonists			
Warfarin (Coumadine)	Initially 5 mg PO or IV per day; Give a lower dose in the geriatric, debilitated patient or patient at high risk of CHF, cirrhosis, or bleeding. In patients well enough to be followed up in an outpatient setting, start with 10 mg PO per day for the first 2 days, according to guidelines.	21-89 hrs	92% excreted with urine Renal dose unnecessary. Adjust the dose with INR

(Table 7) cont.....

Agent	Dosa	Half-Life	Renal Dose
Vitamin K Antagonists			
-	Warfarin should be started simultaneously with heparin (LMWH), and continue for at least 5 days until INR = 2.	-	-

CrCl = creatinine clearance.

Table 8. Thrombolytic regimens and contraindications approved in pulmonary embolism.

Agent	Dosage	Contraindications
t-PA/Alteplase (Actilyse): Standard infusion	100 mg for 2 h infusion	**Exact:** History of stroke of hemorrhagic or unknown etiology Ischemic stroke within 6 months CNS tumor Major trauma or surgery within 3 weeks Bleeding diathesis Active bleeding
t-PA/Alteplase (Actilyse): Accelerated infusion	0.6 mg/kg 15 min (max 50 mg)	
Streptokinase (Streptase, Kabikinase): Standart infusion	250.000 IU 30 min infusion then 100.000 IU/h for 12-24 h infusion	**Relative:** Transient ischemic attack (TIA) within 6 months Using warfarine Pregnancy or the first week after birth Non-compressible vascular puncture
Streptokinase (Streptase, Kabikinase): Accelerated infusion	2 h 1.5 million IU infusion	Traumatic resuscitation Refractory hypertension (systolic BP> 180 mmHg) Liver failure/disease Infective endocarditis Active peptic ulser

After verification of APE, patients can be classified in accord with their clinical status, especially regarding presence of shock and/or hypotension. In the presence of signs and symptoms of clinical instability, the treatment with anticoagulation, will be inadequate and more aggressive therapies such as systemic thrombolysis, catheter-mediated thrombolysis, or surgical embolectomy are warranted depending on the patient factors and the institutional capabilities (Table **9**). The development of multidisciplinary APE response teams has emerged to help facilitate decision-making in these patients (Tak, 2019).

Table 9. Class I and II recommendations in the management of high-risk APE.

Recommendations	Class	Level of Recommendations
Anticoagulation with UFH begins with a bolus adjusted per kilogram.	I	C
Systemic thrombolytics should be used in the treatment of high-risk APE.	I	B
If thrombolysis is not successful in these cases, surgical embolectomy should be performed.	I	C
If thrombolysis is contraindicated or unsuccessful, percutaneous catheter-mediated thrombolysis should be performed in these cases.	Iıa	C
Norepinephrine and/or dobutamine should be considered.	Iıa	C
In addition to all above, ECMO should be considered in patients with refractory shock or cardiac arrest.	Iıb	C

More than 90% of all APE patients benefit from thrombolytics. It is most useful when administered within the first 48 hours of onset of symptoms. However, it can work within 6-14 days in patients with symptoms. Major intracranial hemorrhage can be seen following thrombolytic administration in 1.9%-2.2%, while major extra-cranial bleeding is noted in 6.3%.

Low Molecular Weight Heparin (LMWH)

Low molecular weight heparin (LMWH) is preferred as adjunctive therapy in low-risk outpatients. IV infusion of unfractionated heparin infusion is the first choice in acute treatments, especially those with renal failure, high risk of bleeding, and morbid obesity, whose hemodynamics are not fully stabilized in emergency and ICU settings (Wilbur J, Am Fam Physician. 2017).

Vitamin K antagonists and the New Oral Anticoagulants (NOAC)

Vitamin K antagonists and the New Oral Anticoagulants (NOAC) are also used in both acute and long-term treatment. In cases where PO warfarin is employed, parenteral anticoagulation should be administered simultaneously for at least 5 days. If apixaban or rivaroxaban is chosen, there is no need for anticoagulation with IV/SC heparin. A major advantage of NOACs is that they do not require monitoring of bleeding and coagulation status. Rivaroxaban is ingested with food. However, they can cause bleeding. In case of bleeding, it should be treated with direct antidotes (idarucizumab and andexanet), if not, it should be managed with blood products or PCC in accord with the patient's clinical status. It is reported that 4-factor PCC is more effective than blood products.

Surgical Embolectomy

Surgical embolectomy is an option that should be considered for those with mobile thrombi in the right heart. Inferior vena cava (IVC) filters are recommended for patients who are not candidate for long-term anticoagulants.

Outpatient Treatment of Stable, Low-risk Patients with Verified APE

There are many different considerations on the strategy on the treatment and follow-up of these patients. Very recently, Maughan *et al.* published a systematic review on the issue and reported that these patients can be treated as outpatients, as few patients experienced major adverse outcomes such as mortality, recurrent VTE, or major bleeding within 90 days (Maughan *et al.* 2020). The reported rates of major bleeding were also similar across classes of anticoagulation.

CLUES IN APE FLOWSHEET- SUMMARY

1. In the hemodynamically unstable case, immediately perform bedside POCUS/TTE to distinguish high-risk APE from other vital or non-vital diagnoses.
2. If the suspicion of APE is based on remarkable findings and robust evidence, order anticoagulation immediately (without waiting for the results of the work up).
3. If you order test in accord with proper assessment of PTP, you will avoid unnecessary tests and wasting time.
4. If APE can be diagnosed empirically or there is a high suspicion, the patient's best reperfusion option in the institution should be evaluated: A. IV thrombolytic administration, B. surgical embolectomy C. catheter-mediated thrombolysis.
5. Since the risk of recurrence following APE is high, it may be indicated to continue NOAC therapy, especially with rivaroxaban.
6. CT scan of pregnant women in extremis can be a practical and life-saving option. V/Q scintigraphy should also be evaluated, considering the disadvantages such as transferring to the remote unit for a time-consuming procedure.

REFERENCES

Afonso, L., Sood, A., Akintoye, E., Gorcsan, J., III, Rehman, M.U., Kumar, K., Javed, A., Kottam, A., Cardozo, S., Singh, M., Palla, M., Ando, T., Adegbala, O., Shokr, M., Briasoulis, A. (2019). A doppler echocardiographic pulmonary flow marker of massive or submassive acute pulmonary embolus. *J. Am. Soc. Echocardiogr., 32*(7), 799-806.
[http://dx.doi.org/10.1016/j.echo.2019.03.004] [PMID: 31056367]

Kearon, C. (2008). Antithrombotic therapy for venous thromboembolic disease: American College of Chest Physicians Evidence-Based Clinical Practice Guidelines (8th Edition). *Chest, 133*(6 Suppl), 4548-5458.

Konstantinides, S.V., Meyer, G., Becattini, C., Bueno, H., Geersing, G.J., Harjola, V.P., Huisman, M.V., Humbert, M., Jennings, C.S., Jiménez, D., Kucher, N., Lang, I.M., Lankeit, M., Lorusso, R., Mazzolai, L., Meneveau, N., Ní Áinle, F., Prandoni, P., Pruszczyk, P., Righini, M., Torbicki, A., Van Belle, E., Zamorano, J.L. ESC Scientific Document Group. (2020). 2019 ESC Guidelines for the diagnosis and management of acute pulmonary embolism developed in collaboration with the European Respiratory Society (ERS). *Eur. Heart J., 41*(4), 543-603.
[http://dx.doi.org/10.1093/eurheartj/ehz405] [PMID: 31504429]

Lorenzo, C., Francesca, B., Francesco, P., Elena, C., Luca, S., Paolo, S. (2020). Acute pulmonary embolism in COVID-19 related hypercoagulability. *J. Thromb. Thrombolysis, 50*(1), 223-226.
[http://dx.doi.org/10.1007/s11239-020-02160-1] [PMID: 32474757]

Maughan, B.C., Frueh, L., McDonagh, M.S., Casciere, B., Kline, J.A. (2021). Outpatient treatment of low-risk pulmonary embolism in the era of direct oral anticoagulants: a systematic review. *Acad. Emerg. Med., 28*(2), 226-239.
[http://dx.doi.org/10.1111/acem.14108] [PMID: 32779290]

PIOPED Investigators. (1990). Value of the ventilation/perfusion scan in acute pulmonary embolism. Results of the prospective investigation of pulmonary embolism diagnosis (PIOPED). *JAMA, 263*(20), 2753-2759.
[http://dx.doi.org/10.1001/jama.1990.03440200057023] [PMID: 2332918]

Roy, P.M., Colombet, I., Durieux, P., Chatellier, G., Sors, H., Meyer, G. (2005). Systematic review and meta-analysis of strategies for the diagnosis of suspected pulmonary embolism. *BMJ, 331*(7511), 259.
[http://dx.doi.org/10.1136/bmj.331.7511.259] [PMID: 16052017]

Sekhri, V., Mehta, N., Rawat, N., Lehrman, S.G., Aronow, W.S. (2012). Management of massive and nonmassive pulmonary embolism. *Arch. Med. Sci., 8*(6), 957-969.
[http://dx.doi.org/10.5114/aoms.2012.32402] [PMID: 23319967]

Stein, P.D., Sostman, H.D., Bounameaux, H., Buller, H.R., Chenevert, T.L., Dalen, J.E., Goodman, L.R., Gottschalk, A., Hull, R.D., Leeper, K.V., Jr, Pistolesi, M., Raskob, G.E., Wells, P.S., Woodard, P.K. (2008). Challenges in the diagnosis of acute pulmonary embolism. *Am. J. Med., 121*(7), 565-571.
[http://dx.doi.org/10.1016/j.amjmed.2008.02.033] [PMID: 18589050]

Tak, T., Karturi, S., Sharma, U., Eckstein, L., Poterucha, J.T., Sandoval, Y. (2019). Acute pulmonary embolism: contemporary approach to diagnosis, risk-stratification, and management. *Int. J. Angiol., 28*(2), 100-111.
[http://dx.doi.org/10.1055/s-0039-1692636] [PMID: 31384107]

Tapson, V.F. (2008). Acute pulmonary embolism. *N. Engl. J. Med., 358*(10), 1037-1052.
[http://dx.doi.org/10.1056/NEJMra072753] [PMID: 18322285]

Wells, P.S., Anderson, D.R., Rodger, M., Ginsberg, J.S., Kearon, C., Gent, M., Turpie, A.G., Bormanis, J., Weitz, J., Chamberlain, M., Bowie, D., Barnes, D., Hirsh, J. (2000). Derivation of a simple clinical model to categorize patients probability of pulmonary embolism: increasing the models utility with the SimpliRED D-dimer. *Thromb. Haemost., 83*(3), 416-420.
[http://dx.doi.org/10.1055/s-0037-1613830] [PMID: 10744147]

CHAPTER 8A

Hypertension and Aortic Diseases in The Pandemic Era

Abstract: The term hypertension (HT) is a chronic condition that leads to damage to target organs if untreated expediently. On the other hand, a hypertensive emergency refers to an acute elevation in blood pressure (BP) with evidence of end-organ injury, while hypertensive urgency defines acute BP elevation without progressive target organ dysfunction. Hypertensive emergencies comprise pulmonary edema/left ventricular failure, coronary syndromes, neurological deficits/intracranial hemorrhage, acute kidney injury, retinal hemorrhages, dissecting aortic aneurysm, and eclampsia.

The BP needs to be decreased expediently in the management of hypertensive emergencies. In the rest of the cases, the BP should be reduced in a gradual manner to preclude dangerously reduced cerebral perfusion pressure.

HT is also linked to COVID-19 as a comorbidity linked to a severe clinical course of the infection. On the other hand, dissecting aortic aneurysm (DAA) is most commonly seen after the age of 50 in hypertensive men who smoke. Most emergent aortic diseases appear to be a complication of HT and represents a major threat to public health. Clinicians should be alerted to recognize untreated patient with HT and aortic catastrophes in the emergency setting and primary care institutions.

Keywords: Aortic aneurysm, Aortic diseases, Aortic dissection, Hypertensive emergency, Hypertensive urgency.

HYPERTENSION: BOTH ACUTE AND CHRONIC DISEASE OF THE EMERGENCY DEPARTMENT

Although hypertension (HT) is mostly recognized as a disease that damages specific tissues in the chronic process, these patients can be admitted to the EDs with acute elevations in blood pressure (BP), hypertensive urgencies, and rarely, hypertensive emergencies. When it is presented with end organ damage, it is called hypertensive emergency and requires emergency treatment. HT as a chronic disease, whose prevalence is as high as 8% to 10% common in the society, is frequently encountered in the ED and primary care units.

CLINICAL OUTCOMES OF HT

Chronic persistence of HT from the fourth decade (thirties) causes damage to many organs with advancing age. Renal failure, retinal hemorrhages, intracranial hemorrhage and other forms of stroke, acute coronary syndromes, peripheral artery disease, pulmonary edema are among them.

In the NHANES (National Health and Nutrition Examination Survey) study, which enrolled more than 23.000 patients in the USA, it was reported that more than 50% of mortality due to coronary syndromes and stroke were recorded in hypertensive cases.

BP is an important vital sign which directs clinical decision making processes. Accurate and consistent measurement of BP is a main part of patient assessment in most clinical settings. In general, two values are recorded during the measurement of blood pressure. The first, systolic pressure, represents the peak arterial pressure during systole. The second, diastolic pressure, represents the minimum arterial pressure during diastole (Rehman, 2021). A third value, mean arterial pressure, can be calculated from the systolic and diastolic pressures (Table **1**, Fig. **1**).

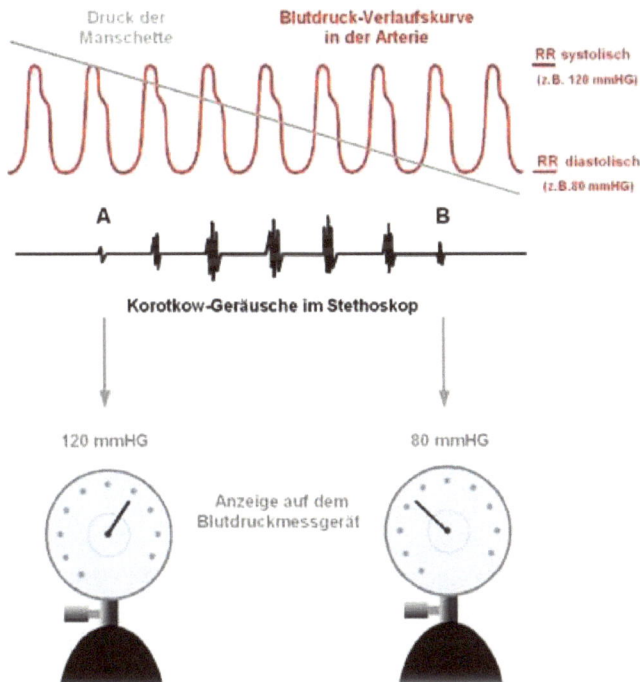

Fig. (1). Schematization of blood pressure evaluation.

Table 1. Definitions in blood pressure measurement.

SBP	Korotkoff Sounds: The First Phase
DBP	Korotkoff sounds: The fifth phase
Pulse pressure	SBP-DBP
Mean arterial pressure (MAP)	DBP + 1/3 Pulse pressure
Mid-BP	Average of DBP and SBP

Hypertensive Emergency

acute, progressive target organ dysfunction with severe BP elevation (> 180/120 mmHg).

Hypertensive Urgency

Acute, severe BP elevation without progressive target organ dysfunction.

How can One Discern HT Emergency and Urgency?

There is no threshold value of BP to distinguish between hypertensive emergency and urgency. The distinctive feature is detection of target organ damage. The diagnosis is made with the patient's clinical status, not figures indicative of the BP.

Findings Compatible with Hypertensive Emergencies

Hypertensive encephalopathy, Ischemic stroke, Intracranial hemorrhage/SAH, pulmonary edema, *de novo* heart failure, Acute MI and other coronary syndromes, Aortic dissection, renal failure, Eclampsia, Sympathetic crisis.

Hypertensive Urgent Situations

BP value higher than Stage II HT and accompanying severe headache, dyspnea, nosebleeds or agitation.

PHYSICAL EXAM AND EVALUATION OF THE HYPERTENSIVE PATIENT

The evaluation for hypertensive conditions varies with the severity of the presentation, *i.e.*, symptoms and signs on admission. The patient should be questioned about if the manifestations suggest an emergency condition, adjunctive studies such as cranial computed tomography (CT), ECG, laboratory markers of damage to kidney and heart, such as urea and creatinine, electrolytes, B type natriuretic peptide (to rule out left ventricular failure), and cardiac enzymes would be important. One should not assume he/she will diagnose every condition with lab and radiological adjuncts, because many serious entities will not affect these ancillary studies. In those with signs and/or symptoms suggestive of hypertensive encephalopathy or intracranial hemorrhage such as neurological deficits, altered mental status, visual abnormalities, and seizures, cranial CT would help expedite diagnosis and management. Likewise, a chest x-ray can be a cheap and effective tool to notice signs of heart failure, cardiomegaly and sometimes AAA/DAA especially in patients with respiratory and/or circulatory compromise. On the other hand, the patient with a suspicion of AAA/DAA or ruptured aorta should undergo thoracic and abdominal CT angiogram to diagnose or exclude a catastrophe immediately, to prepare for a timely intervention (Arbe, 2018).

Pearl Emergency: MAP should be reduced by 20% to 25% within minutes and 1 hour. It should be considered as an intensive care patient Medications are administered *via* IV route.

Urgency

BP should be reduced within 24-48 hours. Observation in ED, outpatient treatment. Oral therapy can be given.

Severe Hypertension with Progressive End-organ Damage

Bedside USG (POCUS), which is non-invasive imaging, is recommended as an alternative method to identify and correct hemodynamic deficits as soon as possible in critically ill patients admitted to the ED (3). Sensitivity of USG in AAA screening is 95% to 100% and specificity is almost 100%.

HT thresholds and classifications are updated within certain timeframes (Table **2**).

Table 2. Hypertension thresholds and classification according to the 2017 guide published 14 years after the JNC VII in 2003 (Whelton, 2018).

Category	Systolic (mmHg)	-	Diastolic (mmHg)
Normal	<120	and	< 80
Levated BP	120-129	and/or	< 80
Grade 1 HT	130-139	and/or	80-89
Grade 2 HT	140-159	and/or	90-99
	≥160	and/or	≥100

Note: If the systolic and diastolic values in the patient's blood pressure belong to different categories, the higher class is accepted.

CAUSALITY OF ACE2 RECEPTORS AND HT

Hoffmann *et al.* demonstrated that SARS-CoV-2 infection depends on the host cell factors ACE2 and the cellular serine protease TMPRSS2 which primes the spike protein of SARS-CoV-2 (Hoffman, 2020). The virus uses the receptor ACE2 to enter the targeted host cell (Fig. **2**).

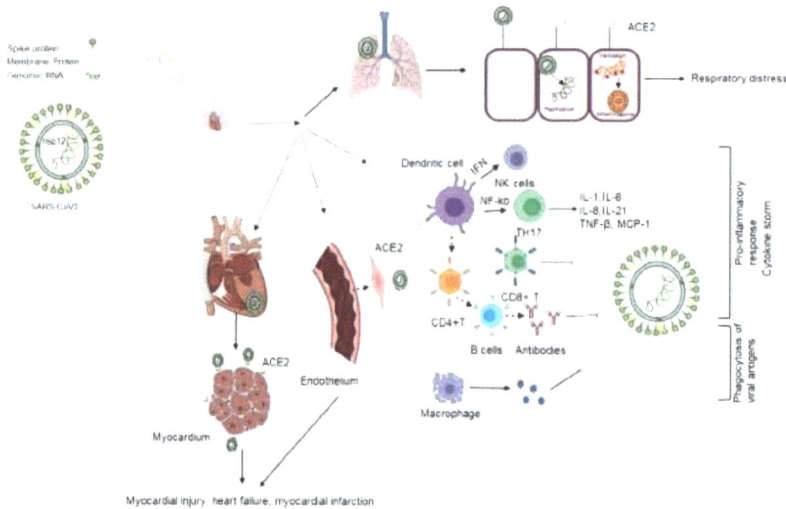

Fig. (2). Schematization of the entry of the virus in the tissues *via* ACE2 receptors and mechanisms of injury to different systems (Adapted from Bandyopadhyay, 2020). Bandyopadhyay D, Akhtar T, Hajra A, Gupta M, Das A, Chakraborty S, Pal I, Patel N, Amgai B, Ghosh RK, Fonarow GC, Lavie CJ, Naidu SS. COVID-19 Pandemic: Cardiovascular Complications and Future Implications. Am J Cardiovasc Drugs. 2020 Aug; 20(4):311-324. doi: 10.1007/s40256-020-00420-2.

ACE2 receptors are abundant in different tissues such as heart, vascular endothelium, lungs (type II alveolar cells) kidney, intestines, which paves the way to rapidly ensuing "multiorgan failure" in afflicted patients (Tikellis, 2012). ACE2 receptors are expressed much more in smokers, elderly, hypertensives, and those with heart failure. Of note, male predominance in death toll and severe disease course has also been attributed to males' susceptibility of increased ACE2 expression (Viveiros, 2020).

IMPACT OF HYPERTENSION ON THE CLINICAL PRESENTATION OF COVID-19

HT is probably the most common comorbidity among the comorbidities in patients with COVID-19. Advanced age (>60 years), male sex, CVD, HT, myocardial injury and thrombocytopenia were the factors which affected mortality significantly in a Chinese sample (Hu, 2020). A total of 29% of non-survivors had been diagnosed with HT, whilst it was present in only 9% in survivors (OR value for HT = 5.5).

Death Relationship with anti-HT Drugs

Bae *et al*. pointed out that use of ACEIs/ARBs was not associated with death in COVID-19 (Bae, 2020). In addition, authors of a meta-analysis reported that use of RAAS inhibitors was accompanied by reduced mortality risk in COVID-19 complicated with HT (Ssentongo, 2020).

Management Principles

High BP or HT is the prominent modifiable risk factor for CVD. In the last decades, guidelines for management of HT set treatment goals lower than before (Whelton, 2017) on the basis of trials that found benefit for CV risk reduction (SPRINT Research Group, 2015) (Albasri, 2021). The 2015 SPRINT trial demonstrated a reduced risk of progression to HF in patients with more intensive BP control with a target systolic BP of 120 mmHg (1.3%) compared with 140 mmHg (2.1%). Proper management of HT is associated with a 64% reduction in the development of HF.

(Figs. **3** - **4**) and Tables **3** - **6** outline basic principles of HT management, characteristics of antihypertensive agents.

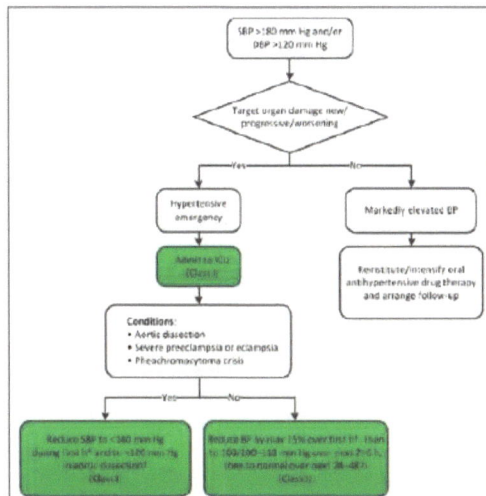

Fig. (3). The strategy to be followed in emergency hypertension treatment.

Table 3. Choice of antihypertensive agents under different circumstances.

Subclinical Organ Injury	Agent of Choice
Left ventricular hypertrophy	ACEI, CA, ARB
Asymptomatic atherosclerosis	CA, ACEI
Microalbuminuria	ACEI, ARB
Kidney dysfunction	ACEI, ARB
Clinical Event	CA, BB, ACEİ,
Stroke	BB, ACEI, ARB
MI history	BB, CA
Angina pectoris	Diuretics, BB, CA, ACEI, ARB, AA
Heart failure	ARB, ACEI, BB, CA
ISH	BB, non-dihydropiridine CA
Atrial fibrillation	CA (never BB)
ESRD	ACEI, ARB, loop diuretics
PAD	CA
Left ventricular dysfunction	ACEI
ISH	Diuretics, CA
Metabolic syndrome	ACEI, ARB, CA
Diabetes Mellitus	

ACEI: ACE inhibitors; CA: calcium antagonists; ARB: angiotensin receptor blockers; BB: Beta-blockers; ISH: isolated systolic hypertension; ESRD: End-stage renal disease; PAD: Peripheral artery disease

Table 4. Antihypertensive agents used in the treatment of hypertensive emergencies *via* IV route.

Class	Agents	Dose	Notes
Calcium channel blockers	Nicardipine	Initial: 5 mg/hour, 2.5 mg/hour increment every 5 minutes, max. 15 mg/hour.	Avoided in severe aortic stenosis; No changes in doses are required in the elderly.
-	Clevidipine	Initial: 1-2 mg/hour, double the dose every 90 seconds-5 minutes to reach the target BP, max. 32 mg/hour, shorter than 72 hours.	Avoided in patients with allergies to soybean and egg. Also not used in patients with lipid metabolism disorders. The lowest dose should be used for geriatric patients.
Vasodilator-nitric oxide	Sodium nitroprusside	Initial: 0,3-0,5 mcg/kg/min, 0.5 mcg/kg/dak increments to reach the target BP max. 10 mcg/kg/min. Stop the treatment in the shortest time possible. Thiosulfate can be considered to give simultaneously if the agent will be infused 4 to 10 mcg/kg/min or longer than > 30 min, to prevent cyanide intoxication.	Invasive arterial lines may be required to avoid hypotension. Dose lowering is necessary for the elderly. Cyanide intoxication in protracted use can lead to irreversible neurological injury and cardiac arrest.

(Table 4) cont.....

Class	Agents	Dose	Notes
-	Nitroglycerine	Initial: 5 mcg/min, 5 mcg/min increment every 3-5 minutes, maximum 20 mcg/min.	It should only be used in cardiac ischemia associated with acute HF. It should not be given to patients with volume deficits.
Direct vasodilators	Hydralazine	Initial: 10 mg by slow IV infusion (maximum initial dose 20 mg); It can be repeated every 4-6 hours when necessary.	BP starts to drop within 10-30 minutes and the effect lasts 2-4 hours. Since the duration of action is long, it should not be the first choice in acute patients.
Adrenergic blocker— beta1 receptor selective blocker	Esmolol	Initial: (Load) 500-1000 mcg/kg in 1 minute. 50 mcg/kg/min infusion is started. If necessary, the bolus dose is repeated and continued in 50 mcg/kg/min increments. The maximum dose is 200 mcg/kg/min.	Don't give the agent to patients receiving concomitant beta-blockers and to those with persistent bradycardia and severe cardiac failure. The patient should be monitored for bradycardia. It can worsen heart failure. High dose beta-blocker may worsen respiratory functions in asthmatic patients.
Adrenergic blocker— combined alpha 1 and non-selective beta blocker	Labetalol	Initial: 0.3-1.0 mg/kg (max. 20 mg) given by slow infusion every 10 minutes. 0.4-1.0 mg/kg/IV infusion per hour up to 3 mg/kg/hour. Cumulative dose 300 mg., which may be repeated in 4 to 6 hours.	Avoided in reactive airway disease and COPD. It is used in hyperallergic situations. It can exacerbate heart failure. Contraindicated in patients with high-degree AV blocks and patients with persistent bradycardia.
Adrenergic blocker— non-selective alpha antagonist	Fentolamine	Initial: IV bolus of 5 mg. Can be repeated every 10 minutes to reach the target BP.	Used in HT emergencies with catecholamine overtness
Dopamine 1 selective receptor antagonist	Fenoldopam	Start with 0.1-0.3 mcg/kg/min; It can be titrated up 0.05-0.1 mcg/kg/min every 15 minutes until the target BP is achieved. Max. infusion rate 1.6 mcg/kg/min.	Avoided in patients with glaucoma and in patients with increased intracranial pressure, and those with sulfide allergy.
ACE inhibitors	Enalapril (only oral in some countries)	The starting dose of 1.25 mg can be given at 5 min intervals. 5 mg can be given every 6 hours if necessary until the target BP is achieved.	Avoided in acute myocardial infarction, bilateral renal artery stenosis and in pregnant patients. It is especially useful in HT emergencies with high plasma renin levels. It acts relatively late.

Table 5. Selected hypertensive emergencies and antihypertensive agents used in these conditions.

Comorbidity	Agents of Choice	Notes-Caution-Interpretations
Acute aortic dissection	Esmolol, labetalol nicardipine, nitroprusside	Systolic BP should be rapidly reduced below 120 mmHg. B-blockers should be given before vasodilators (nicardipine, nitroprusside). Systolic BP should be reduced below 120 mmHg within 20 minutes to control BP and avoid reflex tachycardia and negative inotropic effects.
Acute pulmonary edema	Clevidipine, nicardipine, nitroglycerine nitroprusside	B-blockers are contraindicated in decompensated heart failure.
Acute coronary syndrome	Esmolol, labetalol, nicardipine, nitroglycerine	Nitrates given concomitant with PDE-5 inhibitors (sildenafil) can induce profound hypotension. Beta blockers are contraindicated in LV failure, bradycardia (<60 bpm), hypotension (SBP <100 mm Hg), poor peripheral perfusion, high-degree AV block, and poorly controlled asthma.
Acute renal dysfunction	Clevidipine, nicardipine, fenoldopam	It can be adjusted for other comorbidities. ACEI are to be avoided in severe renal artery stenosis.
Eclempsia ve preeclempsia	Hydralazine, labetalol, nicardipine	Warrants expedient reduction of BP. ACE inhibitors, ARBs, renin inhibitors and nitroprusside are to be withheld.
Intraoperative HT: BP>160/90 mmHg during the operation for at least 15 min	Clevidipine, esmolol, nicardipine, nitroglycerine	Intraoperative HT is most common during anesthesia induction and airway maneuvers. Warrants rapid reduction in BP.
Acute sympathetic discharge and catecholamine surge (feocromacytoma, post-carotid endarterectomy)	Clevidipine, nicardipine, fentolamin	Warrants rapid reduction in BP.
Kidney tx	Clevidipine nicardipine	Warrants rapid reduction in BP. Target BP is below 130/80 mmHg.
Acute intracerebral hemorrhage	No specific recommendation, decisions tailored to the patient	IV drug infusion should be initiated and BP should be monitored in patients with AIH with systolic BP is higher than 220 mmHg. In patients with spontaneous AIH, BP should be rapidly reduced to <140 mmHg.

Comorbidity	Agents of Choice	Notes-Caution-Interpretations
Acute ischemic stroke	No specific recommendation, decisions tailored to the patient	Cases with acute ischemic stroke receiving t-PA, BP needs to be lowered slowly below 185/110 mmHg. It should be maintained below 180/105 within 24 hrs after initiation of drug therapy. Patients with a BP of 220/120 mmHg or higher without IV t-PA or endovascular therapy and no comorbidities requiring acute antihypertensive therapy, the benefit of starting HT therapy within the first 48 to 72 hours is unknown. It may be reasonable to reduce BP by 15% in 24 hours after stroke onset.

Table 6. Anticipated decreases in blood pressure levels with non-pharmacological treatment of chronic severe hypertension.

Intervention	Mean Expected Fall in SBP (mmHg)
Weight loss	5
Healthy diet	11
Sodium restriction	5-6
Increased potassium intake with diet	4-5
Physical activity: Aerobic: Dynamic: Isometric:	5-8 4 5
Anxiolytics or moderate alcohol consumption	4

Hypertensive Neurological Emergencies (HNE), Acute Ischemic Stroke, Seizures

HNE is not very common like pulmonary edema in patients with HT, but is a deadly complication of the disease process. Signs and/or symptoms of HNE or intracranial hemorrhage may include *de novo* focal neurological deficits, altered mental status, visual disturbances (*e.g.* blurred vision), and seizures. Although cranial CT is an important tool for emergency diagnosis and management, unstable patients should be resuscitated firstly, before being transferred to the radiology unit.

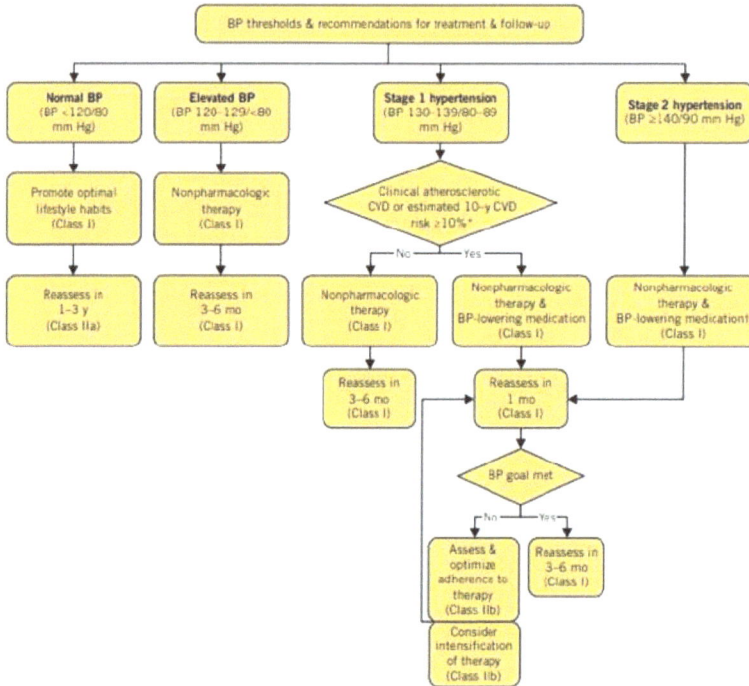

Fig. (4). General management scheme of hypertension.

Treatment of HT and coagulopathy are generally considered basic principles of ICH management, whereas a variety of measures for evacuation of the hematoma, intracranial pressure control can be considered in the emergency circumstances for selected patients.

There is an ongoing debate on the acute management of HT in those with HNE, including intracerebral hemorrhage (ICH). In a meta-analytic study, Lattanzi *et al.* recommended early intensive management of HT as a safe intervention which reduces the hematoma enlargement in patients presenting with acute-onset spontaneous ICH and high BP (Lattanzi *et al.*, 2017) (Algorithm **1**).

In 2015, American Heart Association/American Stroke Association issued a guideline on stroke and cited that: "For ICH patients presenting with SBP between 150 and 220 mm Hg and without contraindication to acute BP treatment, acute lowering of SBP to 140 mm Hg is safe *(Class I)* and can be effective for improving functional outcome *(Class IIa)* (Hemphill *et al.* 2015).

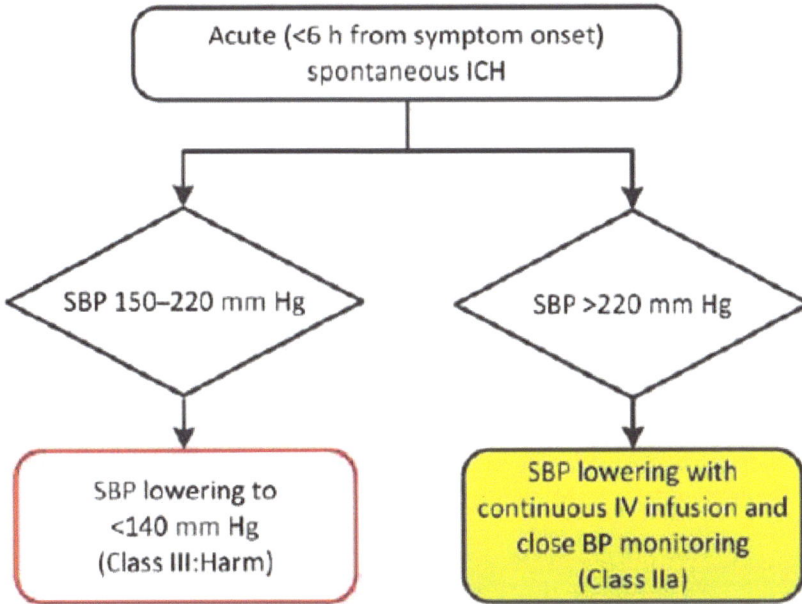

Algorithm 1. Management of HT in the patient with intracranial hemorrhage.

Seizures

Hypertension-related entities including large vessel occlusion and posterior reversible encephalopathy syndrome (PRES) can precipitate seizures *via* various mechanisms. Hypertension-related small vessel disease was shown to be associated with *de novo* epilepsy in adults. PRES is known to be triggered by a HT emergency accompanied by seizures (Gasparini, 2019). PRES and eclampsia share the mechanism characterized by acute hypertensive emergency. In these conditions, rapid alleviation of BP and seizure control must be managed concurrently. The most used drugs include easily titratable IV agents like clevidipine, nicardipine, labetalol, and nitroprusside.

CONCLUSIONS

HT is an important disease which results in injury to target organs: the eyes, heart, kidneys and brain. A clinician should never overlook a possibility of detecting a hypertensive emergency in a patient with elevation in BP, accompanied by certain evidence of end-organ damage. Hypertensive emergencies such as APEd, coronary syndromes, neurologic deficits/intracranial hemorrhage, acute kidney injury, retinal hemorrhages, dissecting aortic aneurysms, and eclampsia must be intervened expediently with hospitalization, medications, monitoring, consultations and other necessary therapeutic strategies.

Most therapeutic agents are administered intravenously in the treatment of emergency conditions, including beta blockers, calcium antagonists, nitrates and others in the emergency setting. BP should not be lowered too rapidly, especially in case of increased intracranial pressure.

HT is definitely associated with a more severe clinical course of COVID-19. Therefore, media campaigns, educative measures and other tools should be employed to augment public awareness to alleviate hazards of HT on COVID-19. Salt-lowering strategies can be launched, for example. Again, individuals with HT should be alerted on the risks they assumed with having HT as a comorbidity in the pandemics.

REFERENCES

Albasri, A, Hattle, M, Koshiaris, C (2021). STRATIFY investigators. Association between antihypertensive treatment and adverse events: systematic review and meta-analysis. *BMJ, 372*, n189.
[http://dx.doi.org/10.1136/bmj.n189]

Alley, W.D., Schick, M.A. (2020). Hypertensive Emergency.*StatPearls.*. Treasure Island, FL: StatPearls Publishing. https://www.ncbi.nlm.nih.gov/books/NBK470371/ Updated 2020 Nov 21 Internet

Arbe, G., Pastor, I., Franco, J. (2018). Diagnostic and therapeutic approach to the hypertensive crisis. *Med. Clin. (Barc.), 150*(8), 317-322.
[http://dx.doi.org/10.1016/j.medcli.2017.09.027] [PMID: 29174704]

Bae, S, Kim, JH, Kim, YJ (2020). Effects of Recent Use of Renin-Angiotensin System Inhibitors on Mortality of Patients With Coronavirus Disease 2019. *Open Forum Infect. Dis., 7*(11), ofaa519.
[http://dx.doi.org/10.1093/ofid/ofaa519]

Bravi, F., Flacco, M.E., Carradori, T., Volta, C.A., Cosenza, G., De Togni, A., Acuti Martellucci, C., Parruti, G., Mantovani, L., Manzoli, L. (2020). Predictors of severe or lethal COVID-19, including Angiotensin Converting Enzyme inhibitors and Angiotensin II Receptor Blockers, in a sample of infected Italian citizens. *PLoS One, 15*(6), e0235248.
[http://dx.doi.org/10.1371/journal.pone.0235248] [PMID: 32579597]

Chobanian, A.V., Bakris, G.L., Black, H.R., Cushman, W.C., Green, L.A., Izzo, J.L., Jr, Jones, D.W., Materson, B.J., Oparil, S., Wright, J.T., Jr, Roccella, E.J. National Heart, Lung, and Blood Institute Joint National Committee on Prevention, Detection, Evaluation, and Treatment of High Blood Pressure; (2003). National High Blood Pressure Education Program Coordinating Committee. (2003). The Seventh Report of the Joint National Committee on Prevention, Detection, Evaluation, and Treatment of High Blood Pressure: the JNC 7 report. *JAMA, 289*(19), 2560-2572.
[http://dx.doi.org/10.1001/jama.289.19.2560] [PMID: 12748199]

DePalma, S.M., Himmelfarb, C.D., MacLaughlin, E.J., Taler, S.J. (2018). Hypertension guideline update: A new guideline for a new era. *JAAPA, 31*(6), 16-22.
[http://dx.doi.org/10.1097/01.JAA.0000533656.93911.38] [PMID: 29762202]

Gasparini, S., Ferlazzo, E., Sueri, C., Cianci, V., Ascoli, M., Cavalli, S.M., Beghi, E., Belcastro, V., Bianchi, A., Benna, P., Cantello, R., Consoli, D., De Falco, F.A., Di Gennaro, G., Gambardella, A., Gigli, G.L., Iudice, A., Labate, A., Michelucci, R., Paciaroni, M., Palumbo, P., Primavera, A., Sartucci, F., Striano, P., Villani, F., Russo, E., De Sarro, G., Aguglia, U. Epilepsy Study Group of the Italian Neurological Society. (2019). Hypertension, seizures, and epilepsy: a review on pathophysiology and management. *Neurol. Sci., 40*(9), 1775-1783.
[http://dx.doi.org/10.1007/s10072-019-03913-4] [PMID: 31055731]

Hemphill, J.C., III, Greenberg, S.M., Anderson, C.S., Becker, K., Bendok, B.R., Cushman, M., Fung, G.L.,

Goldstein, J.N., Macdonald, R.L., Mitchell, P.H., Scott, P.A., Selim, M.H., Woo, D. American Heart Association Stroke Council; (2015). Council on Cardiovascular and Stroke Nursing; (2015). Council on Clinical Cardiology. (2015). Guidelines for the Management of Spontaneous Intracerebral Hemorrhage: A Guideline for Healthcare Professionals From the American Heart Association/American Stroke Association. *Stroke, 46*(7), 2032-2060.
[http://dx.doi.org/10.1161/STR.0000000000000069] [PMID: 26022637]

Hoffmann, M., Kleine-Weber, H., Schroeder, S., Krüger, N., Herrler, T., Erichsen, S., Schiergens, T.S., Herrler, G., Wu, N.H., Nitsche, A., Müller, M.A., Drosten, C., Pöhlmann, S. (2020). SARS-CoV-2 cell entry depends on ACE2 and TMPRSS2 and is blocked by a clinically proven protease inhibitor. *Cell, 181*(2), 271-280.e8.
[http://dx.doi.org/10.1016/j.cell.2020.02.052] [PMID: 32142651]

Hu, H., Yao, N., Qiu, Y. (2020). Comparing rapid scoring systems in mortality prediction of critically ill patients with novel coronavirus disease. *Acad. Emerg. Med., 27*(6), 461-468.
[http://dx.doi.org/10.1111/acem.13992] [PMID: 32311790]

Lattanzi, S., Cagnetti, C., Provinciali, L., Silvestrini, M. (2017). How should we lower blood pressure after cerebral hemorrhage? a systematic review and meta-analysis. *Cerebrovasc. Dis., 43*(5-6), 207-213.
[http://dx.doi.org/10.1159/000462986] [PMID: 28241129]

Mancia, G., De Backer, G., Dominiczak, A., Cifkova, R., Fagard, R., Germano, G., Grassi, G., Heagerty, A.M., Kjeldsen, S.E., Laurent, S., Narkiewicz, K., Ruilope, L., Rynkiewicz, A., Schmieder, R.E., Boudier, H.A., Zanchetti, A. ESH-ESC task force on the management of arterial hypertension. (2007). 2007 ESH-ESC practice guidelines for the management of arterial hypertension: ESH-ESC task force on the management of arterial hypertension. *J. Hypertens., 25*(9), 1751-1762.
[http://dx.doi.org/10.1097/HJH.0b013e3282f0580f] [PMID: 17762635]

Mancia, G., Fagard, R., Narkiewicz, K., Redón, J., Zanchetti, A., Böhm, M., Christiaens, T., Cifkova, R., De Backer, G., Dominiczak, A., Galderisi, M., Grobbee, D.E., Jaarsma, T., Kirchhof, P., Kjeldsen, S.E., Laurent, S., Manolis, A.J., Nilsson, P.M., Ruilope, L.M., Schmieder, R.E., Sirnes, P.A., Sleight, P., Viigimaa, M., Waeber, B., Zannad, F. Task Force Members. (2013). ESH/ESC Guidelines for the management of arterial hypertension: the Task Force for the management of arterial hypertension of the European Society of Hypertension (ESH) and of the European Society of Cardiology (ESC). *J. Hypertens., 31*(7), 1281-1357.
[http://dx.doi.org/10.1097/01.hjh.0000431740.32696.cc] [PMID: 23817082]

Onat, A., Karabulut, A., Yazıcı, M., Can, G., Sansoy, V. (2004). Türk yetişkinlerde hiperkolesterolemi ve hipertansiyon birlikteliği: sıklığına ve kardiyovaskuler riski öngördürmesine ilişkin TEKHARF çalışması verileri. *Turk Kardiyol. Dern. Ars., 32*, 533-541.

Peng, Y.D., Meng, K., Guan, H.Q., Leng, L., Zhu, R.R., Wang, B.Y., He, M.A., Cheng, L.X., Huang, K., Zeng, Q.T. (2020). Clinical characteristics and outcomes of 112 cardiovascular disease patients infected by 2019-nCoV. *Zhonghua Xin Xue Guan Bing Za Zhi, 48*(6), 450-455.
[PMID: 32120458]

Rehman, S., Nelson, V.L. (2020). Blood Pressure Measurement. *StatPearls [Internet].* Reasure Island (FL): StatPearls Publishing.

Ssentongo, A.E., Ssentongo, P., Heilbrunn, E.S., Lekoubou, A., Du, P., Liao, D., Oh, J.S., Chinchilli, V.M. (2020). Renin-angiotensin-aldosterone system inhibitors and the risk of mortality in patients with hypertension hospitalised for COVID-19: systematic review and meta-analysis. *Open Heart, 7*(2), e001353.
[http://dx.doi.org/10.1136/openhrt-2020-001353] [PMID: 33154144]

Tikellis, C., Thomas, M.C. (2012). Angiotensin-converting enzyme 2 (ACE2) is a key modulator of the renin angiotensin system in health and disease. *Int. J. Pept., 2012*, 256294-256294.
[http://dx.doi.org/10.1155/2012/256294] [PMID: 22536270]

Türk hipertansiyon Uzlaşı Raporu. *Türk Kardiyol Dern Arş - Arch Turk Soc Cardiol, 43*(4), 402-409.

Viveiros, A., Rasmuson, J., Vu, J., Mulvagh, S.L., Yip, C.Y.Y., Norris, C.M., Oudit, G.Y. (2021). Sex differences in COVID-19: candidate pathways, genetics of ACE2, and sex hormones. *Am. J. Physiol. Heart*

Circ. Physiol., 320(1), H296-H304.
[http://dx.doi.org/10.1152/ajpheart.00755.2020] [PMID: 33275517]

Wang, D., Hu, B., Hu, C., Zhu, F., Liu, X., Zhang, J., Wang, B., Xiang, H., Cheng, Z., Xiong, Y., Zhao, Y., Li, Y., Wang, X., Peng, Z. (2020). Clinical characteristics of 138 hospitalized patients with 2019 novel coronavirus-infected pneumonia in Wuhan, China. *JAMA, 323*(11), 1061-1069.
[http://dx.doi.org/10.1001/jama.2020.1585] [PMID: 32031570]

Weber, M.A., Schiffrin, E.L., White, W.B., Mann, S., Lindholm, L.H., Kenerson, J.G., Flack, J.M., Carter, B.L., Materson, B.J., Ram, C.V., Cohen, D.L., Cadet, J.C., Jean-Charles, R.R., Taler, S., Kountz, D., Townsend, R.R., Chalmers, J., Ramirez, A.J., Bakris, G.L., Wang, J., Schutte, A.E., Bisognano, J.D., Touyz, R.M., Sica, D., Harrap, S.B. (2014). Clinical practice guidelines for the management of hypertension in the community: a statement by the American Society of Hypertension and the International Society of Hypertension. *J. Clin. Hypertens. (Greenwich), 16*(1), 14-26.
[http://dx.doi.org/10.1111/jch.12237] [PMID: 24341872]

Whelton, P.K., Carey, R.M., Aronow, W.S., Casey, D.E., Jr, Collins, K.J., Dennison Himmelfarb, C., DePalma, S.M., Gidding, S., Jamerson, K.A., Jones, D.W., MacLaughlin, E.J., Muntner, P., Ovbiagele, B., Smith, S.C., Jr, Spencer, C.C., Stafford, R.S., Taler, S.J., Thomas, R.J., Williams, K.A., Sr, Williamson, J.D., Wright, J.T., Jr (2018). 2017 ACC/AHA/AAPA/ABC/ACPM/AGS/APhA/ASH/ASPC/NMA/PCNA guideline for the prevention, detection, evaluation, and management of high blood pressure in adults: executive summary: a report of the American College of Cardiology/American heart association task force on clinical practice guidelines. *Circulation, 138*(17), e426-e483.
[PMID: 30354655]

Whelton, P.K., Carey, R.M., Aronow, W.S., Casey, D.E., Jr, Collins, K.J., Dennison Himmelfarb, C., DePalma, S.M., Gidding, S., Jamerson, K.A., Jones, D.W., MacLaughlin, E.J., Muntner, P., Ovbiagele, B., Smith, S.C., Jr, Spencer, C.C., Stafford, R.S., Taler, S.J., Thomas, R.J., Williams, K.A., Williamson, J.D., Wright, J.T. (2018). 2017 ACC/AHA/AAPA/ABC/ACPM/AGS/APhA/ASH/ASPC/NMA/PCNA guideline for the prevention, detection, evaluation, and management of high blood pressure in adults: executive summary: a report of the American college of cardiology/American heart association task force on clinical practice guidelines. *Hypertension, 71*(6), 1269-1324.
[http://dx.doi.org/10.1161/HYP.0000000000000066] [PMID: 29133354]

Wright, J.T., Jr, Williamson, J.D., Whelton, P.K., Snyder, J.K., Sink, K.M., Rocco, M.V., Reboussin, D.M., Rahman, M., Oparil, S., Lewis, C.E., Kimmel, P.L., Johnson, K.C., Goff, D.C., Jr, Fine, L.J., Cutler, J.A., Cushman, W.C., Cheung, A.K., Ambrosius, W.T. SPRINT research group. (2015). A randomized trial of intensive *versus* standard blood-pressure control. *N. Engl. J. Med., 373*(22), 2103-2116.
[http://dx.doi.org/10.1056/NEJMoa1511939] [PMID: 26551272]

CHAPTER 8B

Aortic Diseases: Abdominal Aortic Aneurysm (AAA) and Dissecting Aortic Aneurysm (DAA)

Abstract: Aneurysmal dilation is most common in the aorta, distal to the kidney vessels and proximal the iliac artery bifurcation. It is much more frequent in males than in females. It most commonly develops in middle aged and geriatric patients, patients with chronic HT, atherosclerosis, smoking history, and those with a genetic propensity for AAA, although none of this is an absolute rule.

The width of the aorta varies depending on the race, body area, gender and age, and the average aortic diameter is between 2.5 and 3.7 cm in general. Aortic diameter measuring 50% more (1.5 times) than expected is considered an aneurysm. If the diameter of the aorta is > 5 cm, the possibility of rupture increases and requires surgical intervention. In the abdominal aorta, which is generally located infrarenal,> 30 mm for both sexes is described as AAA.

In recent years, the term "Acute Aortic Syndrome" has also been used for all aortic emergencies. Signs and symptoms of AAA varies with the patient's physiologic reserves, age and the extent of the disease with resultant organ damage (Table **1**).

Keywords: Abdominal aortic aneurysm, Aortic diseases, Dissecting aortic aneurysm, Hypertension, Management.

If any of the above are found, you should suspect AAA. The patient's abdomen can be gently palpated. Excessive or forceful palpation can lead to rupture.

Crawford classification is used to describe the extent of AAA (Table **2** and Fig. **1**).

A diagnosis of AAA is considered if the ascending aorta has reached 5.5 cm in diameter, or:

• If the diameter of the ascending aorta has increased by 5 mm in the last 6 months.

• If the ascending aorta is 5 cm and the patient has labile hypertension.

• If the descending aorta is 6 cm in diameter or a 5 mm increase in diameter has been noted in the last 6 months.

• If there is compression to any other organ.

• If the abdominal aorta is 5.5 cm or there has been an increase in diameter of 5 mm in the last 6 months.

• In all aneurysms, if there is a suspicion of bleeding, aortic aneurysms should be treated either surgically or by endovascular (interventional) method (EVAR, TEVAR).

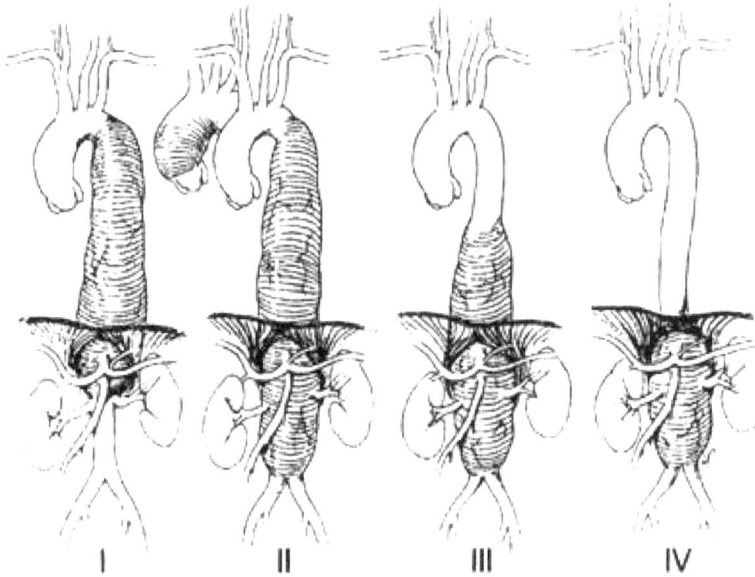

Fig. (1). Crawford classification.

Table 1. AAA signs and symptoms.

• abdominal pain
• back and flank pain
• hypotension
• feeling of defecation due to retroperitoneal bleeding
• pulsatile mass (usually palpable if the diameter of the mass is above 4-5 cm in thin or normal body builds.)
• weak femoral pulse (unilateral or bilateral)
• signs of gastrointestinal bleeding if the aneurysm forms a fistula into the intestines

Table 2. Crawford classification is used to describe the extent of AAA. According to this classification (Fig. 1).

Type I: Aneurysm starts in the proximal descending aorta and ends at the proximal renal artery bifurcation.
Type II: The abdominal aorta is aneurysmatic, from the proximal descending aorta to the distal of the renal arteries.
Type III: The abdominal aorta is aneurysmatic to the distal descending aorta and to the distal of the renal arteries.
Type IV: The abdominal aorta is aneurysmatic starting below the diaphragm, involving the visceral arterial origins.

In most patients with AAA, the clinical manifestation is very mild or even asymptomatic unless the aneurysm is ruptured. Symptomatic patients complain of chest or back pain. The type of pain can be in different ways. Symptoms related to compression to adjacent structures may be remarkable: superior vena cava syndrome, hoarseness, stridor, dysphagia, Horner syndrome, rupture and tamponade-related embolism, CHF, shock. In addition, 16% of the cases have CAD, 10% have peripheral artery disease, and 10% have CVA.

RUPTURED AAA

Anterior intraperitoneal (20%), posterior retroperitoneal (75-80%) rupture can be seen. More rarely, rupture may occur in the form of fistulization to adjacent structures, stomach or intestine. In the case of more frequent retroperitoneal rupture, cardiovascular collapse is delayed due to the buffering effect of surrounding structures, often only temporary syncope/presyncope attack occurs. In anterior intraperitoneal rupture, sudden cardiovascular collapse occurs more rapidly.

A small group of patients may also have chronic rupture. These patients can present with chronic low back or groin pain.

DIAGNOSIS

The sensitivity of palpation in the diagnosis of AAA is around 68%, it can be up to 82% in some large AAA. Therefore, when AAA is suspected, especially in hypertensive men and smokers over 60-65 years of age, it is not satisfactory to complete the physical examination. Bedside USG should be performed and time should not be wasted for more advanced techniques including CT. It should be kept in mind that USG is not sensitive enough for retroperitoneal rupture.

Although contrast-enhanced tomography/angiography is the gold standard in diagnosis, patients with renal insufficiency can be recognized with non-contrast

CT. In vital emergency situations, a calculation of benefits and losses should be done well in administering contrast media. Contrast- enhanced CT can be elicited following the possibility of contrast nephropathy is minimized in patients whose hydration is optimized and does not have other risk factors including DM, advanced age, and HF.

Balloon occlusion of aorta will be a favorable approach that the emergency physician should initiate by contacting intensive care and cardiovascular surgery quickly.

Fluid resuscitation is to be started emergently in the hypotensive patient, together with airway stabilization. If there are signs of instability, such as altered mental status, blood transfusion can take priority to crystalloid fluids.

DISSECTING AORTIC ANEURYSM (DAA)

Although it is most seen after the age of 50 in hypertensive men who smoke, it can also be seen in young people and women. It is also found in other groups such as Marfan and Ehlers-Danlos disease. Hypertension is detected in 3 out of 4 cases.

DAA occurs when only the inner wall of the aorta is ruptured and blood enters there, resulting in sequestration of blood accumulation within the vessel wall. Because of the rupture in the intima, blood dissects the medial layer creating double lumens, that is, true and false lumen. With the increasing pressure in the pseudo-lumen, the flow in the real lumen is gradually obstructed and ischemia occurs in many organs.

Two-thirds of the DAAs involve the ascending aorta. After dissection begins, it can progress to affect the entire abdominal aorta and its branches. DAA can rupture and leak at any time, often bleeding into the pericardial or pleural cavity. Rupture, leakage and/or free hemorrhage results in shock and can lead to cardiac arrest with pulseless electrical activity.

Table **3** summarizes DAA signs and symptoms: Pain is usually expressed as "tearing" or "excruciating". The pain is substernal and may radiate between the scapulae and the back. Palpation of the pulses in the lower extremities may be noted as weak or absent. Blood pressure is usually increased (reflecting long-lasting hypertension), but may be normotensive or in shock if excessive bleeding occurred into the dissection.

Table 3. Common signs and symptoms in aortic dissection.

Sign/Symptom	Explanation	Percentage (%)
Pain	tearing or excruciating, retrosternal	90
Syncope/altered mental status	+++	
Dyspnea	+	
Myocardial infarction	+	1-3
Blood pressure	Elevated in Reduced in	50 20
Asymmetric pulses	Upper and lower extremity	30-50
New diastolic murmur	Aortic auscultation	50
Pericardial /Pleural effusion	+++	
Hemiparesis /hemiplegia	+	5-6
Paraparesis/ paraplegia	+	2-6
Renal or intestinal infarction	+	3-5

Although not expected in every patient, the following can be seen secondary to DAA with the involvement of various arteries and structures;

- Syncope/loss of consciousness
- Signs of stroke or focal neurological deficits (such as speech disorder, hemiplegia, paraplegia, dizziness)
- Different pulse or BP findings in extremities
- Acute heart failure
- Pericardial tamponade
- ACS/AMI (in the case of DAA involving the coronary ostia)
- Abdominal pain, mesentery ischemia
- Acute renal failure, anuria

As a rule, aortic rupture into any body cavity can occur. High flow oxygen is given while trying to calm the patient. Open at least two major IV route on the way to hospital and for the primary survey in the ED with a crystalloid solution, preferably Lactated Ringer's solution (LRS).

Mortality rate is up to 27% in elective surgery, while it is around 50-60% in emergency surgery.

NON-CRITICAL PRESENTATIONS WITH AORTIC SYNDROMES

Absence of hemodynamic compromise or critical organ ischemia defines this phenomenon. This represents the single most common case scenario (four-fifth of patients) in the emergency circumstances. Fulfillment of pre-test probability assessment and clinical gestalt, combined with bedside application of POCUS can take priority to advanced imaging modalities. Cardiothoracic surgery should be consulted and most patients will be discharged with follow-up recommendations.

Diagnosis and Imaging

Since aortic diseases cannot be recognized clearly with physical examination, imaging is used in almost every suspect case. Although most cases can be diagnosed with bedside USG, a definitive diagnosis and CT angiography or arteriography are required to evaluate the extent of the damage (Algorithms **1** and **2**).

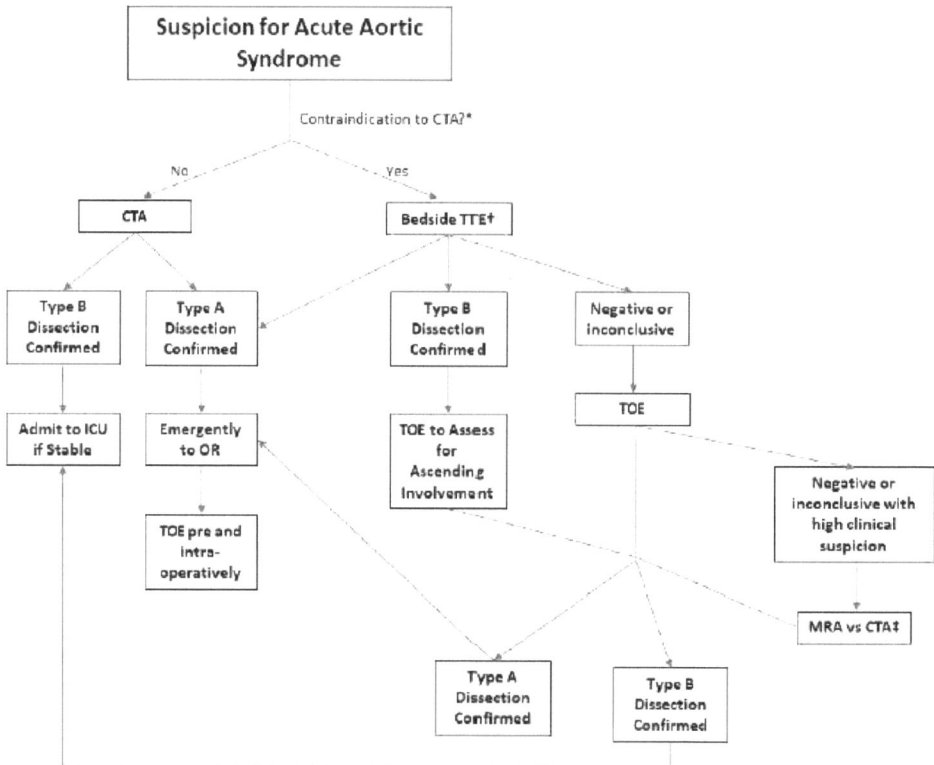

Algorithm 1. Scheme for diagnostic imaging.

The most emphasized biomarker is D-dimer. This marker, which is referenced with a cut-off value of 0.5 ng/mL in systematic reviews and meta-analyzes, has been shown to be successful in excluding DAA. Sensitivity is 98% but specificity is only 40% (Asha, 2015). There is another study that gives these numbers as 95% and 60%, respectively (Watanabe, 2016). Especially when applied to a low-risk population according to AHA criteria, the probability of having DAA decreases to 0.3% despite low D-dimer.

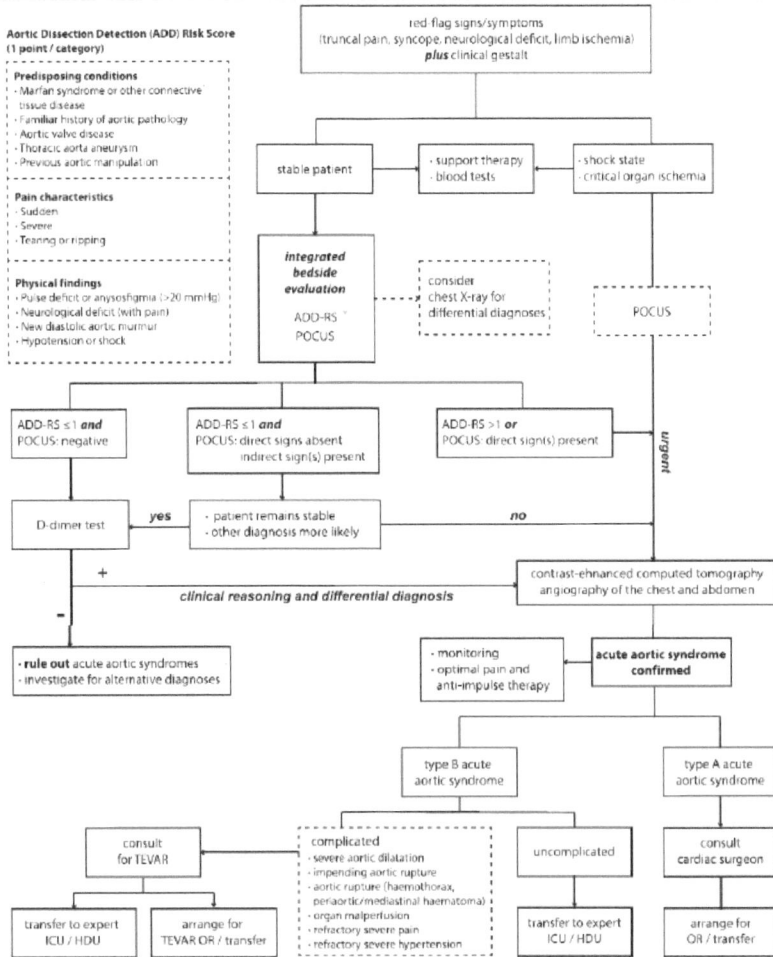

Algorithm 2. A logical workflow for the approach to AAA/DAA. (***ADD-RS*** aortic dissection detection risk score, ***POCUS direct sign***: intimal flap, intramural aortic haematoma or penetrating aortic ulcer detected with point-of-care ultrasonography.

Have COVID-19 affected admissions related to AAA/DAA?

Yes. In a well-designed retrospective registry study in Austria, hospitalizations for ACS, PTE, AAA/AAD were compared to counteracting figures elicited during restrictive measures for COVID-19 (Bugger, 2020). The RR for admissions reflecting the three outstanding deadly conditions were shown to have decreased (RR 0.77; p<0.001) during restrictive measures compared to previous years. On the other hand, in-hospital death rates boosted by 65% (p = 0.041), essentially affected by deaths related to ACS (p = 0.042).

POCUS Indirect Sign

Thoracic aorta dilatation (diameter $\geq$ 4 cm at any level), pericardial effusion/tamponade or aortic valve regurgitation at least moderate detected with POCUS) (Adapted from Morello, 2020).

Ultrasonography/POCUS

Ultrasonography/POCUS has the advantage that it does not require patient transfer and can be performed even in unstable cases (Fig. **2**). It should be known that it is specific even if it is not sensitive. Although it is diagnostic when visualized, it is necessary to order a CT in patients who cannot be displayed well, by providing stabilization without wasting time.

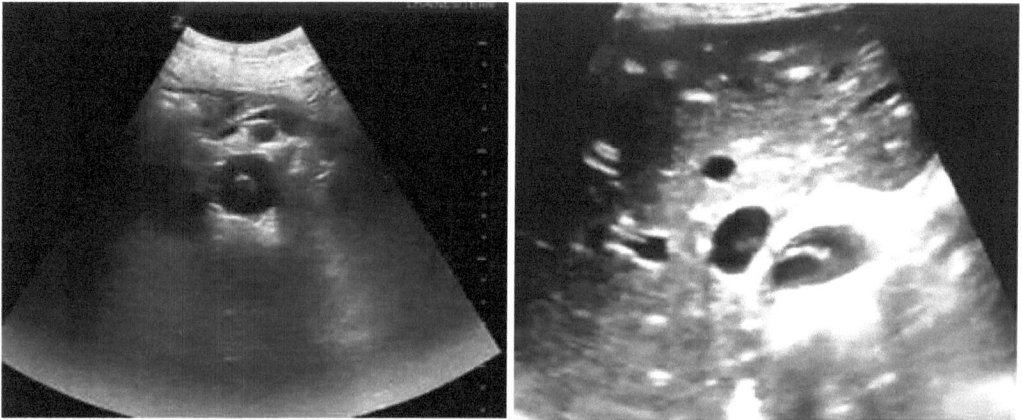

Fig. (2). Intimal flap image on bedside USG.

Contrast-enhanced CT (CT-angiography) is the gold standard in planning the surgery. In vital emergency situations.

Findings on Non-contrast CT

In arterial phase images, the media-intima entrance can be viewed as an intimomedial flap defect. Double aortic lumen may be prominent. In addition, eccentric calcification is seen in the outer wall.

Findings in Contrast-enhanced CT

In the early angiographic phase, the real lumen is enhanced and viewed as smaller than it is in fact. In the venous phase, the false lumen is more easily separated due to thrombosis. CT sensitivity was 90% to 100% and specificity was 87% to 100% in the diagnosis of DAA.

Sensitivity and specificity were reported to be 100% when using multidetector Helical CT.

Classification of DAA

I- Stanford classification:

• Type A: Ascending aorta: Surgery

• Type B: Descending aorta: Primarily medical

II- DeBakey classification:

• Type I: Ascending aorta, aortic arch and descending aorta

• Type II: Ascending aorta only

• Type III: Descending aorta only

Case example. A man in his 68 years of age presented with presyncope and pain in his chest and back (Fig. **3**).

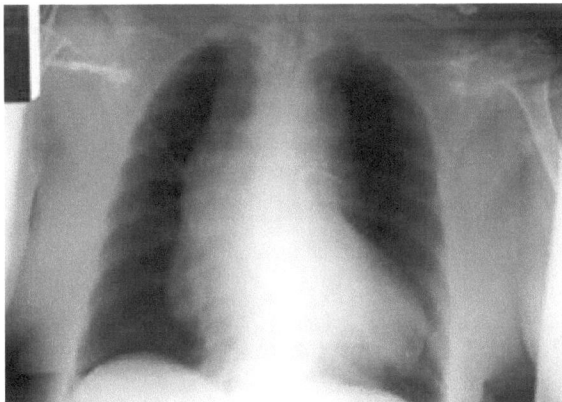

Fig. (3). Chest radiography in mediastinal enlargement is prominent, but it should be known that this is only a 60% sensitive finding for diagnosis.

Case example. Stanford Type B aortic dissection was noted in CT of a man in his

71. He was admitted with chest and back pain (Fig. **4**).

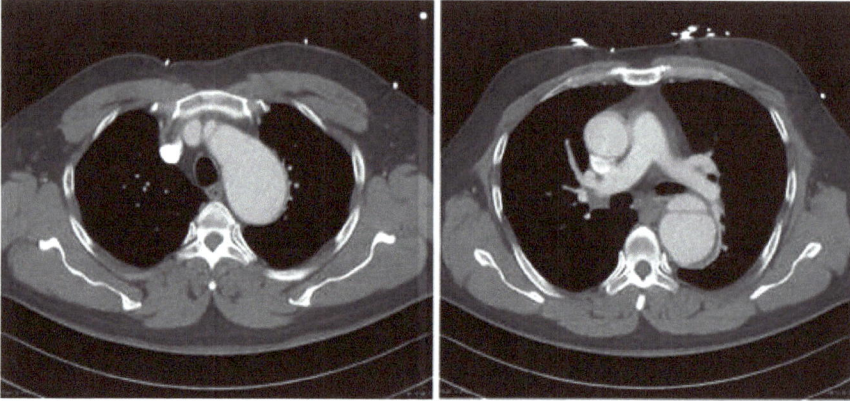

Fig. (4). In the axial image with IV contrast, the intimal flap starting from the subclavian artery branching in the thoracic aorta in the arterial phase to the T10 level is displayed. The largest aortic diameter is measured as 57 mm in the patient without atherosclerotic appearance and pleural effusion.

Case example. Infrarenal involvement in a patient with DAA *via* 3D reconstruction. The patient was admitted with flank and pelvic pain (Fig. **5**).

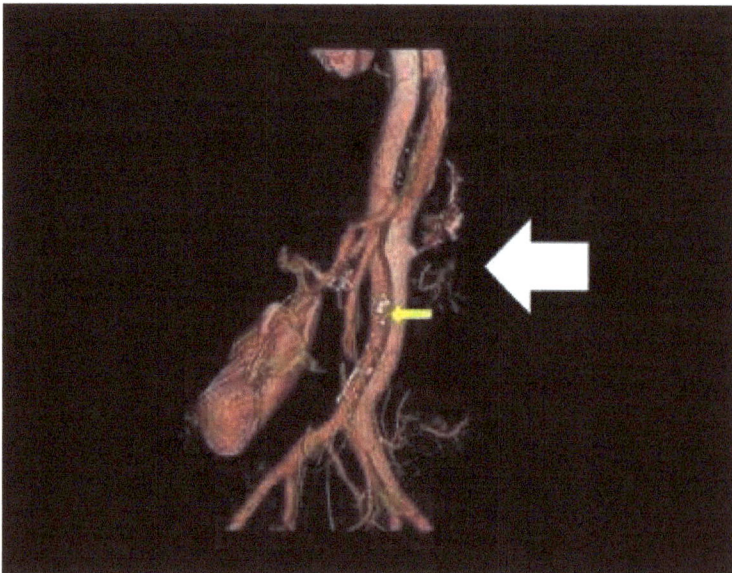

Fig. (5). 3D reconstruction image showing infrarenal involvement in a patient with DAA.

Treatment

In a patient presenting with hypotension, the vascular bed should firstly be filled with adequate fluid resuscitation. It should be aimed to increase the systolic BP to

90 mmHg. Some publications also recommend this as 100 to 120 mmHg. The target heart rate should be 60 to 80 beats/min. Inotropes and vasopressors can also be used for this. If signs of instability such as altered mental status occur, blood transfusion should be performed. If pericardial tamponade has occurred with DAA, its drainage decreases mortality. Extracorporeal support can also be helpful. It has also been shown that adding an ACTH-analogue infusion to standard emergency care results in more favorable outcomes (Noera, 2001).

Severe pain should be relieved with morphine and its derivatives. Beta blockers (BB) (labetalol) are the first choice agents because of their many features. Treatment with metoprolol and esmolol is the priority. Sodium nitroprusside can be administered. IV nicardipine is also an advantageous option among calcium channel blockers.

1. Treatment with beta blockers.
2. If a patient with DAA is high in systolic BP due to pain or other reasons, it should be reduced urgently. If there are no contraindications, BB treatment, which reduces left ventricular contraction power (dP/dt) and has a negative inotropic effect, should be started immediately. In addition to BB therapy, other IV antihypertensive drugs such as nitroprusside should be added to the treatment.

Contraindications for BB drugs may be detected in some patients. BB should be avoided in cases of drug hypersensitivity, asthma attack (or history), heart block, decompensated heart failure, bradycardia below 60 beats per minute, severe COPD, uncontrolled diabetes and persistent hypotension. In a situation such as high- degree heart block, it is recommended to use calcium channel blockers, instead of BBs, to lower the patient's systolic BP.

Metoprolol

Selective beta 1 antiadrenergic agent that alleviates cardiac contraction automaticity. Pulse rate, BP and ECG should be monitored in IV administration. If oral rather than IV therapy is considered, a 2.5 mg oral dose should be given to a 1 mg IV dose.

Trade name: Beloc ampoule (5 mg/5 mL-1 ampoule): 2.5 to 5 mg IV, can be repeated every 2 to 5 min. It can be made up to a total of 15 mg within 15 to 25 min.

Labetalol

It has a reducing effect on both BP and cardiac contractility. It lowers blood pressure by blocking alpha, beta 1 and beta 2 adrenergic receptors. It is a drug that can be used alone as an option for nitroprusside plus BB. 20 mg IV is administered slowly over two minutes. Then 40-80 mg can be given *via* IV route every 10 min. However, a total of 300 mg should not be exceeded. It can also be administered as an infusion of 1-2 mg/min.

Esmolol

It is a very short acting beta 1 blocker ISA (-). It is used with its ability to be stopped immediately and terminate its effect when desired, especially in patients with arterial BP labile undergoing surgery. It can be given together with nitroprusside. It is a safe and easily tolerated agent in those with asthma/COPD and a risk of bronchospasm due to beta 1 blockade. The elimination half-life is around 10 minutes.

Trade name: Brevibloc vial (10 mg/mL 1 vial): 0.25-0.5 mg/kg given slowly IV over 1 minute. Can be infused 0.05-0.1 mg/kg/min., over a 4-minute period. The loading dose can then be repeated, or the dose increased to 0.3 mg/kg/min.

Preference in a patient with severe bronchospasm with DAA; It may be esmolol, metoprolol or verapamil in combination with nitroprusside infusion.

Treatment with Calcium Channel Blockers

These are drugs that reduce BP and cardiac contractility. Diltiazem, one of these; 10-20 mg IV given in two minutes. Dose repetitions and continued infusion are then adjusted to the patient.

Trade name: Diltiazem hydrochloride: Diltizem 25 mg ampoule.

Sodium Nitroprusside

Initially, the vasodilator drug of choice is IV nitroprusside infusion. Nitroprusside is a drug that reduces peripheral resistance by triggering peripheral vasodilation directly acting on venous and arteriolar smooth muscles. Both the vial and the serum set must be wrapped in aluminum foil as it is very light-sensitive. The vial whose color has changed since it is not protected from light should never be used. Before starting nitroprusside therapy, BB therapy should be administered first to prevent reflex tachycardia induced by this drug.

Contraindications for Nitroprusside Infusion

Drug hypersensitivity, impaired cerebral perfusion, impaired coronary perfusion. It is not a suitable drug for direct injection, it is given as an infusion after diluting with normal saline, RL or 5% dextrose.

Trade name: Nipruss Ampoule (60 mg, 5 mL ampoule): initial dose; 0.3-0.5 mcg/kg/min IV infusion. Its dosage can be increased up to 3-4 mcg/kg/minute to ensure proper effect. However, the dose should not exceed 10 mcg/kg/min.

Example: 0.5 mcg/kg/min is 35 mcg/min for a 70 kg patient (2.1 mg/hour).

1 ampoule-60 mg Nipruss is put into 500 mL of saline. The infusion starts at approximately 17 mL/hour.

Pain Relief: Another important problem in medical treatment is pain control. Cessation of pain should be essential in quality patient care. Pain relief is necessary to ensure patient comfort, provide pulmonary toilet and prevent exacerbation of tachycardia and HT. Most patients are hypertensive and require pain control. In hypotensive patients, pain control can be performed by titrating according to the patient's clinical status and consciousness. In pain control, opiate analgesics with marked effects on increased blood pressure and heart rate should be preferred. Opiates can be given safely, as their effects are reversible with naloxone. For this purpose, mostly morphine sulfate and fentanyl are used. IV morphine/fentanyl therapy is an appropriate approach to protect the patient from tachycardia and hypertension attacks. Morphine reduces the patient's cardiac contractility and aortic pressure. Thus, it delays the progress of DAA and rupture. Fentanyl is advantageous in that it has a shorter effect and a reliable side effect profile.

Intravenous: Morphine 2.5-15 mg/70 kg is infused within 3-5 minutes, the same dose can be repeated every 4 hours.

Fentanyl, on the other hand, is infused 2-3 mcg/kg in a few minutes and the infusion or boluses are continued depending on the effect.

Hypotension Treatment: Hypovolemia resulting from blood loss and hemorrhage leads to hypotension in patients with DAA. Conditions such as rupture of the aorta from anywhere, pericardial tamponade, rupture into the pleura, acute aortic valve insufficiency, cardiac ischemia due to coronary dissection should be ruled out emergently in such a situation. Nitroprusside, beta blockers and calcium channel blockers have no place in the treatment of such a patient with hypotension, even in presence of DAA. In patients with hypotension with DAA, blood pressure should be normalized with volume support. In addition, if necessary, vasopressor drugs can be added to the treatment. Inotropic drugs increase ventricular contractility and rate. It should be borne in mind that these drugs may cause further progression of the false lumen. Pericardiocentesis performed for hemopericardium due to DAA may cause recurrent pericardial hemorrhages in the patient and result in mortality. It should be noted that pericardiocentesis is only recommended in case of acute type A intramural hematoma in many publications. As a result, it is recommended that patients with hypotension or shock should be taken into operation immediately.

The International Registry of Acute Aortic Dissection (2018-IRAD) highlighted diagnostic and therapeutic principles of type A and B DAA (Table **4**).

Table 4. Key messages and summary (from The International Registry of Acute Aortic Dissection (2018-IRAD).

• Sudden onset, excruciating/never-before-experienced pain is the most important indicator for early recognition of DAA.
• DAAs are visualized below (more caudal) the cut-off points accepted for surgery in a significant percentage of patients. This indicates that better genetic, biomarker, and imaging tests should be found and used for earlier diagnosis.
• ECG and radiographs are not as helpful as thought for early diagnosis. On the other hand, IRAD reported that when thoracic aortic dilatation is added to the radiographic findings, sensitivity in early diagnosis increases up to 98%.
• D-dimer is a highly sensitive marker (0.5 mcg/mL cut-off value), but a specific marker is required.
• Type B mortality is more stable, it is seen that TEVAR is beginning to replace surgery in complicated patients.
• Partial thrombosis development in the false lumen is an indicator of poor prognosis in Type B DAAs.
• Intramural hematoma in the ascending aorta suggests acute type A DAA, indicating poor prognosis.

The DAA treatment algorithm can be summarized as follows:

1) If the patient has no hypotension or shock; IV BB should be given immediately (should there be contraindications to BB drugs, CCB; diltiazem or verapamil can be administered). Pain control should be provided with IV opiates. If the patient's systolic BP is above 120 mmHg; IV vasodilators are titrated until BP is below 120 mmHg. If the patient's systolic BP is below 120 mmHg; It should be checked whether the dissection is progressing from the ascending aorta or not. If it is advanced, an operative or interventional approach should be provided. If it has not progressed, systolic BP is to be maintained at 120 mm Hg and below.

2) If the patient has a state of hypotension or shock; the approach and strategy depend on the anatomical characteristics of DAA.

a- If Type A dissection is detected; surgical consultation should be requested immediately for the operation. In addition, IV fluids should be given until the MAP is 70 mmHg or until euvolemia is achieved. If hypotension continues despite fluid therapy, IV vasopressor agents should be initiated. In addition, imaging studies should be pursued in search for tamponade, ongoing rupture and severe aortic regurgitation.

b- If Type B dissection is visualized; again, fluid therapy should be given. IV bolus fluid therapy is given until the MAP is 70 mmHg or the euvolemia is achieved. If hypotension continues despite fluid therapy, IV vasopressor agents should be initiated and the etiology of hypotension should be investigated. Transthoracic echo (TTE)/POCUS, and surgical consultation should be requested for imaging and assessment of cardiac function to demonstrate ongoing rupture. If the etiology of hypotension can benefit from surgery, the patient should be taken into operation. However, if it is thought that it will not benefit from surgery, medical treatment that will ensure systolic BP to be 120 mmHg and below should be continued.

3) Whether the patient has hypotension or shock condition or not, if problems such as malperfusion syndrome, progress in dissection, aneurysm enlargement, uncontrolled hypertension develop in the follow-up; operation or interventional approach to the patient must be provided.

Endovascular repair is a contemporary approach with the collaboration of interventional radiology/cardiovascular surgery. Endovascular repair is increasingly used in AAA and in the treatment of thoracic aortic aneurysm. For the endovascular repair procedure, a guidewire passed *via* the femoral artery is advanced into the involved part of the aorta. The stent-graft is placed in the catheter over the guidewire and advanced to the aneurysm area. Here the catheter is retracted and the stent-graft expands like a spring on both side of the aneurysm. The aneurysm will recover over time as the pressure within the aneurysmatic vessel will be normalized. Recovery is supported with measures such as exercise, quitting smoking, regulating additional problems such as blood pressure, diabetes, and kidney failure.

ADDITIONAL ADVANTAGES OF ENDOVASCULAR REPAIR

• The procedure typically takes 1 to 3 hours

• You can be discharged a few days after the procedure.

• Compared to open surgery, smaller incisions are adequate, so recovery is easier and quicker.

• Most patients return to their normal life within 2 to 6 weeks.

Hospitalization and Discharge

Patients who are newly diagnosed with DAA should be hospitalized. Patients with chronic AAA are discharged if there is no suspicion of leakage, bleeding and/or rupture. They can be followed up on an outpatient basis if the pain is under control, if the aortic diameter is below 5 cm in the widest part, if there is no new kidney or heart failure, if BP is under control with medication, diet or lifestyle.

CONCLUSIONS

Misdiagnosis and delayed diagnosis of AAA/DAA represent significant considerations in the management of these patients. A CT-angiography can expedite diagnosis in critically ill patients, although instability can preclude some patients' transfer to radiology units. Bedside USG/POCUS can be life-saving adjunct which will aid timely recognition of the patient in extremis. In addition, ancillary studies such as ECG, CXR, glucose, d-dimer and complete blood count are mandatory to rule in or out alternative or overlapping diagnoses. A logical algorithm should incorporate clinical probability assessment, POCUS and other adjuncts to skip cumbersome studies and commence life-saving treatments.

Acute treatment options include morphine or fentanyl (and/or benzodiazepines in selected patients) and antihypertensive agents (a beta-blocker and a nitrate derivative), to alleviate and maintain heart rates around 60 bpm and systolic BP around 100 and 120 mmHg. Aortic catastrophes inflicting the ascending aorta can be viewed as candidates for emergent surgery, and complicated type B syndromes (severe aortic dilatation, impending or frank rupture, organ malperfusion, refractory pain, severe HT) necessitate evaluation for TEVAR. Meanwhile, optimal medical therapy is more suitable for those with uncomplicated type B AAA.

REFERENCES

Asha, S.E., Miers, J.W. (2015). A Systematic review and meta-analysis of D-dimer as a rule-out test for suspected acute aortic dissection. *Ann. Emerg. Med., 66*(4), 368-378.
[http://dx.doi.org/10.1016/j.annemergmed.2015.02.013] [PMID: 25805111]

Bugger, H., Gollmer, J., Pregartner, G., Wünsch, G., Berghold, A., Zirlik, A., von Lewinski, D. (2020). Complications and mortality of cardiovascular emergency admissions during COVID-19 associated restrictive measures. *PLoS One, 15*(9), e0239801.
[http://dx.doi.org/10.1371/journal.pone.0239801] [PMID: 32970774]

Carroll, B.J., Schermerhorn, M.L., Manning, W.J. (2020). Imaging for acute aortic syndromes. *Heart, 106*(3), 182-189.
[http://dx.doi.org/10.1136/heartjnl-2019-314897] [PMID: 31822571]

Clouse, W.D., Hallett, J.W., Jr, Schaff, H.V., Spittell, P.C., Rowland, C.M., Ilstrup, D.M., Melton, L.J., III

(2004). Acute aortic dissection: population-based incidence compared with degenerative aortic aneurysm rupture. *Mayo Clin. Proc., 79*(2), 176-180.
[http://dx.doi.org/10.4065/79.2.176] [PMID: 14959911]

Evangelista, A., Isselbacher, E.M., Bossone, E., Gleason, T.G., Eusanio, M.D., Sechtem, U., Ehrlich, M.P., Trimarchi, S., Braverman, A.C., Myrmel, T., Harris, K.M., Hutchinson, S., O'Gara, P., Suzuki, T., Nienaber, C.A., Eagle, K.A. IRAD Investigators. (2018). Insights from the international registry of acute aortic dissection: A 20-Year experience of collaborative clinical research. *Circulation, 137*(17), 1846-1860.
[http://dx.doi.org/10.1161/CIRCULATIONAHA.117.031264] [PMID: 29685932]

Hiratzka, L.F., Bakris, G.L., Beckman, J.A. (2010). 2010 guidelines for the diagnosis and management of patients with thoracic aortic disease. *Circulation, 121*, e266-e369.
[PMID: 20233780]

Katzen, B.T., Dake, M.D., MacLean, A.A., Wang, D.S. (2005). Endovascular repair of abdominal and thoracic aortic aneurysms. *Circulation, 112*(11), 1663-1675.
[http://dx.doi.org/10.1161/CIRCULATIONAHA.105.541284] [PMID: 16157785]

Mancini, M.C. (2020). *Aortic Dissection.* http://emedicine.medscape.com/article/2062452-overview

Mészáros, I., Mórocz, J., Szlávi, J., Schmidt, J., Tornóci, L., Nagy, L., Szép, L. (2000). Epidemiology and clinicopathology of aortic dissection. *Chest, 117*(5), 1271-1278.
[http://dx.doi.org/10.1378/chest.117.5.1271] [PMID: 10807810]

Morello, F., Santoro, M., Fargion, A.T., Grifoni, S., Nazerian, P. (2021). Diagnosis and management of acute aortic syndromes in the emergency department. *Intern. Emerg. Med., 16*(1), 171-181.
[http://dx.doi.org/10.1007/s11739-020-02354-8] [PMID: 32358680]

Mussa, F.F., Horton, J.D., Moridzadeh, R., Nicholson, J., Trimarchi, S., Eagle, K.A. (2016). Acute aortic dissection and intramural hematoma: a systematic review. *JAMA, 316*(7), 754-763.
[http://dx.doi.org/10.1001/jama.2016.10026] [PMID: 27533160]

Nienaber, C.A., Powell, J.T. (2012). Management of acute aortic syndromes. *Eur. Heart J., 33*(1), 26-35b.
[http://dx.doi.org/10.1093/eurheartj/ehr186] [PMID: 21810861]

Noera, G., Lamarra, M., Guarini, S., Bertolini, A. (2001). Survival rate after early treatment for acute type-A aortic dissection with ACTH-(1-24). *Lancet, 358*(9280), 469-470.
[http://dx.doi.org/10.1016/S0140-6736(01)05631-8] [PMID: 11513913]

Schwartz, S.A., Taljanovic, M.S., Smyth, S., O'Brien, M.J., Rogers, L.F. (2007). CT findings of rupture, impending rupture, and contained rupture of abdominal aortic aneurysms. *AJR Am. J. Roentgenol., 188*(1), W57-62.
[http://dx.doi.org/10.2214/AJR.05.1554] [PMID: 17179328]

Tsai, T.T., Nienaber, C.A., Eagle, K.A. (2005). Acute aortic syndromes. *Circulation, 112*(24), 3802-3813.
[http://dx.doi.org/10.1161/CIRCULATIONAHA.105.534198] [PMID: 16344407]

Watanabe, H., Horita, N., Shibata, Y., Minegishi, S., Ota, E., Kaneko, T. (2016). Diagnostic test accuracy of D-dimer for acute aortic syndrome: systematic review and meta-analysis of 22 studies with 5000 subjects. *Sci. Rep., 6*, 26893.
[http://dx.doi.org/10.1038/srep26893] [PMID: 27230962]

Wu, J., Zafar, M., Qiu, J., Huang, Y., Chen, Y., Yu, C., Elefteriades, J.A. (2019). A systematic review and meta-analysis of isolated abdominal aortic dissection. *J. Vasc. Surg., 70*(6), 2046-2053.e6.
[http://dx.doi.org/10.1016/j.jvs.2019.04.467] [PMID: 31204217]

CHAPTER 9

Supraventricular Arrhythmias and Their Management in the Emergency Setting: PSVT and AF

Abstract: Supraventricular tachycardia (SVT) is a type of tachyarrhythmia with a narrow QRS complex and regular rhythm (heart rate >100 bpm). These patients are often symptomatic and present to the emergency department (ED) in acute attacks called paroxysmal SVT (PSVT). Most SVTs are regular rhythms. It starts suddenly with the reentry mechanism in the majority of patients. 60% of the patients have reentry with Atrioventricular (AV) node, and 20% have reentry *via* bypass pathways. Coronary artery disease, anginal chest pain and dyspnea occur in patients due to tachycardia. Heart failure and pulmonary edema may occur with left ventricular dysfunction. Vagal maneuvers and adenosine appear to be the treatments of choice for termination of stable SVT.

Keywords: Adenosine, Paroxysmal supraventricular tachycardia, Supraventricular tachycardia, Tachyarrhythmia, Vagal maneuvers.

IN MULTIFOCAL ATRIAL TACHYCARDIA (MAT)

On the other hand at least 3 different P wave morphologies originating from the atrium are observed in the ECG tracks. There are also variable PP, PR and RR ranges. Treatment is to correct the underlying disease. Specific antiarrhythmic therapy is rarely required.

PATIENTS WITH ATRIAL FLUTTER (AFL)

Also clearly sense that the attack has started, and they tend to come to the ED with more unstable findings. It may also accompany acute coronary syndromes.

Atrial fibrillation (AF) is the term used to define the inactive 'worm bag-like' oscillations of the atria, which means there is no true atrium contraction. Ruling out atrial or ventricular thrombi with echocardiography/POCUS is important to avoid embolization. Priority should be given to hemodynamic stability and determination of factors that trigger the underlying disease. IV beta-blocker and diltiazem or verapamil are the drugs of choice for acute rate control in AF with rapid ventricular response.

SUPRAVENTRICULAR TACHYCARDIAS

Supraventricular tachycardia (SVT) is a type of arrhythmia with a narrow QRS complex (<120 msec) and regular rhythm. Heart rate is over 100 per minute. In its pathophysiology, it has been shown that the factor causing arrhythmia is impulse formation and abnormalities in the conduction pathways. The most common mechanism is the reentry mechanism. Patients may present with asymptomatic, minor palpitations or severe symptoms. They are often symptomatic and present to the emergency department (ED) in acute attacks called paroxysmal SVT (PSVT).

Epidemiology

The incidence of SVT is approximately 1 to 3/1000. Its prevalence has been reported as 2.25/1000 and the number of new cases seen each year as 35/100000. Its prevalence increases with age. Atrioventricular (AV) Nodal Reentrant Tachycardia (AVNRT) is most common in middle age and older, while SVT with accessory conduction is more common in young adults. PSVT can also be seen in patients who present with previous myocardial infarction (MI), mitral valve regurgitation (MVR), rheumatic heart disease, pericarditis, pneumonia, chronic obstructive pulmonary disease (COPD) and intoxications *via* alcohol/caffeine/energy drink, apart from healthy individuals.

Ectopic SVT usually originates in the atrium and the atrial velocity is 100-250 bpm (most often 140 to 200 bpm). Regular P waves may be misdiagnosed as atrial flutter or 2: 1 AV block, sinus rhythm. Reentrant SVT is seen in most patients with SVT. A total of 60% of the patients have reentry with AV node, and 20% have reentry *via* bypass pathways. The normal heart tolerates the typical SVT rate of 160-200 bpm in days or hours. However, cardiac output is generally decreased and may lead to signs of heart failure (HF) in the intact myocardium in those with high heart rates.

Pearl: The rhythm is considered supraventricular if the QRS complex is narrow (<0.12 seconds), or if the QRS is wide in the setting of a previously known branch/fascicular block or rate-dependent aberrant conduction.

Reentrant SVT usually starts when the AV node encounters an ectopic atrial impulse while the AV node is in the partial refractory period (Fig. **1**). From here, the impulse proceeds with two different functional parallel arms. The node is below the ventricular ending and above the atrium. In the case of AV nodal reentry, QRS complexes usually hide the P waves and are not visible. These have a 1: 1 message and QRS complexes are normal.

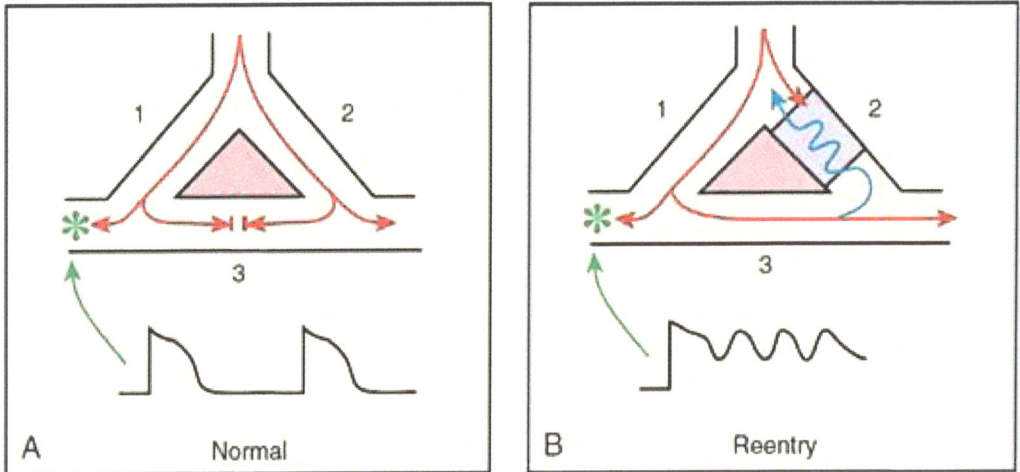

Fig. (1). Cardiac conduction in SVT. A goes down from normal depolarization pathways 1 and 2 and fades away at 3 (repolarization). B, Reentrant pathway. 1: Normal conduction; 2: there is delay/slowing down due to unilateral block; 3: normal conduction pathway.

Symptomatology

Most patients with SVT are symptomatic (Table **1**). The most common symptom is palpitations. Complaints can last from a few minutes to hours. Patients can sometimes present with shortness of breath, air hunger or chest pain. There may be dizziness, lightheadedness and rarely fainting. Dizziness and syncope are more common in those with a heart rate above 170. Syncope in SVT is mostly related to vasovagal factors. Although symptoms such as loss of consciousness and syncope increase the risk, SVT is generally not a serious or life-threatening condition. However, if any of these symptoms develop, they should be investigated with close monitoring.

Table 1. Clinical symptoms and percentages of patients presenting with PSVT.

Symptom	%
Palpitation	96
Dizziness/lightheadedness	75
Dyspnea	47
Chest pain	35

(Table 1) cont.....

Symptom	%
Fatigue, weakness	23
Syncope attack	20
Diaphoresis	17
Nausea	13

Pearl: Ectopic SVT can be seen in patients with acute MI, chronic lung disease, pneumonia, alcohol or digoxin intoxication (often associated with AV block). atrial tachycardia with block is also frequently (75%) associated with digoxin toxicity. Reentrant SVT is mostly associated with normal heart or rheumatic heart disease, acute pericarditis, MI, and MVR.

Clinical Course And Findings

Coronary artery disease, anginal chest pain and dyspnea occur in patients due to tachycardia. Heart failure and pulmonary edema may occur with decreased left ventricular function. Decrease in diastolic filling period and subsequent decrease in cardiac output may not be tolerated in the patient with left ventricular failure. Tachycardia is usually the only finding in those with normal hemodynamic reserve. In the presence of right heart failure, tachypnea, hypotension, third heart sound (S3), jugular venous distension (JVD) and hepatomegaly may be observed. Murmurs of underlying heart disease may be heard.

Evaluation And History

Time of onset, trigger mechanism, previous arrhythmia episodes and treatments received, previous medical and cardiac history should be noted in detail. Since the hypotensive event and episode of hypoxia may have triggered the arrhythmia, the history should be extended in terms of diseases such as gastrointestinal bleeding, ruptured ectopic pregnancy, carbon monoxide poisoning and pneumonia, especially in cases presenting with the first attack. Drugs such as nitrate or diuretic, phosphodiesterase inhibitors (PDEI)-5 (sildenafil), alpha blocker that may cause new onset hypotension should also be questioned in the history.

Most SVTs are regular rhythms.It starts suddenly with the reentry mechanism. Although there is a triggering cause such as excessive coffee consumption, exertion, and anxiety in some cases, this may not be the case in most of the attacks.Differentiation of SVT should be performed in accord with the origin of dysrhythmia. Atrial tachyarrhythmias should be distinguished from atrioventricular tachyarrhythmias since treatment approaches will differ (Table **2-4**)

Laboratory

Further examination of the patients who are stable at admission and have been converted to NSR immediately is unnecessary in the emergency setting. Cardiac enzymes should be evaluated in patients with risk factors for MI, those presenting with chest pain, unstable patients and patients with HF, hypotension, and APEd. Electrolyte abnormalities should be searched for. A complete blood count (CBC) is useful in showing anemia that can cause ischemia or tachycardia. Thyroid function tests can be used to seek for hyperthyroidism. Serum level should be measured in patients using digoxin.

Table 2. Differentiation of SVT according to the origin of dysrhythmia.

Atrial Tachyarrhythmias	Atrioventricular Tachyarrhythmias
Sinus tachycardia Inappropriate sinus tachycardia (IST) Sinus nodal reentrant tachycardia (SNRT) Atrial tachycardia Multifocal atrial tachycardia (MAT) Atrial flutter Atrial fibrillation	Atrioventricular nodal reentrant tachycardia (AVNRT) AV reentrant tachycardia (AVRT) Junctional ectopic tachycardia (JET) Nonparoxysmal junctional tachycardia (NPJT)

ECG is the most used test in diagnosis. Some ECG findings may provide information about the anatomical location and type of tachycardia.

Imaging

Triggering diseases and infections such as edema and pneumonia can be displayed on chest radiography. Point-of-care ultrasound (POCUS)/echocardiography may be useful in suspected structural heart disease.

Table 3. The differential diagnosis of narrow QRS tachycardia with ECG findings in patients presenting with PSVT.

Tachycardias	ECG FINDINGS
Sinus tachycardia	Heart rate> 100/min Sinus rhythm (P waves) Regular PR intervals
Inappropriate sinus tachycardia (IST)	Similar to sinus tachycardia Sinus rhythm (P waves)
Sinus nodal reentrant tachycardia	Sudden start and end Sinus rhythm (P waves)

(Table 3) cont.....

Tachycardias	ECG FINDINGS
Atrial tachycardia	Heart rate 120-250/min P waves with different configurations Prolonged PR interval
Multifocal atrial tachycardia	Heart rate> 100-200/min 3 different P wave morphologies
Atrial flutter	Atrial rate 200-300/min Sawtooth flutter waves AV conduction ratio 2: 1 or 4: 1
Atrial fibrillation	Irregular rhythm P waves are not visible
Atrioventricular nodal reentrant tachycardia	Heart rate 150-200/min P wave inside or immediately after the QRS complex Short PR interval in typical AVNRT Long PR interval in atypical AVNRT
Atrioventricular reentrant tachycardia	Heart rate 150-250/min Narrow QRS complexes in orthodromic conduction Wide QRS complexes in antidromic conduction P waves after the QRS complex

Table 4. SVT differentials according to the PR interval.

Tachycardias with short PR intervals	Tachycardias with long PR intervals PR
• Typical AV nodal reentrant tachycardia (AVNRT) • AV reentrant tachycardia (AVRT) • Junctional ectopic tachycardia • Nonparoxysmal junctional tachycardia	• Sinus tachycardia • Sinus nodal reentrant tachycardia • Atrial tachycardia • Atrial flutter • Atypical AVNRT • Permanent junctional reciprocal tachycardia

If the reentry circuit is within the atrial myocardium; atrial fibrillation, atrial flutter, and some types of atrial tachycardia may occur. In this situation, AV node suppressing agents slow down the tachyarrhythmia but do not convert it.

In some re-entry tachycardias, the reentry circuit is in the AV node. These arrhythmias, which are characterized by a sudden onset and end, are recognized with a resting heart rate of over 150.

- AV nodal reentry tachycardia (AVNRT) occurs when both arms of the reentry circuit are in the AV node; The typical finding is that P waves cannot be discerned in this form.
- One arm of the reentry circuit is in the accessory pathway and the other is in the AV node, called "AV reentry tachycardia" (AVRT).

- AVNRT and AVRT are both PSVT.
- If at least one branch of the circuit is in the AV node, AV node suppressing agents will have a chance to terminate the arrhythmia.
- Group 3 SVT is called automatic tachycardias. These are linked to an excited automatic stimulus focus, including ectopic atrial tachycardia, MAT and junctional tachycardias. Termination of these will be more gradual and slower.
- Automatic tachycardias do not respond to electrical cardioversion (ECV), furthermore, these are arrhythmias for which ECV is contraindicated. These are treated with rate control with agents that slow down AV conduction.

Multifocal Atrial Tachycardia (MAT)

There are at least 3 different P wave morphologies originating from the atrium in the ECG tracks. There are also variable PP, PR and RR ranges. The heart rate is above 100 beats per minute and the rhythm is irregular. It can be mistakenly interpreted as AF. It is frequently seen in elderly patients with chronic lung disease. Treatment is to correct the underlying disease. Specific antiarrhythmic therapy is rarely required. It has been reported that standard antiarrhythmics are ineffective in suppressing multiple atrial ectopias and these agents may have toxic effects. Also, digoxin depresses the AV node and slows the ventricular rate. In the management, magnesium sulphate 2 g IV is given within 60 seconds; followed by administration of 1-2 g/hr with a constant infusion rate. It has been shown to reduce conversion to sinus rhythm and ectopia. Verapamil slows down the ventricular response with 5-10 mg IV administration, reduces ectopias in some patients, and provides conversion to sinus rhythm in many patients.

Treatment

Vagal maneuvers (VM) and adenosine appear to be the "plan A" for termination of stable PSVT. For other SVTs, VM and adenosine may be partially beneficial, reducing the pulse but they do not provide termination.

The first approach should be drug-free, simple, noninvasive, easy-to-use maneuvers. The most common applications for this purpose among the context of VM include carotid sinus massage (CSM) and Valsalva. Apart from these, there are also techniques such as cold water immersion and massage on the eyeball, which used to be more common in the past.

The VM slows down the AV node and lengthens the refractory period within the node. It also has a negative inotropic effect on the ventricular myocardium. VM is also indicated for the examination of cardiac murmurs. It has been shown in some documents that it can also be useful in terminating stable ventricular tachycardia (VT), but it is not a rule.

VALSALVA MANEUVER AND SIMPLIFIED MODIFIED VALSALVA (SMV)

Valsalva maneuver is the most used VM because it is easy and practical. In most guidelines, it is primarily recommended for regular tachycardia treatment with narrow QRS. It is more successful in AVRT than AVNRT. Valsalva should not be administered to patients whose hemodynamic stability is not attained, those with known aortic stenosis, those who have had a recent MI, and those who have diseases in which an increase in venous pressures may be dangerous.

Different percentages (19% to 54%) are reported for clinical success rate. Although a Cochrane review recently announced that there is insufficient evidence to support or refute its effectiveness, it is widely used all over the world (Smith, 2015). In a recent multi-center controlled study in China, SMV was found to be 43% successful and standard Valsalva 17% successful in terminating PSVT.

How To Perform The Procedure

For standard Valsalva, the patient with stable narrow QRS and regular tachycardia sits in a comfortable position. After inspiration with normal tidal volume, it is asked to try to move the piston for 15 seconds by blowing into the injector with a 10 or 20 ml needle removed (trying to reach a pressure of 40 mmHg). It is desired to blow as strong as possible and can be measured with a manometer. We can understand that a strong enough maneuver is made by the fullness of the neck veins and the flushing of the face.

In SMV, in the standard method that starts in a semi-sitting position, after blowing for 15 seconds, supination is started and the legs are passively lifted at the same time. After waiting in this way for 15 seconds, 30 seconds. The rest period starts and the process is completed within 1 minute (Fig. **2**).

On the other hand, CSM is applied under monitoring in the supine position, unilaterally with the neck facing the opposite side and in extension. At the point where the carotid pulsation is taken (just caudal to the corner of the mandible), rubbing is performed with cranial-caudal movements.

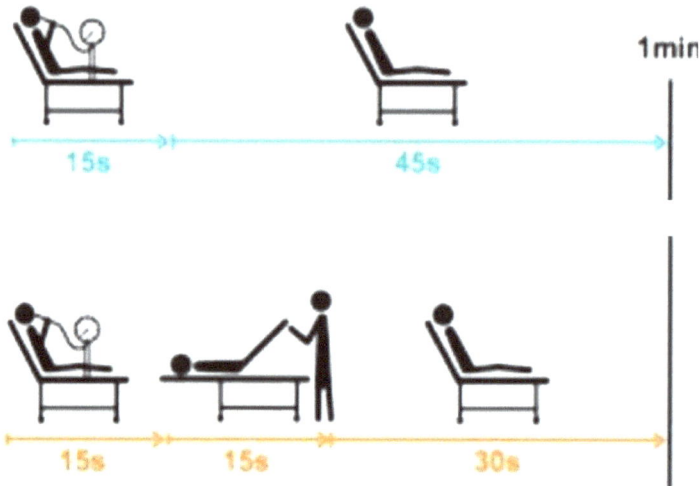

Fig. (2). A. Standard Valsalva, B. Simplified Modified Valsalva method.

The process is completed in 5 seconds. Double-sided procedure is absolutely contraindicated. It is not attempted in patients with a history of TIA, stroke and a murmur on the carotid artery area.

Pearl: CSM is applied to clarify the diagnosis, especially in syncope work up, in people who are thought to have a sensitive carotid sinus. Hypersensitive carotid sinus findings comprise persistent asystole or a drop in systolic blood pressure> 50 mmHg, lasting for at least 3 seconds just after CSM.

Adenosine

Administer 6 mg IV adenosine IV push in patients with PSVT unresponsive to the vagal maneuver (Class I, LOE B). Then flush 20 mL of IV SF *via* the same vein. If sinus rhythm does not return within 1-2 minutes, repeat 12 mg of the agent. Submit IV fluid flush again, to increase the success rate. Conversion of the rhythm is achieved in most patients with an average of 6 mg (Brugada, 2019).

Maintain continuous ECG monitoring which will help in rhythm analysis, with or without sinus rhythm conversion. Rapid ventricular rate AF can be triggered in patients with WPW.

In case of continuation of SVT or triggering of AF/Flutter, non-dihydropyridine group CCB (diltiazem or verapamil) (Class IIa, LOE B) or beta-blocker (metoprolol) should be administered (Class IIa, LOE C) to slow down the AV node for a long time. CCB should not be given in cases of decompesated HF or wide-complex tachycardia in adults and in young children (Fig. **3**).

If PSVT with preexcitation such as WPW or LGL is considered, extreme caution should be exercised. The aforementioned agents may not be beneficial in these patients, and they may trigger fatal arrhythmias by increasing the ventricular rate. (Class III, LOE C). It will be correct to ask for a consultation.

Combined use of the aforementioned AV nodal blocking agents should also be avoided and caution should be exercised. They can cause severe bradyarrhythmias. Agents such as amiodarone, procainamide, sotalol can provide rate control in AF/flutter, and sometimes they can cause sinus rhythm. Care should be taken in terms of thromboembolic complications.

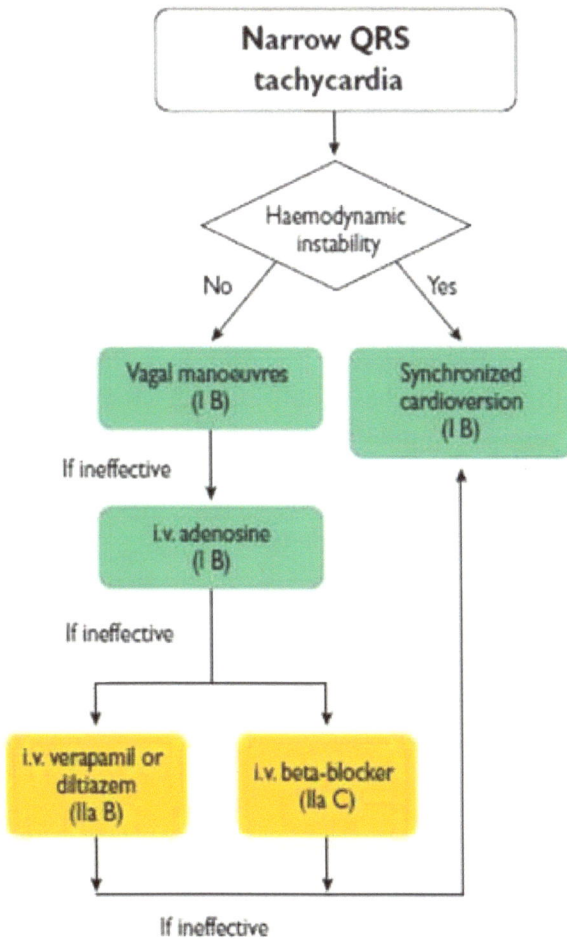

Fig. (3). Algorithm for emergency treatment of narrow-QRS tachycardia in the absence of previously established diagnosis.

ATRIAL FIBRILLATION: CLASSIFICATION, DIAGNOSIS AND TREATMENT

Case presentation: 52-year-old male teacher; comes with palpitations that started in the morning. He is taking drugs for hyperthyroidism. The cardiology consultant had reported beforehand in the shift that the echocardiography device is out of order and the cardiologist is on annual leave. TA: 120/80, HR: 124 bpm, ECG is given in Fig. (**4**).

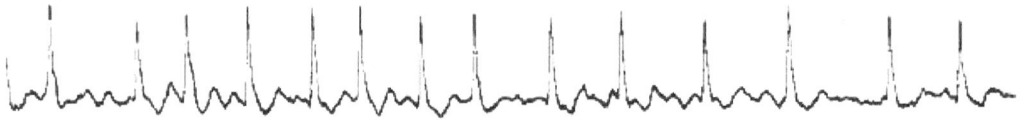

Fig. (4). Atrial fibrillation with rapid ventricular rate.

The third-year resident administered 5 mg IV metoprolol after establishing vascular access from the left antecubital and monitoring the patient. There was no wall motion defect, and no atrial thrombus was observed in the bedside USG. Aortic diameters are normal. After metoprolol, the pulse was 102 bpm, and he appeared to be relaxed. The team decided to proceed with electrical cardioversion after consulting the cardiologist. 300 mg ASA was chewed and swallowed. ECV was performed with a 150 J biphasic defibrillator, after administration of 100 mcg of fentanyl and 20 mg of etomidate, while the Ramsay sedation scale score was 3 to 4. Work up revealed that TSH value was quite low and Troponin and BNP were within normal limits. The patient was discharged after institution of outpatient treatment for hyperthyroidism.

Definition

Atrial fibrillation (AF) is the term used to define the inactive 'worm bag-like' oscillations of the atria, which means there is no true atrium contraction. Different electrical vectors move in different directions simultaneously from the atrial myocardium, causing irregular and rapid impulses. The result is rapid and irregular vibrations in every part of the atria. A regular atrial activity is not recorded in AF. There are no P waves and no sawtooth/flutter waves. There are only waves called F waves.

Although the atrial rate is around 400, it is limited by the refractory period and can be very variable. The distance between the QRS complexes (RR) is unequal, thus it is an irregular rhythm. Acute AF, which brings patients to the ED and is therefore common in the emergency, is often discloses a high ventricular rate.

As the age increases, AF is encountered more frequently, with a male predominance. AF is the most common rhythm disorder encountered and managed by emergency physicians following only sinus tachycardia. Majority of patients with AF and atrial flutter (AFL) can be treated and discharged in the ED without the need for hospitalization.

AF can be acute or chronic. Patients with acute AF (AAF) mostly present with a rapid ventricular response, that is, more than 100 beats per minute.

In chronic AF, the ventricular response can be in 3 ways. So heart rate can be normal, high or low (Fig. **5A** and **B**).

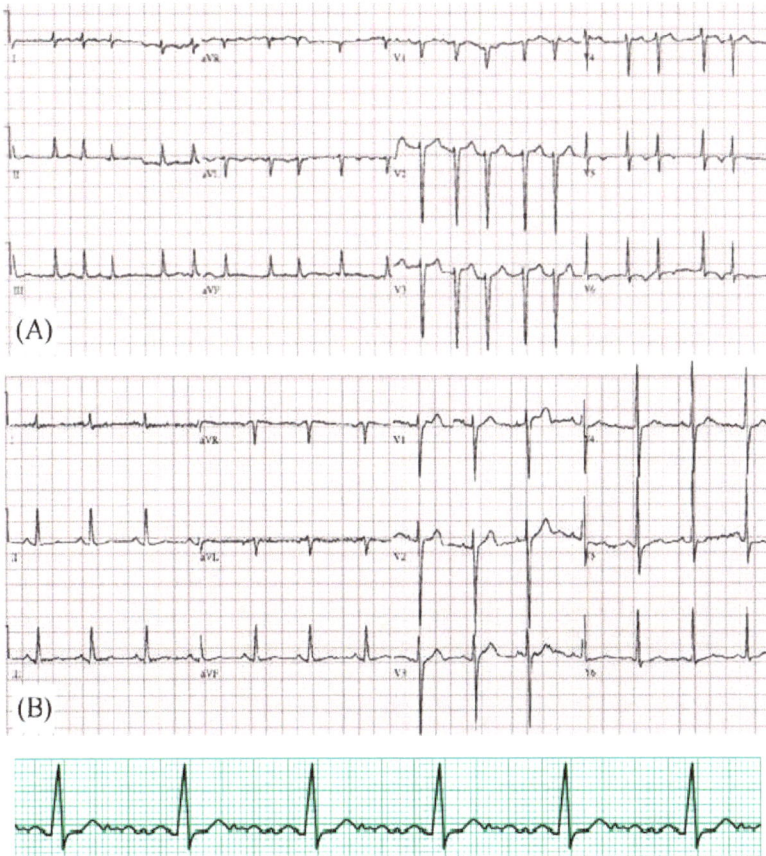

Fig. (5). Atrial fibrillation with normal rapid ventricular response **(A)** and after spontaneous conversion to sinus rhythm **(B)**. Atrial fibrillation with normal ventricular response **(C)**.

AAF is the term used for AF that lasted no longer than 48 hours from the onset of an attack. It is an entity triggered by many reasons; poor outcomes of AAF arise mostly due to hemodynamic instability and thromboembolic events. The most common causes are mitral valve diseases, ACS/ischemic heart disease and thyrotoxicosis (Table **5**).

What happens when you have AF? In AF, HF may ensue because the heart cannot achieve pump activity as it did normally before, especially at high ventricular rates. Patients with AF is also predisposed to peripheral venous and atrial embolism with the risk of pulmonary and systemic arterial embolism. 5% to 15% of patients with chronic AF can be expected to have thromboembolism once a year. Therefore, patients with chronic AF should regularly use anticoagulant medication.

Table 5. Triggering causes of AAF and predisposing factors to acute or chronic AF.

Causes that Trigger AAF	Factors Predisposing to Acute or Chronic AF
structural cardiac abnormalities/cardiomyopathies/valvular diseases, mainly mitral	atrial enlargement, congestive heart failure vagal stimulation, atherosclerosis hyperthyroidism refractory period differs in various parts of the atrium.
inflammation/infections/fever (may or may not affect the heart directly	
Fluid/electrolyte disorders, dehydration	
Strenous exercise/athletic training	
hormonal and autonomic nervous system disorders	
ACS/atherosclerosis/coronary heart disease	
Intoxications: carbon monoxide/alcohol	
Hypoxemia	
pulmonary embolism	
Overt release/intake of thyroid hormones	

Clinical Status

Priority should be given to hemodynamic stability and determination of factors that trigger the underlying disease. The onset of arrhythmia should be especially questioned and understood, with special regard to acute/chronic distinction. In doubtful cases, it should be treated as chronic AF and presence of thrombi should be assumed. Stroke risk should be evaluated with validated scores.

In patients with AAF a pulse rate of around 180 bpm which may cause instability, is recorded frequently, and in rare cases, it may pose a danger by exceeding 200 bpm. In cases with Wolff-Parkinson-White (WPW) syndrome, which has an aberrant conduction pathway, extremely high heart rates can be life-threatening because of by-passed AV node.

Approximately half of the patients presenting with AAF return to sinus rhythm within 48 hours. This rule is especially true for those whose etiology is highlighted and treatment is commenced.

AF frequently accompanies hypertension. In contrary to the developed countries, AF is also common in the setting of rheumatic heart diseases, especially with mitral stenosis in developing countries. Loss of atrial contractions, especially in cases of left ventricular failure, may lead to the acute exacerbation or worsening of HF.

Common complaints in patients with AF are fatigue, palpitations, chest pain, and shortness of breath. The reason for these is that the ejection fraction is reduced due to AF. Another important consequence of AF is that it predisposes to stroke and peripheral acute artery occlusions as a result of formation of atrial thrombi. Troponin-positive coronary artery disease was detected in 5% of the patients who presented to the ED with AAF. Acute-onset AF, especially, should be considered ACS until proven otherwise.

Differential Diagnosis

Differential diagnosis of AAF includes entities such as AFL, PSVT, sinus rhythm, and AV nodal tachycardia. These diseases can be easily differentiated from each other basically both with their clinical features and their ECGs.

Clinical Distinction

Unlike the clinical features of AAF outlined above, PSVT cases describe the onset of the arrhythmia very clearly. Most of the cases have gained experience and are knowledgeable about CSM, Valsalva maneuver, and rhythm correcting agents, and some even present to the ED only after failing to treat themselves with maneuvers. Its findings are more stable, serious findings are rarely detected. Pharmacological cardioversion (PCV) with agents such as metoprolol and diltiazem is generally uneventful. Of these, verapamil is used less frequently than before, due to its side effect profile. Electrical cardioversion (ECV) is required in a small group, ECV can be applied with low doses such as 50 J.

Patients with Afl (Flutter)

Also clearly sense that the attack has started, and they tend to come to the ED with more unstable findings. It may accompany AMI and unstable angina pectoris. Digoxin overdose has also been encountered in these cases. Chest pain, dyspnea and hypotension are more common in this group, compared to AF. The ventricular rate, or pulse rate, changes according to the degree of AV block, which directly affects the clinical status and stability. Since the atrial rate is generally around 300 bpm, the ventricular rate is often recorded as 75, 100 or 150 bpm, which exactly correspond to 1: 2, 1: 3, 1: 4 blocks. For ECV, 30J to 50 J with monophasic defibrillators is usually sufficient.

Multifocal Atrial Tachycardia (MAT)

MAT is mostly seen in advanced stages of chronic lung diseases and critical HF. It has also been reported in cases of theophylline poisoning and those who consume caffeine excessively. Atrial rhythm is usually between 100 and 180 bpm. ECV is not indicated in this entity.

Differential Diagnosis by ECG

In a patient whose clinic is suitable for the diagnosis of MAT, at least 3 different p wave structures and variable P-P, P-R, and R-R intervals are sought in the ECG tracing. In AFL, around 300 atrial velocity, regular waves called saw tooth (seesaw), characterized by the absence of isoelectric line, are seen. Findings are best observed in limb leads II, III, and aVF.

The presence of fibrillation (f) waves replacing the isoelectric line in the ECG in patients with AF, the absence of a consistent and continuously traceable p wave, are observed as 'irregular irregular' rhythm characterized by the inequality of R-R intervals. As a rule, QRS waves are normal, ie narrow. Delta waves and short PR should be investigated for concomitant WPW syndrome.

Imaging and Laboratory

The purpose of imaging in AAF cases under emergency conditions is to collect information about differential diagnoses and triggering causes, and more importantly, to anticipate and prevent thromboembolic events.

There are no 'routine' laboratory examinations to be ordered in every case of AF, instead, a cost-effective list of work up can be culminated for each individual patient. For example, pulmonary embolism can be distinguished by POCUS-computed tomography-angiography. Other diseases associated with or triggering AF can be sought for *via* chest radiography; findings compatible with pneumonia, congestive heart failure, enlargement of the heart chambers, chronic pericarditis, aneurysm can be investigated. Carboxyhemoglobin (COHb) level is critical in guiding the treatment in cases where carbon monoxide poisoning is thought to be the trigger for AAF attack. ECG, troponin and creatine kinase levels can yield vital findings in terms of acute ischemic heart disease. Hemoglobin and hematocrit should be requested in terms of acute hemorrhagic losses, blood urea nitrogen and creatinine levels should be requested for uremic pericarditis or RF. Oxygenation should be measured under emergency conditions with pulse oximetry, hypoxemia should be excluded and corrected, if any. In cases such as diabetic ketoacidosis or COPD, arterial blood gas analysis should be used. In a recent study, it was determined that patients with NT-proBNP levels below 450 pg/ml mostly reverted to sinus rhythm during their hospital stay, whereas patients with values above 1800 pg/ml were persistent patients with AF (Buccelletti, 2011). For this reason, BNP level should also be requested in patients with dyspnea and to be distinguished from heart failure and lung disease. If thyroid diseases such as thyrotoxicosis, Basedow-Graves disease, multinodular goiter are considered as triggering causes, T3, T4 and thyroid stimulating hormone levels help.

It is vital to exclude pericardial tamponade due to trauma and patients with suspected cardiac arrest (asystole or pulseless electrical activity) despite electrical activity on the ECG under emergency conditions. In addition, POCUS/echocardiography evaluates the size and motion of the heart chambers, the presence of a heart-related mass, valve problems and the presence of intracardiac thrombus. In this way, important information can be obtained with a low cost, simple application at the bedside.

The most important limitation of the technique is that its reliability and accuracy are dependent on the experience and ability of the operator. Since the results can also change with the position that can be given to the patient, there is a limitation in cases who cannot easily change position or those with obesity.

For ideal cardiac USG/POCUS, lowering the pulse is important. For this, depending on the condition of the patient with atrial tachyarrhythmia, beta-blocker or calcium channel blocker agents can be used.

Beta-blockers (metoprolol) may be preferred in young people with anxiety, coronary artery disease or hyperthyroidism, and calcium channel blockers in other groups and in patients who are contraindicated to beta blockers such as asthma. PO/IV Metoprolol should be preferred for beta blockade and IV esmolol in more urgent cases. Diltiazem, one of the calcium channel blockers, is the first choice due to its more positive side effect profile than verapamil. Concomitant administration of metoprolol and calcium channel blocker in selected cases is acceptable, but attention should be paid to dose adjustment and titration to effect.

Echocardiography can be performed by transesophageal (TEE) or transthoracic (TTE) methods in patients with AF. Since TEE is performed using the esophageal probe, it both takes images from the window closer to the heart anatomically and gives a more accurate result as it eliminates the blocking effect of the chest and ribs. However, in some cases it is difficult to tolerate and may take longer. TTE is a faster diagnostic tool chosen under emergency conditions. TEE is more sensitive in showing the left atrium, left atrial appendix (LAA), atrial septum, and aortic arch. For example, potential sources of cardiac embolism that may be overlooked by TTE in stroke cases can be determined by TEE.

The cause of cardiac embolism can be found in nearly 80% of the cases with TEE in patients with uncertain cause of stroke. With TTE, this rate is lower, between 15% to 40%. TTE is often chosen in elderly patients with a known cardioembolic cause. TEE yields better results in patients under 50 years of age for whom the cause of stroke cannot be determined.

In a detailed echocardiographic examination to be performed in patients with AF, hemodynamic variables such as mean diastolic mitral gradient, pulmonary artery pressure, mitral valve area, tricuspid and mitral regurgitation, left atrial diameter should be measured and given quantitatively. In addition, the Wilkins mitral valve score is calculated. For example, in different studies, the mitral valve score and tricuspid valve involvement among those with mitral stenosis were found to be higher in patients with AF than those with sinus rhythm, indicating the prevalence of rheumatic activity.

Echocardiographic findings are closely related to the clinical course. For example, in studies examining the variables that affect the conversion of AF cases to sinus rhythm, the duration of AF attack less than 24 hours, young age, left atrial diameter and absence of primary heart disease appear as independent variables. Dogan *et al*. found only the duration of AF as an effective factor on conversion (Dogan, 2003). In this study, the mean left atrium diameter of patients presenting with AF was found to be 39.0 mm.

In recent years, after correction of AF with ECV, attention has been drawn to the 'stunning' phenomenon and related TTE findings have been underlined. Decreased LAA flow rates, decreased LAA discharge fraction, decreased transmitral inflow rates, and the appearance of spontaneous echo contrast have been reported as findings indicating atrial stunning.

Current Management

In cases presenting with AAF, the treatment of the underlying disease, to eliminate pain and anxiety, to provide oxygenation and to correct the hemodynamics are primary and mandatory goals to achieve. After this treatment, a return to sinus rhythm can be accomplished without any other intervention in most cases.

Apart from this basic principle, there are three mainstays in the treatment of AF cases.

1- Provision of normal sinus rhythm and maintaining its stability.

2- Although AF is not terminated, reducing the heart rate to a normal/acceptable level.

3- Prevention of formation of mural thrombi.

Pearl: If AF is one of rapid ventricular rate and the patient has symptoms related to rate (HF, pulmonary edema, dyspnoea, impaired consciousness, ischemic chest pain), rate control should be provided immediately. As with flutter, agents such as diltiazem, verapamil or beta blocker (propranolol or metoprolol) can be used. ECV should be considered in those with acute hemodynamic compromise.

When AAF cases are considered to be hemodynamically stable, one of two ways is chosen in treatment. These two options, known as rhythm control or rate control, are selected and applied in accord with the patient's clinical characteristics. Stiell *et al.* in their population-based study in Canada, examined whether the methods conducted in different centers differed from each other (Stiell, 2011). It was observed that rhythm control strategy was applied to approximately 60% of 1018 AAF and AFL cases, and ECV was performed primarily for 40% of them. In total, 83% of the patients were discharged from the ED successfully. The variables that affect the choice of rhythm control strategy and the decision of ECV independently from other factors were determined as age, previous ECV history, presence of HF, and the center admitted the patient. Case example. A woman presents with AF with rapid ventricular rate (Fig. **6**).

In general, treatment strategies can be divided into conservative (preparation for elective ECV after rate control and anticoagulation) and aggressive (performing cardioversion as ECV or chemical/pharmacological cardioversion (PCV) in appropriate patients under safety precautions in the ED). It has been reported that there are important differences between physicians and disciplines in terms of approach to AAF.

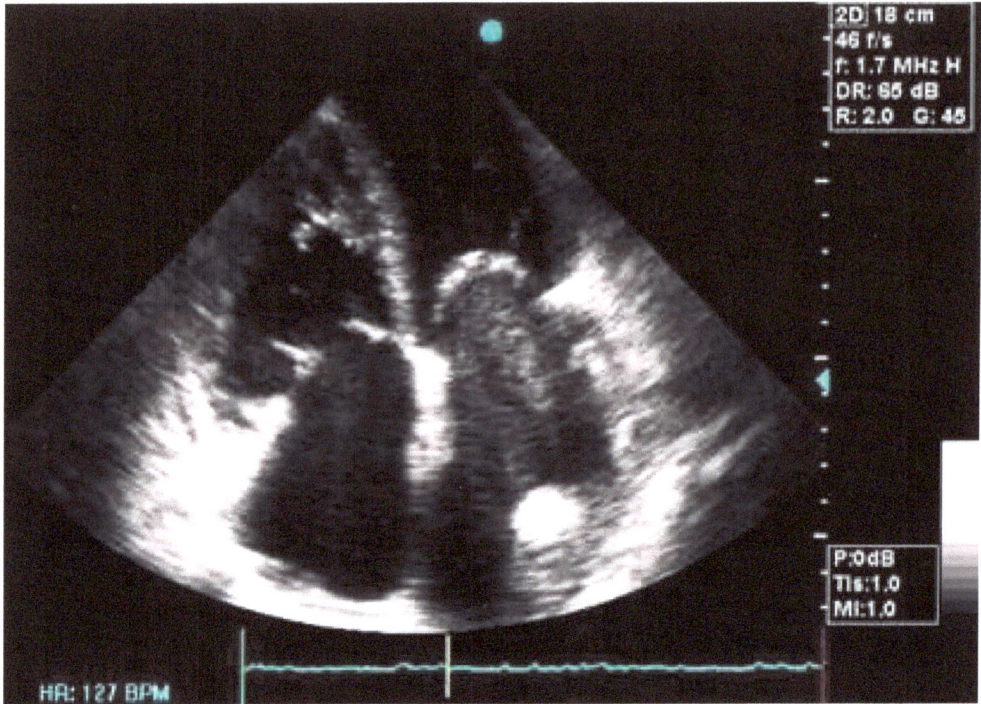

Fig. (6). Left atrial thrombus appearance in POCUS/ECHO in the patient with AF . The patient's condition was improved with medical therapy, diltiazem infusion, and thus electrical cardioversion was abandoned.

Rhythm Control And Cardioversion (Conversion To Sinus Rhythm)

ECV or PCV can be applied under emergency conditions to provide the conversion of AAF to sinus rhythm. The difference of cardioversion performed under emergency conditions from elective procedure is that the rhythm is returned to normal without anticoagulation in emergency practice, whereas in elective procedure, it would be clarified that there is no thrombus and other contraindications are excluded, and the cardioversion procedure is performed.

Therefore, it should be ensured as much as possible that less than 48 hours have passed from the onset of AAF for ECV and that the patient does not pose a high risk for embolic stroke. If you cannot be sure how long has passed, a rate control strategy should be adopted at first. Therapeutic anticoagulation should be commenced to these cases 3 weeks before and 4 weeks following ECV.

Pearl: Ruling out atrial or ventricular thrombi with echocardiography/POCUS is important to avoid embolization. In some cases, 3-week anticoagulant regimens may be required, in others, vitamin K antagonists (Coumadin) is warranted. Expert consultation is usually recommended.

In a very recent study, Bellone *et al.* randomized 247 patients to these two groups (ECV vs PCV). The success rate of ECV was higher (89% *versus* 73%). The mean time spent in the ED is also much shorter in the ECV group (180 vs 420 minutes). Side effects and adverse events occurred in a short time and in very small subgroups. Similarly, Cristoni *et al.* published a study in 2010, which showed that by establishing a short observation unit linked with the ED, these cases could be effectively treated without the need for hospitalization. In this study, they were randomized to ECV (n = 171) and PCV (n = 151) groups, and discharge in sinus rhythm was achieved in 93% and 51%, respectively. During the 6-month follow-up, 2 patients in the ECV group had stroke. As a result, the treatment of AAF cases can be safely performed by applying ECV in the short observation unit.

More than 60% of patients return to normal sinus rhythm with 100 J and more than 80% with 200 J.

Drugs used in PCV are predominantly Class IC and III, according to Vaughan-Williams classification. Recently, Conti *et al.* reported that, flecainide, propafenone or amiodarone were administered in a total of 378 patients in a non-randomized design for PCV in the Italian EDs, and 87% of the total group returned to sinus rhythm within 6 hours. The success rates of the 3 drugs were 72%, 55% and 30%, respectively. Conversion times were also sorted by the same sequence, with an average of 178, 292 and 472 minutes. They postulated that IC group antiarrhythmics (flecainid, propafenone) are apparently more efficacous than Class III drugs (amiodarone) and should be selected first for PCV.

Propafenone 150 mg tablets, which are commercially available in most places from the Ic group, can be administered orally as 300 or 600 mg, and as we have also seen in our experience in Turkey, PCV can be safely and successfully administered in the ED.

In a Croatian study published in 2008, data on 140 patients were shared. It has been reported that a success rate close to 100% has been achieved *via* PCV by administering three drugs from different pharmacological classes consecutively within a certain protocol.

Class I agents that produce antiarrhythmic effects by blocking sodium channels are divided into groups IA, IB and IC. Class IC drugs are one of the groups with the highest potential to terminate AAF *via* PCV. Propafenone, which is frequently used for this purpose in many centers, is also in this group. It should be selected in young patients with AF without structural heart disease. Bradycardia and heart failure, which can be life-threatening, can be seen rarely with this agent.

Although amiodarone (Class III; blocking sodium and potassium channels) is one of the most effective antiarrhythmic agents, it is less effective in termination of AAF by PCV. A feature that does not exist in other drugs is that it can be used safely in individuals with poor general condition, elderly and/or those with underlying structural heart disease.

Use of Amiodarone for PCV: IV: infused primarily 150 mg/10 minutes. Then 1 mg/min is infused for 6 hours, 0.5 mg/min for 18 hours. The maximum total dose is 10 g. It can be continued orally (100-200 mg/day).

Can the patients terminate AF themselves? Yes. One approach that can also be seen as a variant of the rhythm control strategy is that individuals with infrequent attacks are given a certain training, and these individuals immediately receive PCV by taking the appropriate medication right next to them. This approach, also known as the "drug in the pocket" concept, can be used very beneficially in selected patient groups.

In an Austrian study, Hirschl *et al.* reported that flecainide (95%) and ibutilide (76%) were the most effective drugs used for PCV in 376 patients with AAF in the ED. Amiodarone, digoxin and diltiazem have very low success rates. A striking result is the observation that patients presenting with low blood pressure and who had a short period of time from the onset of AF to treatment revert to sinus rhythm with higher success.

Pearl: Procedure recommendation: For PCV, propafenone from group Ic can be used for conversion of AF to NSR. For this purpose, 600 mg propafenone (4x150 mg tb) is administered orally at a time and the patient is expected to convert within a few hours. This procedure is only recommended in the hospital.

ECG monitoring is recommended because a prolonged period of asystole, rarely syncope or prolonged bradyarrhythmias may occur during 'successful' conversion.

Synchronized/Simultaneous Cardioversion

Explained in the chapter for 'Electrotherapies' When midazolam and fentanyl are administered at recommended doses and under appropriate conditions, the side effect profile is at an acceptable level. In the presence of signs of opioid overdose that may occur, albeit very rarely, naloxone should be used by titrating at the recommended doses in Table **6**. Ketamine, which is widely used for sedoanalgesia in other indications, is not preferred in this group of cases as it may have tachycardic effects.

Table 6. Sedatives and narcotics, doses, duration of action and expected side effects for sedoanalgesia used in ECV procedure in the ED. The drugs are used by an experienced emergency physician or anesthesiologist, titrated with respect to the response of the patient.

Medication	Starting dose (adult ~ 70 kg)	Dose/kg (for titration)	Duration of effect	Side effect
Midazolam (for sedation, anxiolysis)	1-2 mg IV	0.04-0.06 mg/kg (IV/ IM)	60-90 min	Respiratory depression, hypotension (very rare at recommended doses)
Etomidate (for sedation, anxiolysis)	15-20 mg IV	0.2-0.3 mg/kg IV	20-30 min	Myoclonus, adrenocortical suppression in long-term administration
Fentanyl (for analgesia)	1-2 mcg/kg IV	0.5-1.0 mcg/kg IV	1-2 hrs	Respiratory depression, chest wall rigidity (very rare at recommended doses)
Naloxone (Narcotic antagonist)	0.2-0.4 mg IV (up to 2 mg)	0.4 mg IV	2-3 hrs	Tachycardia

Rate Control

Rate control strategy is a treatment approach that can be preferred in cases where the AF attack is thought to recur especially in those with structural heart disease, coronary artery disease, elderly *etc.* It is aimed to improve the symptoms by

reducing the heart rate. Patients who are not selected/unsuitable for ECV are evaluated in the rate control group.

Agents such as beta blockers (metoprolol), calcium channel blockers (diltiazem), and amiodarone are widely used for rate control. The serious toxic effects of amiodarone on many organs and systems limit its use. Digoxin is also a frequently used agent in the past, but it is rarely recommended in contemporary practice.

Current Recommendation

IV beta-blocker and nondihydropyridine CCB (diltiazem) is the drug of choice for acute rate control in AF with rapid ventricular response (Class IIa, LOE A).

Digoxin and amiodarone can be used for rate control in patients with CHF + AF. However, after the use of amiodarone, the risk of return to sinus rhythm and resultant embolization should be taken into account.

A large complex, irregularly irregular rhythm may reflect a AF with pre-excitation (WPW/LGL). Expert consultation should be obtained early.

• Adenosine, CCB, digoxin and β-blocking agents that cause AV nodal block should be avoided, as they pose a risk of increasing the ventricular rate.

• These cases are often converted to NSR with emergency ECV. If this is unavailable, other than abovementioned objectionable agents can be tried.

Procainamide

Procainamide is a widely used agent in most parts of the world for PCV. In a study in which the "Ottawa Aggressive Protocol" put forward in Canada in the last decade was tested, 660 AAF (4.9% AFL) cases were taken as a cohort (Stiell IG, 2010). If it could not be understood whether the AAF attack lasted longer than 48 hours, the presence of mural thrombus was examined by TEE. Initially IV procainamide was given to all cases, a conversion rate of 58.3% was achieved. ECV procedure was performed in all remaining 243 cases, it was successful in 91.7% of them. Recurrent attacks were observed in 8.6% of the cases within 7 days. The patients stayed in the ED for an average of 4.9 hours (3.9 hours in patients with PCV, 6.5 hours in patients with ECV) and 96.8% were discharged from the ED.

Antithrombotic-Antiaggregant Treatment in Patients With AF

In AF cases in whom effective contractions do not occur, blood may undergo stasis and turn into clots, especially in the left atrium. This phenomenon is clearly seen in AF patients lasting for 48 hours and older. The delivery of these clots to the arterial circulation *via* the aorta occurs most often during the conversion of AAF to normal sinus rhythm, so it is important to demonstrate that there is no clot for ECV/PCV of chronic AF. Arterial circulation may stop in any part of the body with this event called thromboembolism of mural thrombi. Acute arterial occlusion, renal infarction, acute mesenteric embolism may occur, but the most important morbidity is that it causes cerebral thromboembolism, or stroke.

Warfarin (Coumadine) and heparin are agents that prevent fibrin formation, they are in the anticoagulant group. Acetyl salicylic acid (ASA, Aspirin) and clopidogrel (Plavix) or ticagrelor (Brillinta) are antiaggregant or antiplatelet agents. The combined use of P2Y12 inhibitor and ASA is called dual antiplatelet treatment (DAPT). Among these, warfarin prevents clot formation in the most efficient way, provides full effectiveness within a few days after its use, and requires monitoring with prothrombin time (PT) and INR level every 4-8 weeks. In recent years, the "triple antiplatelet therapy" (TAPT) method has been in question, with the addition of an agent from the DOAC group (such as dabigatran/rivaroxaban) to the DAPT regimen.

As of the update in January 2019, the following recommendations are in effect (Kirolos I, *et al*. 2019):

- If the CHA2DS2-VASc score is> = 2 in AF + ACS cases, warfarin (vitamin K antagonist-VKA) "triple therapy/triple therapy" (TAPT) is recommended in addition to the DAPT (aspirin + P2Y12 inhibitor) regimen.

- Double therapy in the form of warfarin (vitamin K antagonist) with P2Y12 inhibitor + dose adjustment after stenting is an acceptable treatment.

- P2Y12 inhibitor (clopidogrel or ticagrelor) + oral anticoagulant rivaroxaban, dabigatran or VKA with dose adjustment can be given as an alternative (Dewilde WJ, *et al*. Lancet 2013; 381: 1107-15 .; Lamberts M, *et al*. J Am Coll Cardiol 2013; 62: 981-9 .; Braun OÖ, *et al*. Thromb Res 2015; 135: 26-30.).

Does AF in my patient cause a cerebrovascular accident?

Yes, it can. In NVAF, we use the CHA2DS2-VASc Score and Risk criteria in recent years instead of the CHADS2 criteria in 2001 in order to predict this more clearly (Tables **7-9**).

Table 7. CHA2DS2-VASc Score and Risk criteria.

Score	CHA$_2$DS$_2$-VASc Risk Criteria
1	CHF
1	Hypertension
2	Age ≥75
1	Diabetes mellitus
2	Stroke/TIA/Thromboembolic event
1	Vascular disease (MI, PAH, aortic disease)
1	Age 65 to 74
1	Woman

Table 8. CHA2DS2-VASc Score and Annual Stroke Risks.

CHA$_2$DS$_2$-VASc Score	Annual Stroke Risk, (%, per year)
0	0
1	1.3
2	2.2
3	3.2
4	4.0

(Table 8) cont.....

CHA$_2$DS$_2$-VASc Score	Annual Stroke Risk, (%, per year)
5	6.7
6	9.8
7	9.6
8	6.7
9	15.2

Table 9. Treatment recommendations based on the CHA2DS2-VASc score

CHA$_2$DS$_2$-VASc Score	Recommendation
0	No treatment
1	No treatment or aspirin or OAC
>=2	OAC

How is Emergency Anticoagulation Done Before ECV?

If PCV or ECV is planned in a patient with AF that is thought to last longer than 48 hours, one of the following three regimens should be started:

- emergency IV (unfractionated) heparin (target PTT, 60 s).

- or LMWH (in DVT therapeutic dose).

- or VKA/warfarin for at least 5 days (target INR, 2.5).

When no thrombus is seen and ECV/PCV is successful, anticoagulation is continued for another 4 weeks (target INR, 2.5). If thrombus is seen, ECV/PCV is delayed. TEE should be repeated before each ECV attempt.

At the earliest period in a hemodynamically unstable case with an suspected ECV.

- emergency IV (unfractionated) heparin (target PTT, 60 s).

- or LMWH (at DVT therapeutic dose) should be initiated.

After successful cardioversion, VKA/warfarin (target INR, 2.5) is continued for at least 4 weeks. Long-term anticoagulation will depend on the patient's risk status, previous cardioversions or other embolism status. For example, maintenance with rivaroxaban, one of the NOACs, is more suitable for those who have had pulmonary embolism.

The above regimens are also valid in cases with flutter (grade 2C).

The following agents were found to be effective in cases where treatment with OAC was considered:

• Warfarin, (with the target INR in the range of 2 to 3).

• Dabigatran

• Rivaroxaban

• Apixaban

• Edoxaban

I am treating the patient with OAC. Do I cause a bleed in the patient?

Yes, maybe. There is a risk of bleeding. HAS-BLED score is the best tool developed for this. This term acronym consists of the initials of the criteria "Hypertension, Abnormal liver/renal function, Stroke history, Bleeding predisposition, Labile INR, Elderly, Drug/alcohol usage" (Table **10-11**).

Table 10. HAS-BLED score has been devised to evaluate risk of bleeding when the physician prescribes OACs for the patient. The following are the variables to score the patients. The total number of the variables present in a given patient constitutes the HAS-BLED score.

Variable	Score
Hypertension	1
renal failure (dialysis, transplant, creatinine> 2.26 mg/dL or 200 μmol/L)	1
liver diseasae (cirrhosis or bilirubin> 2x normal + AST/ALT/ALP> 3x normal)	1
a history of stroke	1
a previous history of significant bleeding from any area	1
labil INR (unstable/high INR, time within the therapeutic range <60%)	1
age> 65	1
use of drugs such as aspirin, clopidogrel, NSAID that may cause bleeding tendency	1
alcohol use (≥8 times a week)	1

Table 11. HAS-BLED score of the patients and their relation with major bleeding risk, percentage of pts with a bleeding annually and due recommendation for them.

HAS-BLED Score	Risk group	major bleeding risk (%)	Percentage of pts with a bleeding annually	recommendation
0	Low	0.9	1.13	Anticoagulation can be considered
1		3.4	1.02	
2	Moderate	4.1	1.88	Anticoagulation can be considered
3	High	5.8	3.72	Alternatives for anticoagulation can be considered
4		8.9	8.70	
5		9.1	12.50	
>5	Very high	-	-	Think about individualized options

CONCLUSION AND SUMMARY

AF is an important public health problem because it is a common arrhythmia and causes high morbidity. It causes serious consequences through hemodynamic complications and thromboembolic problems such as stroke and acute arterial occlusion. POCUS/Echocardiography is vital in patients with AF because it shows potential thromboembolism at its source and reveals cardiac functions, valve and chamber problems. Safe and effective pharmacological or electrical cardioversion (PCV/ECV) and other contemporary treatments by emergency physicians and cardiologists, especially in cases with acute AF, will directly increase the quality of patient care. Emergency physicians should not look for a template to apply to every case, but should be aware of the characteristics of specific agents for the patient and the situation. In addition, it is more appropriate to conduct management and follow-up from cardiology outpatient clinics in more stable and elective cases.

REFERENCES

Arendts, G., Krishnaraj, M., Paull, G., Rees, D. (2010). Management of atrial fibrillation in the acute setting--findings from an Australasian survey. *Heart Lung Circ., 19*(7), 423-427. [http://dx.doi.org/10.1016/j.hlc.2010.01.009] [PMID: 20362506]

Bellone, A., Etteri, M., Vettorello, M., Bonetti, C., Clerici, D., Gini, G., Maino, C., Mariani, M., Natalizi, A., Nessi, I., Rampoldi, A., Colombo, L. (2012). Cardioversion of acute atrial fibrillation in the emergency department: a prospective randomised trial. *Emerg. Med. J., 29*(3), 188-191. [http://dx.doi.org/10.1136/emj.2010.109702] [PMID: 21422032]

Braun, O.Ö., Bico, B., Chaudhry, U., Wagner, H., Koul, S., Tydén, P., Scherstén, F., Jovinge, S., Svensson, P.J., Gustav Smith, J., van der Pals, J. (2015). Concomitant use of warfarin and ticagrelor as an alternative to triple antithrombotic therapy after an acute coronary syndrome. *Thromb. Res., 135*(1), 26-30. [http://dx.doi.org/10.1016/j.thromres.2014.10.016] [PMID: 25467434]

Buccelletti, F., Gilardi, E., Marsiliani, D., Carroccia, A., Silveri, N.G., Franceschi, F. (2011). Predictive value

of NT-proBNP for cardioversion in a new onset atrial fibrillation. *Eur. J. Emerg. Med., 18*(3), 157-161.
[http://dx.doi.org/10.1097/MEJ.0b013e328342f2bf] [PMID: 21183856]

Conti, A., Del Taglia, B., Mariannini, Y., Pepe, G., Vanni, S., Grifoni, S., Abbate, R., Michelucci, A., Padeletti, L., Gensini, G.F. (2010). Management of patients with acute atrial fibrillation in the ED. *Am. J. Emerg. Med., 28*(8), 903-910.
[http://dx.doi.org/10.1016/j.ajem.2009.05.005] [PMID: 20825922]

Cristoni, L., Tampieri, A., Mucci, F., Iannone, P., Venturi, A., Cavazza, M., Lenzi, T. (2011). Cardioversion of acute atrial fibrillation in the short observation unit: comparison of a protocol focused on electrical cardioversion with simple antiarrhythmic treatment. *Emerg. Med. J., 28*(11), 932-937.
[http://dx.doi.org/10.1136/emj.2009.083196] [PMID: 20947916]

Dankner, R., Shahar, A., Novikov, I., Agmon, U., Ziv, A., Hod, H. (2009). Treatment of stable atrial fibrillation in the emergency department: a population-based comparison of electrical direct-current *versus* pharmacological cardioversion or conservative management. *Cardiology, 112*(4), 270-278.
[http://dx.doi.org/10.1159/000151703] [PMID: 18815445]

Decker, W.W., Stead, L.G. (2011). Selecting rate control for recent-onset atrial fibrillation. *Ann. Emerg. Med., 57*(1), 32-33.
[http://dx.doi.org/10.1016/j.annemergmed.2010.08.041] [PMID: 21183084]

Dewilde, W.J., Oirbans, T., Verheugt, F.W., Kelder, J.C., De Smet, B.J., Herrman, J.P., Adriaenssens, T., Vrolix, M., Heestermans, A.A., Vis, M.M., Tijsen, J.G., van 't Hof, A.W., ten Berg, J.M. WOEST study investigators. (2013). Use of clopidogrel with or without aspirin in patients taking oral anticoagulant therapy and undergoing percutaneous coronary intervention: an open-label, randomised, controlled trial. *Lancet, 381*(9872), 1107-1115.
[http://dx.doi.org/10.1016/S0140-6736(12)62177-1] [PMID: 23415013]

Doğan, A.O., Ergene, C., Nazlı, O. (2003). Yeni Atrial Fibrilasyonda Kendiliğinden Sonlanma Belirleyicileri ve Propafenon ile Uzun Süreli Sinüs Ritminin İdamesi. *Turk Kardiyol. Dern. Ars., 31*, 392-399.

Hirschl, M.M., Wollmann, C., Globits, S. (2011). A 2-year survey of treatment of acute atrial fibrillation in an ED. *Am. J. Emerg. Med., 29*(5), 534-540.
[http://dx.doi.org/10.1016/j.ajem.2009.12.016] [PMID: 20825828]

Kirolos, I., Ifedili, I., Maturana, M., Premji, A.M., Cave, B., Roman, S., Jones, D., Gaid, R., Levine, Y.C., Jha, S., Kabra, R., Khouzam, R.N. (2019). Ticagrelor or prasugrel *vs.* clopidogrel in combination with anticoagulation for treatment of acute coronary syndrome in patients with atrial fibrillation. *Ann. Transl. Med., 7*(17), 406.
[http://dx.doi.org/10.21037/atm.2019.07.41] [PMID: 31660305]

Lamberts, M., Gislason, G.H., Olesen, J.B., Kristensen, S.L., Schjerning Olsen, A.M., Mikkelsen, A., Christensen, C.B., Lip, G.Y., Køber, L., Torp-Pedersen, C., Hansen, M.L. (2013). Oral anticoagulation and antiplatelets in atrial fibrillation patients after myocardial infarction and coronary intervention. *J. Am. Coll. Cardiol., 62*(11), 981-989.
[http://dx.doi.org/10.1016/j.jacc.2013.05.029] [PMID: 23747760]

Milicevic, G., Gavranovic, Z., Bakula, M., Pazur, V., Frank, B. (2008). Successful conversion of recent-onset atrial fibrillation by sequential administration of up to three antiarrhythmic drugs. *Clin. Cardiol., 31*(10), 472-477.
[http://dx.doi.org/10.1002/clc.20268] [PMID: 18855351]

Smith, G.D., Fry, M.M., Taylor, D., Morgans, A., Cantwell, K. (2015). Effectiveness of the Valsalva Manoeuvre for reversion of supraventricular tachycardia. *Cochrane Database Syst. Rev., 2015*(2), CD009502.
[http://dx.doi.org/10.1002/14651858.CD009502.pub3] [PMID: 25922864]

Stiell, I.G., Clement, C.M., Brison, R.J., Rowe, B.H., Borgundvaag, B., Langhan, T., Lang, E., Magee, K., Stenstrom, R., Perry, J.J., Birnie, D., Wells, G.A. (2011). Variation in management of recent-onset atrial fibrillation and flutter among academic hospital emergency departments. *Ann. Emerg. Med., 57*(1), 13-21.

[http://dx.doi.org/10.1016/j.annemergmed.2010.07.005] [PMID: 20864213]

Stiell, I.G., Clement, C.M., Perry, J.J., Vaillancourt, C., Symington, C., Dickinson, G., Birnie, D., Green, M.S. (2010). Association of the Ottawa Aggressive Protocol with rapid discharge of emergency department patients with recent-onset atrial fibrillation or flutter. *CJEM, 12*(3), 181-191.
[http://dx.doi.org/10.1017/S1481803500012227] [PMID: 20522282]

Xavier Scheuermeyer, F., Grafstein, E., Stenstrom, R., Innes, G., Poureslami, I., Sighary, M. (2010). Thirty-day outcomes of emergency department patients undergoing electrical cardioversion for atrial fibrillation or flutter. *Acad. Emerg. Med., 17*(4), 408-415.
[http://dx.doi.org/10.1111/j.1553-2712.2010.00697.x] [PMID: 20370780]

CHAPTER 10

Agents Used in the Treatment of Arrhythmias and Advanced Cardiovascular Life Support

Abstract: Advanced Cardiovascular Life Support (ACLS) guidelines recommend certain drugs for hemodynamic stabilization, prevention of collapse, stabilization of a perfusing rhythm, improving peripheral resistance and cardiac output, and restoration of organ perfusion. It is known that no antiarrhythmic agent increases the percentage of patients discharged with good neurological status. For this reason, the commencement of medications and establishing vascular access should not delay high-quality CPR.

ACLS guidelines recommend drug adrenaline in the asystole algorithm and in those with cardiac arrest due to ventricular fibrillation (VF). For pulseless electrical activity (PEA)-related cardiac arrest, adrenaline and, in some cases, sodium bicarbonate is recommended. The drugs used in VF and pulseless VT (PVT) apart from adrenaline are vasopressin, amiodarone, lidocaine, esmolol, magnesium, and procainamide in selected situations. This chapter provides a brief outline of arrhythmias commonly encountered in routine clinical practice, together with principles of ACLS and indications and usage of resuscitative agents employed in these situations.

Keywords: Adrenaline, Advanced Cardiovascular Life Support, Amiodarone, Antiarrhythmics, CPR, Lidocaine, Sodium bicarbonate, Ventricular fibrillation.

INTRODUCTION

According to the ACLS guideline, the recommended drug in the asystole algorithm is adrenaline. For pulseless electrical activity (PEA)-related cardiac arrest (CA), adrenaline and, in some cases, sodium bicarbonate are recommended. The drugs used in ventricular fibrillation (VF) and pulseless VT (PVT) are adrenaline and/or vasopressin, amiodarone, lidocaine, esmolol, magnesium, and procainamide in certain situations.

DRUGS IN ACLS CAN BE EXAMINED UNDER TWO SUBHEADINGS

1. Those used for ACLS at the moment of CA manifested with VF/PVT, Adrenaline, lidocaine, and amiodarone are in this group. ACLS providers should bear in mind that it is unlikely that a perfused rhythm can be instituted merely by drug administration without a high-quality CPR.

Ozgur KARCIOGLU

2. Those used in post-arrest management (that is after ROSC is achieved): Beta-blockers (esmolol) and lidocaine infusion can be used in this context. Evaluation should be made case by case basis. These agents are not recommended routinely for every post-arrest patient. *(Class IIb, LOE C-LD).*

Amiodarone OR Lidocaine may be considered in the treatment of persistent VF and PVT where defibrillation fails to convert to a perfusing rhythm. These drugs are particularly effective when the duration of administration is short, for example, in witnessed arrests due to VF/PVT (Class IIb, Level B-R).

In adult CA, routine use of magnesium is not recommended. (Class III: No Benefit, LOE C-LD). Magnesium is recommended for Torsades de pointes (polymorphic VT accompanying the long QT interval) (Class IIb, LOE C-LD).

Inotropic Support: 70% of CA cases show myocardial dysfunction after ROSC is achieved. Therefore, positive inotropic support should be given in patients with hypotensive patients despite adequate fluid therapy (Marcolini, 2017).

EXTRACORPOREAL CPR (ECPR)

ECPR is bypassing the patient's physiological cardiopulmonary system and providing extracorporeal circulation and oxygenation. For this, cannulation of a large artery and vein and venoarterial extracorporeal circulation and oxygenation are required. The purpose of ECPR is to provide vital organ perfusion if the underlying conditions are deemed reversible.

ECPR is a complex intervention that requires a well-trained and organized team, specialized equipment, and multidisciplinary support within the healthcare system. So far, there are no randomized controlled trials (RCT) that investigate the effects of the use of ECPR for in-hospital or OHCA. Some observational studies have shown that ECPR when used for selected patient groups, increases survival with good neurological outcomes.

Should ECPR be performed? According to the 2019 updates:

1. There is currently insufficient evidence to recommend ECPR in the routine management of CA.

2. ECPR may be a rescue therapy for selected patients when the traditional CPR fails if it can be performed immediately by the specially trained healthcare provider (Class 2B, Level of Evidence C-LD).

END-TIDAL CO$_2$ (ETCO$_2$) MONITORING

ETCO$_2$ value is the partial pressure of the CO$_2$ exhaled at the end of expiration. CO$_2$ production is directly affected by alveolar ventilation and pulmonary blood flow.

In meta-analyses and other studies which recent guidelines are based on, it has been reported that ETCO$_2$ monitoring can predict the clinical course after CA. It is best viewed by waveform capnography. The capnograph curve shows the partial ETCO$_2$ pressure (PETCO$_2$) exhaled after intubation in the vertical axis in mmHg. After the patient is intubated, a significant amount of CO$_2$ exhaled through the tube is detected, confirming the correct placement of the tracheal tube. The value of the PETCO$_2$ varies through the respiration, the highest point being at the end of expiration.

In the study we conducted in 1997 in patients with nontraumatic CA, we demonstrated that the ETCO$_2$ value at the time of arrest can be an important tool in predicting the survival of CA cases (Karcioglu, 2000).

Apart from ineffective CPR, low ETCO$_2$ values may also result from bronchospasm, trachea, bronchial or tubular obstruction, air leakage in the ventilation circuit, pulmonary edema, and hyperventilation. ETCO$_2$ measurement gives incorrect values in patients in whom supraglottic airway device is inserted, or BVM is attempted. There are not enough studies on this situation, and ETCO$_2$ should not be solely used as a guide (Class III: Harm, LOE C-EO).

ETCO$_2$ levels below 10 mmHg after intubation means there is insufficient CPR or ventilation. If the patient still has a low value after 20 minutes of CPR, the patient's poor clinical course (death) is almost certain (Class IIb, LOE C-LD). On the other hand, initial values above 20 mmHg predict a good clinical course (Ahrens 2001).

ETCO$_2$ may not provide reliable information if the factors above are not excluded. Therefore, caution should be exercised and not interpreted alone (Class IIb, LOE C-LD).

How are the Drugs Given?

The essential route of drug administration within the context of ACLS is IV administration. IO route is the first option when IV administration is not secured in 3 consecutive trials or 90 seconds. Different approaches are also recommended in the literature. If IV or IO administration is not possible, some drugs can be administered *via* the endotracheal tube (ETT) (Table 1). In this application, the drugs are given at a dose of 2-2.5 times and diluted with NS to 10 mL. Then, the lungs are ventilated with bag-valve-mask (BVM) and the agents pass from the alveolocapillary membrane to the capillaries of the bloodstream.

Table 1. Drugs that can be given *via* ETT (NAVEL).

Naloxone
Atropin
Valium (diazepam)
Epinephrine
Lidocaine

In IV administration from the arm or leg, the limb should be elevated as much as possible and sustained there. If this is impossible, then the IV route can be flushed with 20 mL of IV saline. Otherwise the agent will stuck in the peripheral vein and would not reach at the central circulation.

Vasopressor Use in Cardiac Arrest

The ILCOR working group conveyed the following evaluations for vasopressors in the 2019 update.

Standard Dose Epinephrine

Epinephrine is thought to have beneficial effects in the case of CA due to its α-adrenergic effects. With these effects, administration of epinephrine in CPR may increase perfusion pressure in the brain and coronary arteries.

Recommendation

- Epinephrine administration is recommended in case of CA. (Class I, LOE B-R).
- In the light of the protocols used in clinical studies, it is appropriate to administer 1 mg every 3 to 5 minutes (Class IIA; LOE C-LD).

The use of epinephrine in patients with CA is associated with a significant positive difference in 30-day survival and survival at discharge and return of spontaneous circulation (ROSC).

It has not been clearly shown that epinephrine increases survival with a favorable neurological outcome. It has been observed that there is a possible benefit for those who have asystole or PEA as the first detected rhythm.

"High-dose epinephrine" are doses in the range of 0.1-0.2 mg/kg.

Recommendation

• Routine use of high-dose epinephrine is not recommended in the case of CA (Class 3, Level of Evidence B-R).

The undesirable effects of high-dose epinephrine such as tachycardia and increased intracranial pressure in the period following ROSC surpasses its advantages during CA.

Vasopressin - Epinephrine Vasopressin is a non-adrenergic peripheral vasoconstrictor that also causes coronary and renal vasoconstriction (shows its effect *via* V1 receptors in the smooth muscle).

Recommendation

Vasopressin can be considered in the case of CA, but it is not advantageous against epinephrine. (Class 2b; Level of Evidence C-LD)

Epinephrine with Vasopressin or Epinephrine Only?

Epinephrine + Vasopressin can be considered in patients with CA, but it does not provide any advantage against epinephrine. (Class 2B, Level of Evidence C-LD), when to Administer Epinephrine. There is no randomized controlled study specifically investigating the optimal time of epinephrine administration.

In non-shockable rhythms, epinephrine should be administered as soon as possible in addition to high quality CPR. Epinephrine use and appropriate timing may differ when a reversible cause of non-shock arrest is immediately identified and addressed.

In terms of timing, it is acceptable to administer epinephrine as soon as possible in non-shockable rhythm cardiac arrests (Class 2A, Level of Evidence C-LD). In terms of timing in CA with shockable rhythm, it is acceptable to administer epinephrine after the first defibrillation attempt has failed (Class 2B; Level of Evidence C-LD).

Action potential (AP) cycle of antiarrhythmics and their effects were demonstrated in Fig. (**1**). The "Class" of an antiarrhythmics delineate its main paharmacological properties, effects and side effects, thus categorizations should be taken into account.

Class 1a agents   Class 1b agents   Class 1c agents

Class I a. Prolongs AP

Class I b. Shortens AP

Class I c. No impact on AP

Class II agents   Class III agents   Class IV agents

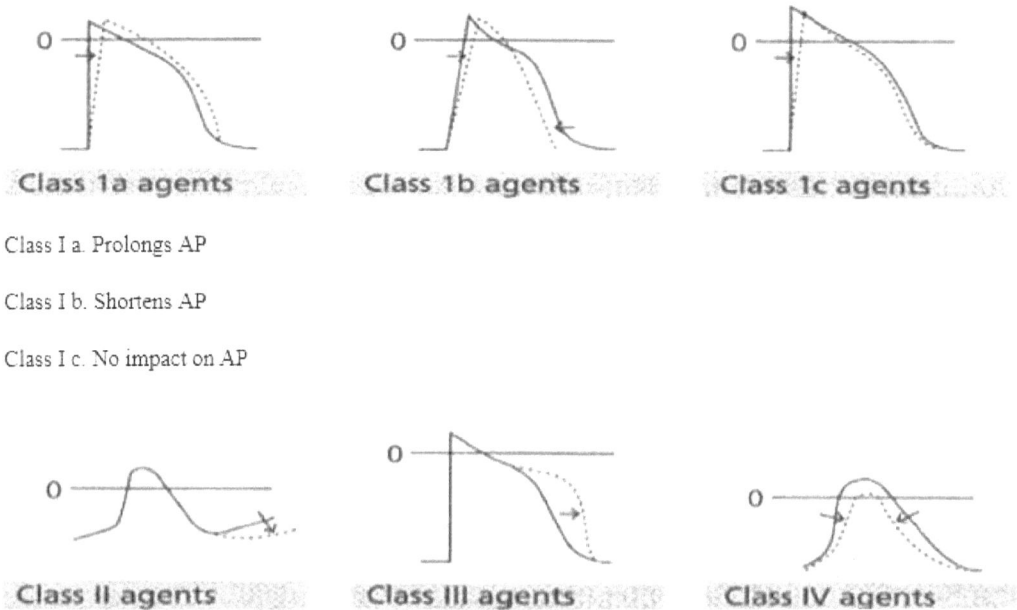

Fig. (1). Action potential (AP) cycle of antiarrhythmics and their schematized effects on SA-AV nodes in accord with Vaughan Williams classification (summary).

Class II (Beta-blockers). It is primarily effective on SAN.

Class III. Prolongs AP.

Class IV (Calcium channel blockers). It is primarily effective on AVN.

Characteristics of some ACLS drugs.

I. Adrenaline (The Chief of the Resuscitation)

Mechanism of Action

It is an endogenous catecholamine from the class of adrenergic amines that has alpha (α) and beta (β) adrenergic agonistic activity. Its primary indications are anaphylactic shock and CA. It is also used in the treatment of hemodynamic instability due to overdoses of various drugs (beta-blockers, calcium antagonists and other cardiac depressants). Its beneficial effects in CA are mostly related to its α-adrenergic effect and thus it has the advantage of increasing myocardial and cerebral blood flow. It also increases peripheral resistance and restores coronary artery perfusion pressure. The β-adrenergic effects of adrenaline lead to an increase in heart rate, contractility and conduction velocity. It accelerates the AV nodal conduction and decreases the refractory period in the myocyte membrane.

Adrenaline increases systemic vascular resistance, systolic and diastolic blood pressure, electrical activity in myocardium, coronary and cerebral blood flow, myocardial contractions, myocardial O2 requirement and automaticity (Table **2**).

Table 2. Adrenaline indications and levels of evidence, according to the 2019 update.

1- **Adrenaline is indicated in CA.** (Class 1; LOE B-R).
2- **Adrenaline is indicated 1 mg every 3-5 minutes in CA.** (Class 2a; LOE C-LD).
3- **High-dose adrenaline** (0.1-0.2 mg/kg) is not recommended routinely in CA. (Class 3; LOE B-R).
4- **Timing:** it should be administered as soon as possible in CA. (Class 2b; LOE C-LD).
5- **Timing:** it should be administered following defibrillation attempt fails in CA with a shockable rhythm (Class 2b; LOE C-LD).
6- **In case of CA,** vasopressine administration may be considered, but it has no advantage against epinephrine (Class 2b; LOE C-LD). The same holds true for a comparison of epinephrine against epi + VP administration.
7- **In symptomatic bradycardia:** Signs of instability (altered mental status, heart failure, hypotension, shock) atropine is the 1st choice (Class IIa, LOE B). If unresponsive to atropine, aminergic agents such as dopamine or adrenaline are administered, transcutaneous pacing is prepared (Class IIa, LOE B).
8- **In severe hypotension:** It can be a rescue therapy *via* its adrenergic effects, however, be cautious for it can be malicious with increased O2 demand of the myocardium in the presence of ACS.
9- **Anaphylaxis and severe allergic reactions:** It is the primary therapeutic option, combined with fluid replacement, O2 supplement, corticosteroids and antihistaminics.

It was revealed that there was significantly more ROSC (25% *versus* 40%) in patients who were treated with adrenaline infusion compared to the others, but there was no difference in 1-year survival rates. In post-hoc analysis, the negative relationship between adrenaline use and neurological outcome was reported (Olasveengen 2009 and 2012).

In recent RCT and meta-analyzes, it has been determined that adrenaline increases ROSC in patients with CA but does not improve neurological outcomes. In non-shockable rhythms, the increase in the 3-month favorable neurological outcome rate with the use of adrenaline approaches the statistical significance (PARAMEDIC 2 study, 2018).

Finally, AHA ACLS updates were published by Panchal *et al.* in 2019 (Circulation.2019; 140: 00--00. DOI: 10.1161/CIR.0000000000000732). In this document, the administration of epinephrine in CA is recommended as Class 1, LOE B-R. Its use every 3-5 minutes is at Class 2a, LOE-LD level. High-dose epinephrine administration is not recommended because it is Class III, LOE-B-R.

Route of administration: IV/IO is recommended. IM use has priority in anaphylaxis. Intracardiac or SC use is not recommended.

In adult VF and PVT, 1 mg adrenaline is administered every 3-5 minutes *via* IV/IO route, (Class 2a, LOE-LD).

Many studies on the use of adrenaline in resuscitation have highlighted that there is no clear effect on survival to discharge from hospital (Table 3). Sanghavi *et al.* reported in 2015 that patients who received no ACLS drugs including adrenaline had better survival (Sanghavi 2015).

Table 3. Effect of the use of adrenaline in resuscitation: Adjusted OR values change as a function of timing of administration and the dosages. In accord with the CA phases, the favorable effect of adrenaline was observed on the survival in the first 9 minutes, whereas the effect approached to zero as longer time passed.

Treatment	Adjusted OR (95% CI)
Time to epinephrine dose	
< 9 min	0.54 (0.32–0.91)
10–15 min	0.33 (0.20–0.56)
16–22 min	0.23 (0.12–0.43)
> 22 min	0.17 (0.09–0.34)
Total epinephrine dose	
1 mg	0.48 (0.27–0.84)
2-5 mg	0.30 (0.20–0.47)
> 5 mg	0.23 (0.14–0.37)

OR = odds ratio; CI = confidence interval.

Dosage: The standard dose of adrenaline is 1 mg in adults, regardless of weight. It is known that the survival rate in asystole and PEA is low with or without the use of adrenaline.

It is recommended to administer 1 mg in shock-resistant VF. Because high dose adrenaline produces β-adrenergic effect, it is likely to be harmful (Class III). In patients with VF/PVT, high doses of adrenaline may increase the rate of ROSC, especially in the first minutes after CA. However, it is not recommended after resuscitation, as it does not improve long-term rate of survival and neurological outcomes. Adrenaline infusion may be helpful in institution of vasopressor response in patients with cardiogenic shock and resistant collapse who have not developed CA (prearrest situations). Initially, a dose of 2 to 10 mcg/min should be commenced and titrated according to the desired hemodynamic response.

Attention! It should not be mixed in the same bag or vial with alkaline solutions and drugs such as sodium bicarbonate. Adrenaline can trigger myocardial ischemia. It may cause hypokalemia, hypophosphatemia, hyperglycemia and leukocytosis due to its β-adrenergic effects. It triggers or exacerbates ventricular ectopic rhythms in patients using digital.

II. ESMOLOL (The Emerging Star)

In emergency conditions, it is one of the most commonly used drugs as the rapid-onset Beta-1 selective agent. The elimination half-life is 9 minutes. The commercial preparation contains 10 mg/mL esmolol HCl.

Esmolol infusion is recommended after the 3rd defibrillation, 3 mg Epinephrine and 300 mg amiodarone in resistant VF patients with CA.

In these conditions, IV Esmolol 500 mcg/kg loading dose has been reported to cause an increase in ROSC. It is continued with 50 mcg/kg/min infusion and titrated in accord with the effect in the patient. Although this is often sufficient, doses up to 200 mcg/kg/min can be climbed at.

It can be increased up to 300 mcg/kg/min in the management of emergency hypertension.

It is also indicated in SVT and resistant sinus tachycardia (when noncardiac causes are ruled out). It is also used in emergency rate control of atrial fibrillation or flutter.

It is also indicated in the treatment of periintubation temporary tachycardia/hypertension. However, prophylactic administration is not recommended.

New findings on efficacy: A recent meta-analysis was conducted by Miraglia *et al.* to assess the effectiveness of esmolol on pre-hospital refractory VF/pVT, compared with standard of care (Miraglia, 2020). Only two studies comprising 66 patients were eligible for the analysis. They have cited that although the evidence is inconclusive, esmolol was likely associated with an increased rate of survival to discharge.

Esmolol can be given with dextrose or isotonic serum. Side effects may occur in varying proportions. Hypotension without clinical significance is noted in up to 25%, symptomatic hypotension in 12%. Nausea, light-headedness, drowsiness can be noted in 3 to 7%.

Precautions and attention points:

- Simultaneous use with calcium channel blockers may lead to CA in case of depressed myocardial functions.
- It should be used after excluding hypovolemia.
- It is not used in decompensated-severe heart failure and patients wit bronchosm (asthma).
- Caution should be exercised in case of Prinzmetal's angina and diabetes. Precautions should also be taken against the development of hyperkalaemia.
- Untoward effects such as hypotension and bradycardia end in minutes upon discontinuation of the drug and fluid replacement.

III. LIDOCAINE

Lidocaine is a sodium channel blocker, local anesthetic and Class Ib antiarrhythmic agent according to Vaughan Williams antiarrhythmic classification. It is used to control ventricular tachyarrhythmias. It is also used in ventricular arrhythmias due to intoxications of digoxin, cyclic antidepressants, stimulants and theophylline. Lidocaine is not effective against atrial arrhythmias, SVT and should not be used in these entities. It is never used in bradyarrhythmias (*e.g.* idioventricular rhythm, reperfusion arrhythmias), even if they are ventricular.

Its main pharmacological effects are as follows: suppressing ventricular arrhythmias by decreasing automaticity, reducing ventricular ectopias by slowing phase 0 action potential in myocytes during post-AMI period. First, it depresses phase 4 (automaticity). It ends reentry ventricular arrhythmias. It prolongs the refractory period in ischemic tissue. Suppresses ventricular ectopia in myocardial tissue in acute coronary ischemia.

Indications, Dosage And Administration

1. Shock-resistant VF/PVT: Its use has been recommended as Class IIa, together with amiodarone in CA due to refractory VF/VT.	1 to 1.5 mg/kg given in 2 to 3 min (slow IV bolus).
2. In hemodynamically stable monomorphic VT: Using Lidocaine is Class IIb.	1 to 1.5 mg/kg; repeat dose of 0.5 to 0.75 mg/kg in 5-10 min; max. total 3 mg/kg; 1 to 4 mg/dak infusion if necessary
3. It can be used to treat ventricular arrhythmias in acute AMI and during cardiac surgery at the specified doses.	

Dose: In CA due to VF/VT; the initial dose is 1 to 1.5 mg/kg IV. In refractory VF, an additional dose of 0.5-0.75 mg/kg IV push can be given, it can be repeated in 5-10 minutes, up to the maximum total dose at 3 mg/kg. In tracheal administration, it should be diluted into 10 mL normal saline (NS), given at a dose of 2 to 4 mg/kg and insufflated with BVM.

In patients with reperfusion arrhythmia after AMI: In stable VT, wide complex tachycardia of unknown type or severe ectopia; 1 to 1.5 mg/kg IV push is given. 0.5 to 0.75 mg/kg IV push in 5-10 minutes can be administered, up to a total of 3 mg/kg.

Infusion: It can be titrated at a dose of 1 to 4 mg/min (30-50 µg/kg/min) in regard to clinical requirement and plasma lidocaine concentration.

Attention! The use of "prophylactic lidocaine" is not recommended in AMI. Caution should be exercised in hypotensive patients due to cardiac depressant effects of the agent. The maintenance dose should be reduced if the patient has liver failure or left ventricular dysfunction.

AMIODARONE

Mechanism of Action

It is a Class III antiarrhythmic. It is a noncompetitive blocker of α and β receptors and also a negative inotropic agent. It suppresses automaticity in sinoatrial and AV nodes while inhibiting potassium channels and influx of the ion. Most important effect of the agent is prolongation of the action potential duration and ventricular effective refractory period in all cardiovascular tissues. It is used in the treatment of atrial and ventricular arrhythmias in patients with cardiac structural abnormalities and ventricular dysfunction. The incidence of proarrhythmic effects is low in these patients. Amiodarone is shown as the antiarrhythmic agent of choice in VF/PVT together with lidocaine in 2019 guidelines (Class IIa).

Antiarrhythmic drugs have not been shown to improve survival to hospital discharge, regardless of defibrillation. The effects of antiarrhythmic drugs have been shown only for short-term results (such as ROSC ratio). IV amiodarone can be recommended as Class IIa for the treatment of persistent or recurrent VF/PVT. The drug is administered after three or more shocks and an adrenergic agent (adrenaline) which fail to convert the rhythm to a perfusing one. Although amiodarone increased the rate of hospitalization (early survival) in VF-related CA patients, it was not found to be superior to lidocaine and placebo in healthy discharge from the hospital.

In a meta-analysis comparing the efficacy of amiodarone and nifekalant in the treatment of shock-resistant VF and PVT, the results of 33 studies were pooled and evaluated (Sato S, *et al.*, 2017). Nifekalant has also been shown to be comparably effective in improving survival and preventing major cardiac events in the short and long term.

Indications

1. Refractory/Recurrent VF/ PVT: Its use is IIa following third shock, adrenaline and 4th shock, in patients with **refractory/recurrent VF/ PVT**.
2. In atrial fibrillation (AF) and atrial flutter: Its use is Class IIa in the conversion of AF and atrial flutter rhythm in patients with normal cardiac function with an arrhythmia duration shorter than 48 hours.   It is Class IIb for use in both rate and rhythm control in patients with shorter than 48 hours of arrhythmia or in patients with impaired ventricular function (for example, in patients with a history of congestive heart failure or with an ejection fraction below 40%). Emergency electrical cardioversion is appropriate in these patients.
3. Stable narrow complex tachycardias: In the paroxysmal supraventricular tachycardia (PSVT) developed by reentry mechanism, amiodarone can be used if the arrhythmia continues despite adenosine administration, vagal maneuvers and AV node blockade. Its use is Class IIa in those with normal ventricular function, and Class IIb in those with impaired ventricular function. Its use in narrow complex tachycardias (such as junctional tachycardia, ectopic or multifocal atrial tachycardia) developed by the automaticity mechanism in those with normal or impaired ventricular function is Class IIb.
4. Stable monomorphic VT: It is used in stable monomorphic VT whether ventricular function is normal or impaired (Class IIb). Procainamide or sotalol should be preferred in patients with normal ventricular function (Class IIa). Its use in patients with polymorphic VT with a normal basal QT interval is Class IIb, regardless of cardiac function.

Dose: In VF/PVT, the dose is 300 mg IV infusion (diluted with 20-30 mL of 5% dextrose). In recurrent or refractory VF/PVT, 150 mg additional dose can be given in 3-5 minutes. Then 1 mg/min for 6 hours and 0.5 mg/min for 18 hours can be ordered. The maximum total dose is 2.2 g in 24 hours.

Wide complex tachycardias (VT with a pulse), stable AF and atrial flutter; 150 mg IV is given over 10 minutes (15 mg/minute). Then, infusion is started from 1 mg/minute for 6 hours. After that, a maintenance infusion is started at 0.5 mg/min for 18 hours. If necessary, in case of recurrent or refractory arrhythmia, 150 mg IV rapid infusion can be repeated every 10 minutes.

4. Attention! The most important adverse effects are hypotension and bradycardia. It may lead to pulmonary fibrosis in the long term. It is not used with other drugs with similar adverse effects, as it prolongs the QT interval. Concomitant use with Vaughan-Williams Class I agents may cause torsades de pointes (polymorphic ventricular tachycardia).

5. Attention! Amiodarone infusion should be administered with 5% dextrose solution. In infusions of longer than 2 hours, plastic bags (mediflex) can adhere the amiodarone compound. For this reason, glass bottles should be preferred.

Dilution with dextrose is not mandatory under arrest conditions.

MAGNESIUM

Mechanism of Action

Magnesium is an enzymatic cofactor that takes part in biochemical pathways. It is also a cation that directly affects the sodium-potassium ATPase pump in the cardiac and nervous tissues. Magnesium deficiency usually occurs in patients who are on diuretics, have chronic diseases, and have chronic alcoholism or malnutrition. On the other hand, severe magnesium deficiency can cause cardiac arrhythmias such as refractory VF, heart failure and sudden cardiac arrest 3. Magnesium is not routinely used in in-hospital cardiac arrest (IHCA). When used routinely, it has been noted that it does not increase the 24-hour survival and successful resuscitation rates for hospital discharge from the hospital.

Indications

1- Magnesium is used in stable polymorphic VT with baseline prolonged QT interval (Class IIb).
2- It is also used in refractory or recurrent VF/PVT due to a known hypomagnesemic condition (Class IIb).
3- Routine prophylactic use in AMI is controversial. Although some studies indicate that it reduces mortality from arrhythmia and heart failure, larger randomized studies fails to prove that it reduces mortality.

Dose

- In refractory or recurrent VF/PVT, which develops depending on the known hypomagnesemic condition, 1 to 2 grams are diluted with 10 mL of 5% dextrose and given in 1 to 2 minutes.

- 1 to 2 grams is given IV in polymorphic VT with basal prolonged QT interval (torsades de pointes) in 5 to 60 minutes with 50 to 100 mL 5% dextrose. Then 0.5 to 1 g/hour can be titrated.

- In AMI due to hypomagnesemia, the loading dose is given by IV in 1 to 2 grams, 50 to 100 mL 5% dextrose in 5 to 60 minutes. Then 0.5 to 1 gr/hour infusion can be administered up to 24 hours.

CONSIDERATIONS

It is not recommended for routine use in CA, it is recommended only in case of arrhythmia or torsades de pointes due to magnesium deficiency. If infused rapidly, it will cause a reduction in blood pressure. It should be used with caution in patients with kidney failure and is contraindicated in heart blocks and bradycardia.

SODIUM BICARBONATE

Mechanism of Action

The use of $NaHCO_3$ under ACLS is only appropriate in certain situations. In the past, it that routine administration of sodium bicarbonate was recommended during closed cardiac compressions, considering that it would buffer hydrogen ions (acidemia) produced during metabolism in arrest situation. Sodium bicarbonate itself contains a high concentration of CO_2 (260 to 280 mmHg). CO_2 released in plasma causes a paradoxical increase in intracellular CO_2 and a decrease in intracellular pH. Intracellular CO_2 elevation in the heart muscle cells lowers cardiac contractility, cardiac output and blood pressure. Sodium bicarbonate causes a shift to the left in the oxygen-hemoglobin curve. It inhibits the release of oxygen.

Indications

1- It is used in patients with asystole developing due to known hyperkalemia (Class I).
2- It is used in overdoses of tricyclic antidepressants, salicylates, chlorpropamide, herbicides, phenobarbital *etc.* and in patients with known acidosis that responds to bicarbonate (Class IIa).
3- Administration of $NaHCO_3$ after intubation may be beneficial in patients with a long arrest interval before intubation (Class IIb). Its use in long-term arrest is also Class IIb.
4- Administration of $NaHCO_3$ to non-intubated patients with hypercarbic acidosis can be both ineffective and harmful (Class III). Its use in hypoxic lactic acidosis is also stated as Class III.

Dose

The treatment dose is 1 to 2 mEq/kg IV bolus depending on the condition of the patient. It reverses cardiac effects such as widened QRS and hypotension when used as an antidote in tricyclic antidepressant poisoning.

Notes

Unnecessary use of $NaHCO_3$ can cause metabolic alkalosis, hypernatremia and hyperosmolarity. It is dangerous due to excessive sodium overload in case of HF and hypertension.

ATROPIN SULPHATE

Mechanism of Action

It is an agent that exerts an anticholinergic effect in the heart and augment atrioventricular (AV) conduction and sinus node automaticity *via* direct vagolytic effect. It is used in the treatment of symptomatic bradycardia due to an increase in parasympathetic tonus. It is also used in the treatment of cholinergic overdoses such as organophosphate and carbamate poisoning and Clitocybe and Inocybe mushroom poisoning.

Increased parasympathetic tone in the damaged myocardium is dangerous as it will precipitate conduction disturbances or asystole. Atropine may convert the rhythm to normal AV nodal conduction in patients with grade I AV block or Mobitz (second-degree) Type I AV block. Atropine is not required unless there are signs of bradycardia, hemodynamics, ischemia and ventricular ectopia. According to the bradycardia algorithm, atropine is recommended in absolute (heart rate below 60 bpm) and relative bradycardia (depending on the underlying physiological condition).

It should not be used in PEA and asystole as there is insufficient data in the case of non-shockable CA. Although there are conflicting data in the literature, it has no routine indication for use in patients with CA (Dumot 2001, van Walraven 1998). (Class IIb, LOE B).

Indications

1- Its use in symptomatic sinus bradycardia is Class I recommendation (0.5 mg IV), and it is the first drug to be used in preparation for TCP.
2- It is used in high-degree nodal AV blocks (Class IIa). It is recommended against bradycardia with severe symptoms and signs. Atropine is often given in infranodal (type II) AV block or 3rd degree AV block with acutely developed wide QRS. But in the absence of increased parasympathetic tone, these are rarely effective in arrhythmias.
3- It is not routinely used in asystole and PEA-related CA. (Class IIb, LOE B).

Dose

0.5 to 1 mg IV is repeated every 3-5 minutes in patients with bradycardia AND clinical signs and symptoms related to low cardiac output. The total dose should not exceed 0.04 mg/kg within around 8 hours.

If the vascular access cannot be found, 2 to 3 mg of atropine can be diluted with 10 mL of normal saline and administered *via* an intraosseous line or endotracheal tube.

CONSIDERATIONS

Since atropine increases the demand for myocardial oxygen (O_2), caution should be exercised in myocardial ischemia, hypoxia and hypothermic patients. It should not be used especially in patients with infranodal Mobitz type II AV block and in third degree blocks with a wide QRS complex. Paradoxical bradycardia may also develop when giving atropine at a dose lower than 0.5 mg. If the His-Purkinje system is abnormal, atropine can increase the degree of AV block. Repeated doses of atropine should be avoided in patients with ischemic heart disease.

Incorrectly high amounts of atropine can cause anticholinergic toxidrome characterized by delirium, tachycardia, coma, flushing, hot skin, ataxia, and blurred vision.

Other drugs in VF/PVT: bretylium, nifekalant, or sotalol: ALS Task Force has too few evidence to conclude to recommend the use of bretylium, nifekalant, or sotalol in case of resistant VF/PVT (Panchal, 2018) (Table **4**).

Table 4. Grouping and characteristics of cardiac electrophysiological active agents after updates in accord with the Vaughan Williams classification.

Class	Molecular Mechanisms of Action	Clinical Indication - Notes
0	Cyclic nucleotide-dependent canal blockers activated *via* hyperpolarization	-
Ivabradin	I f, I Kr antagonism and slowed AV conduction, reduction in SAN automaticity	stable angina and chronic HF with heart rate ≥70/min; A potential new treatment in some tachyarrhythmias
I	Voltage- dependent Na+ canal blockers	-
Quinidine (Ia)	I to, I Kr, I Ks, I K1, I KATP, I Ca, Class Ia antagonism; autonomic α-adrenergic , and cholinergic blockade.	Supraventricular tachyarrhythmias, especially recurrent AF; VT, VF (including SQTS and Brugada syndrome).
Dysopiramide (Ia)	Class Ia antagonism and I to, I Kr, I K1, I KATP, and cholinergic antagonism; (negative inotropic without α- and/or β adrenergic effects).	
Procainamide	Class Ia antagonism and I Kr, I K1, I KATP antagonism plus autonomic ganglion blockade.	-

(Table 4) cont.....

Lidocaine and Mexiletine (Ib)	No I K effect; Diminihes ectopic ventricular automaticity Reduces DAD-induced activity and converts unidirectional block to bidirectional block and reduces reentrant arrhythmia tendency especially in ischemic, partially depolarized myocardium.	especially post-AMI VT and VF
Flecainide and Propafenone (Ic)	Class Ic antagonism and I Kur, I Kr, I Ca and ryanodin receptor 2 (RyR2) antagonism Diminishes ectopic ventricular/atrial automaticity Reduces DAD-induced activity Converts unidirectional block to bidirectional block and reduces reentrant arrhythmia tendency Alleviates excitability and slows conduction especially in case of tachycardias blocking reentrant pathways	Supraventricular tachyarrhythmias (atrial tachycardias, AFlu, AF, and tachycardias with accessory pathways) ventricular tachyarrhythmias (ventricular premature contractions, catecholaminergic polymorphic VT) resistant to other treatments in the absence of structural heart disease
Encainide	Class Ic, I Kur and I Kr antagonism	-
Ranolazine (Id)	Class Ic, I Kr antagonism Shortens AP recovery duration Reduces EAD-induced triggered activity	Potential new class agents in the management of stable angina, VT; tachyarrhythmias
II	Autonomic inhibitör and activators	-

(Table 4) cont.....

Carteolol (IIa)	Artmış nitrik oksid üretimi; Class IIa antagonism	Sinus tachycardia or supraventricular arrhythmias (AF, AFlu, atrial tachycardia), Rate control in AF and ventricular tachyarrhythmias (VT, ventricular premature contractions) Note: atenolol, propranolol, and nadolol are also used in LQTS; nadolol is used in catecholaminergic polymorphic VT. Reduces SAN automaticity Reduces AVN automaticity Alleviates ectopic ventricular/atrial automaticity Reduces EAD-/DAD-induced triggered activity Diminishes SAN reentry Slows AVN conduction Stops reentries
Carvedilol (IIa)	Probable antioxidant activity; Class IIa antagonism and I CaL, ryanodin receptor 2 (RyR2)-Ca^{2+} canal, and α1 - adrenergic antagonism	
Propranolol (IIa)	Class IIa and I Na antagonism	
Betaxolol (IIa)	Class IIb and I CaL antagonism	
Celiprolol (IIa)	Augmented production of nitric oxide, Class IIb antagonism and partial β2 - adrenergic agonist, and weak α2 - adrenergic antagonist effects	
Nebivolol (IIa)	Class IIb antagonism and augmented production of nitric oxide	
Esmolol (IIa)	Increased adenylyl kinase activity and [cAMP]i; inhibition of adrenergic-induced Gs protein-mediated efficacy Reduced *I*f and *I*ca resulting in slowed rate of SAN pacemaker;	
Metoprolol (IIa)	Reduced ICaL resulting in prolonged AVN conduction duration, and reduced activity triggered by SAN pacing. Reduced RyR2-mediated SR Ca^{2+} release and triggered activity; Prolongation of RR and PR intervals	
Isoproterenol (IIb) Nonselective β-adrenergic receptor activators	Increased adenylyl kinase activity and [cAMP]I resulting in activation of adrenergic-induced Gs-protein effects; Shortening of RR and PR intervals	To increase the rate of ventricular escape rhythm in complete AV block prior to insertion of definitive pacemaker Acquired, commonly drug-related bradycardia-dependent torsades de pointes
Muscarinic M2 receptor inhibitors (IIc): Atropine, anisodamin, hyoscine, scopolamine	Increased SAN automaticity Increased AVN conduction	Mild-to-moderate symptomatic sinus bradycardia; Supra-His, AVN, conduction blocks, *e.g.*, acute inferior wall MI or vagal syncope
Muscarinic M2 receptor activators (IId): Carbachol, pylocarpine, metacholine, digoxin	Reduced SAN automaticity Reduced SAN reentry Slowed AVN conduction, Inhibited reentries	Sinus tachycardia or supraventricular tachyarrhythmias

(Table 4) cont.....

Adenosine, ATP; Aminophyline: Adenosine A1 receptor activators	SAN automaticity sinde reduction AVN iletiminde reduction , reentry sonlandırma; EAD-/DAD induced activity reduction	Emergency blockade of AVN tachycardia and cAMP-mediated triggered VTs; Distinguishing sinus and atrial tachycardia
III	K⁺ canal blockers and openers	-
Amiodaron (IIIa, Nonselective K+ canal blockers)	I Kr, I Na, I Ca, I to, I Ks, I K1, I KACh, α- and β-adrenergic antagonism; reduced automaticity; prolongation in AP recovery duration and refractory period, reduced reentrant tendency	Patients with VT in the absence of structural heart disease; tachyarrhythmias in Wolff-Parkinson-White syndrome AV conduction in AF *via* accessory pathway; Ventricular premature contractions following VF Supraventricular arrhythmias and AF
Dronedarone (IIIa, nonselective K+ canal blockers)	I Kr, I Ks and β1-adrenergic antagonism	
Dofetilid (IIIa)	"Pure" I Kr blocker	Patients with VT in the absence of structural heart disease; tachyarrhythmias in Wolff-Parkinson-White syndrome; AF *via* AV conduction accessory pathways; Ventricular premature contractions following VF Supraventricular arrhythmias and AF
Ibutilid (IIIa)	I Na activation and I Kr antagonism	
Sotalol (IIIa)	I Kr and I to, I K1, and β-adrenergic antagonism	
Vernakalant	I NaL, I Kur antagonism; Atrium-specific effects: increase in AP recovery duration and refractory period; reduced reentrant tendency	Emergency (pharmacological) cardioversion in acute AF
Nicorandil (IIIb),	I KATP antagonism and effects of vasodilator nitrates on vascular smooth muscles; Potential reduction in AP recovery duration	Stable angina treatment (second line)
IV	Modulators of Ca²⁺ metabolism	-
Bepridil (IVa, nonselective)	Cardiac I CaL antagonism (bradycardic effects) and tachycardic effects on vascular smooth muscles; Reduced late after-depolarization	Angina pectoris; Treatment of SVT (potential).
Phenylalkylamines (*e.g.*, verapamil), benzothiazepines (*e.g.*, diltiazem)	Blockade of Ca²⁺ influx (*I*Ca), resulting in inhibition of SAN pacing and AVN conduction, prolonged ERP and AP recovery durations, increased refractory period, reduced repolarization reserve, and depressed intracellular Ca²⁺ signal; prolonged PR intervals	Supraventricular arrhythmias in the absence of structural heart disease and VT; Rate control in AF

(Table 4) cont.....

Flecainide, Propafenon (IVb)	Reduced SR Ca^{2+} release: reduced cytosolic and SR $[Ca^{2+}]$	Catecholaminergic polymorphic VT
VII	Upstream target modulators	-
Kaptopril, enalapril, delapril, ramipril, quinapril, perindopril, lisinopril, benazepril, imidapril, trandolapril, Cilazapril	Diminished AP conduction Improvement in structural and electrophysiological remodeling changes leading to increased reentrant tendency	Management of hypertension and symptomatic HF; Potential application: Reduction in arrhythmic substrates
Losartan, kandesartan, eprosartan, telmisartan, irbesartan, olmesartan, valsartan, saprisartan		
Omega-3 fatty acids:		Risk reduction in post–AMI cardiac death, AMI, stroke, and abnormal cardiac rhythm
Statins		

Note: Class V and VI are excluded as they are not used in clinical practice.
SR: Sarcoplasmic reticulum.
AP: Action potential; APD, action potential duration; AVN, atrioventricular node; CaMKII, calcium/calmodulin kinase II; DAD, delayed afterdepolarization (delayed post-depolarization).
EAD: Early afterdepolarization.
SAN: Sino-atrial node.
SQTS: Short-QT syndrome.
LQTS: Long-QT syndrome.

CONCLUSIONS

In fact, 2020 ACLS Guidelines carry no essential differences from 2016, 2017, 2018, and 2019 guidelines to new generations. Main themes remain the same: perform high-quality CPR/BLS, give evidence-based drugs only when really necessary.

One of the critical factors of efficient ACLS is to be ready for different patient scenarios to be encountered in routine practice. Firstly, the clinician has to assess and manage a patient in CA who has one of the four lethal arrhythmias: PEA, asystole, VF or PVT.

ACLS guidelines recommend certain agents to ensure hemodynamic stabilization, prevention of collapse, stabilization of a perfusing rhythm, improving peripheral resistance and cardiac output, and ROSC. It is known that no antiarrhythmic agent increases the percentage of patients discharged with good neurological status. For this reason, high-quality CPR takes priority to all maneuvers performed against death. Of note, administration of epinephrine and/or other resuscitative agents can only be succesful with concurrent high-quality CPR especially in patients with nonshockable rhythms.

It should not be overlooked that CA events are not identical, not only for their diagnostic challenges, but also in terms of management strategies. To achieve optimal patient outcome, individualized treatment pathways and specialized management is necessary for many conditions. The drugs used in VF and pulseless VT (PVT) apart from adrenaline are vasopressin, amiodarone, lidocaine, esmolol, magnesium and procainamide in selected situations.

New high-quality evidence can modify current knowledge on how to resuscitate patients from lethal arrhythmias. Until then, ACLS providers will be responsible to master the 2020 protocols to perform the best care for their patients.

REFERENCES

Abriel, H. (2010). Cardiac sodium channel Na(v)1.5 and interacting proteins: physiology and pathophysiology. *J. Mol. Cell. Cardiol., 48*(1), 2-11.
[http://dx.doi.org/10.1016/j.yjmcc.2009.08.025] [PMID: 19744495]

Ahrens, T., Schallom, L., Bettorf, K., Ellner, S., Hurt, G., O'Mara, V., Ludwig, J., George, W., Marino, T., Shannon, W. (2001). End-tidal carbon dioxide measurements as a prognostic indicator of outcome in cardiac arrest. *Am. J. Crit. Care, 10*(6), 391-398.
[http://dx.doi.org/10.4037/ajcc2001.10.6.391] [PMID: 11688606]

Al-Khatib, S.M., Stevenson, W.G., Ackerman, M.J. (2017). AHA/ACC/HRS guideline for management of patients with ventricular arrhythmias and the prevention of sudden cardiac death. *Circulation*.https://www.ahajournals.org/   doi/10.1161/CIR.0000000000000548?url_ver=Z39.88-2003&rfr_id=ori:rid:crossref.org&rfr_dat=cr_pub%3dpubmed

American Heart association focused update on advanced cardiovascular life support use of antiarrhythmic drugs during and immediately after cardiac arrest. *Circulation, 138*, e740-e749.

Amin, A.S., Asghari-Roodsari, A., Tan, H.L. (2010). Cardiac sodium channelopathies. *Pflugers Arch., 460*(2), 223-237.
[http://dx.doi.org/10.1007/s00424-009-0761-0] [PMID: 20091048]

Belardinelli, L., Giles, W.R., Rajamani, S., Karagueuzian, H.S., Shryock, J.C. (2015). Cardiac late Na^+ current: proarrhythmic effects, roles in long QT syndromes, and pathological relationship to CaMKII and oxidative stress. *Heart Rhythm, 12*(2), 440-448.
[http://dx.doi.org/10.1016/j.hrthm.2014.11.009] [PMID: 25460862]

Biel, M., Wahl-Schott, C., Michalakis, S., Zong, X. (2009). Hyperpolarization-activated cation channels: from genes to function. *Physiol. Rev., 89*(3), 847-885.
[http://dx.doi.org/10.1152/physrev.00029.2008] [PMID: 19584315]

Capel, R.A., Terrar, D.A. (2015). The importance of Ca(2+)-dependent mechanisms for the initiation of the heartbeat. *Front. Physiol., 6*, 80.
[http://dx.doi.org/10.3389/fphys.2015.00080] [PMID: 25859219]

Chadda, K.R., Jeevaratnam, K., Lei, M., Huang, C.L. (2017). Sodium channel biophysics, late sodium current and genetic arrhythmic syndromes. *Pflugers Arch., 469*(5-6), 629-641.
[http://dx.doi.org/10.1007/s00424-017-1959-1] [PMID: 28265756]

DiMarco, J. (2004). Adenosine and digoxin. In: Zipes, D., Jalife, J., (Eds.), *Cardiac Electrophysiology: From Cell to Bedside.* (4th ed., pp. 942-949). Philadelphia, PA: Saunders.
[http://dx.doi.org/10.1016/B0-7216-0323-8/50105-6]

Dobrev, D., Nattel, S. (2010). New antiarrhythmic drugs for treatment of atrial fibrillation. *Lancet, 375*(9721), 1212-1223.
[http://dx.doi.org/10.1016/S0140-6736(10)60096-7] [PMID: 20334907]

Dorian, P., Cass, D., Schwartz, B., Cooper, R., Gelaznikas, R., Barr, A. (2002). Amiodarone as compared with lidocaine for shock-resistant ventricular fibrillation. *N. Engl. J. Med, 346*(12), 884-890.
[http://dx.doi.org/10.1056/NEJMoa013029] [PMID: 11907287]

Dumot, J.A., Burval, D.J., Sprung, J., Waters, J.H., Mraovic, B., Karafa, M.T., Mascha, E.J., Bourke, D.L. (2001). Outcome of adult cardiopulmonary resuscitations at a tertiary referral center including results of "limited" resuscitations. *Arch. Intern. Med., 161*(14), 1751-1758.
[http://dx.doi.org/10.1001/archinte.161.14.1751] [PMID: 11485508]

Fuster, V., Rydén, L.E., Cannom, D.S., Crijns, H.J., Curtis, A.B., Ellenbogen, K.A., Halperin, J.L., Kay, G.N., Le Huezey, J.Y., Lowe, J.E., Olsson, S.B., Prystowsky, E.N., Tamargo, J.L., Wann, L.S. (2011). 2011 ACCF/AHA/HRS focused updates incorporated into the ACC/AHA/ESC 2006 Guidelines for the management of patients with atrial fibrillation: a report of the American College of Cardiology Foundation/American Heart Association Task Force on Practice Guidelines developed in partnership with the European Society of Cardiology and in collaboration with the European Heart Rhythm Association and the Heart Rhythm Society. *J. Am. Coll. Cardiol., 57*(11), e101-e198.
[http://dx.doi.org/10.1016/j.jacc.2010.09.013] [PMID: 21392637]

Gillis, A. (2004). Class I anti-arrhythmic drugs: quinidine, procainamide, disopyramide, lidocaine, mexiletine, flecainide and propafenone. In: Zipes, D., Jalife, J., (Eds.), *Cardiac Electrophysiology: From Cell to Bedside.* (4th ed., pp. 911-917). Philadelphia, PA: Saunders.
[http://dx.doi.org/10.1016/B0-7216-0323-8/50102-0]

https://www.acls.net/acls-tachycardia-algorithm-stable.htm

Huang, C.L. (2017). Murine electrophysiological models of cardiac arrhythmogenesis. *Physiol. Rev., 97*(1), 283-409.
[http://dx.doi.org/10.1152/physrev.00007.2016] [PMID: 27974512]

Iwasaki, Y.K., Nishida, K., Kato, T., Nattel, S. (2011). Atrial fibrillation pathophysiology: implications for management. *Circulation, 124*(20), 2264-2274.
[http://dx.doi.org/10.1161/CIRCULATIONAHA.111.019893] [PMID: 22083148]

January, C.T., Wann, L.S., Alpert, J.S., Calkins, H., Cigarroa, J.E., Cleveland, J.C., Jr, Conti, J.B., Ellinor, P.T., Ezekowitz, M.D., Field, M.E., Murray, K.T., Sacco, R.L., Stevenson, W.G., Tchou, P.J., Tracy, C.M., Yancy, C.W. American College of Cardiology/American Heart Association Task Force on Practice Guidelines. (2014). 2014 AHA/ACC/HRS guideline for the management of patients with atrial fibrillation: a report of the American College of Cardiology/American Heart Association Task Force on Practice Guidelines and the Heart Rhythm Society. *J. Am. Coll. Cardiol., 64*(21), e1-e76.
[http://dx.doi.org/10.1016/j.jacc.2014.03.022] [PMID: 24685669]

January, C.T., Wann, L.S., Alpert, J.S., Calkins, H., Cigarroa, J.E., Cleveland, J.C., Jr, Conti, J.B., Ellinor, P.T., Ezekowitz, M.D., Field, M.E., Murray, K.T., Sacco, R.L., Stevenson, W.G., Tchou, P.J., Tracy, C.M., Yancy, C.W. ACC/AHA Task Force Members. (2014). 2014 AHA/ACC/HRS guideline for the management of patients with atrial fibrillation: a report of the American College of Cardiology/American Heart Association Task Force on practice guidelines and the Heart Rhythm Society. *Circulation, 130*(23), e199-e267.
[http://dx.doi.org/10.1161/CIR.0000000000000041] [PMID: 24682347]

Jeevaratnam, K., Guzadhur, L., Goh, Y.M., Grace, A.A., Huang, C.L. (2016). Sodium channel haploinsufficiency and structural change in ventricular arrhythmogenesis. *Acta Physiol. (Oxf.), 216*(2), 186-202.
[http://dx.doi.org/10.1111/apha.12577] [PMID: 26284956]

Karcıoğlu, Ö., Karcıoğlu, Y. (2000). Role of end-tidal CO_2 monitoring in patients intubated and resuscitated in the emergency department. *Turk. J. Med. Sci., 30*(5), 475-478.

Lei, M., Zhang, H., Grace, A.A., Huang, C.L. (2007). SCN5A and sinoatrial node pacemaker function. *Cardiovasc. Res., 74*(3), 356-365.
[http://dx.doi.org/10.1016/j.cardiores.2007.01.009] [PMID: 17368591]

Mangoni, M.E., Nargeot, J. (2008). Genesis and regulation of the heart automaticity. *Physiol. Rev., 88*(3), 919-982.
[http://dx.doi.org/10.1152/physrev.00018.2007] [PMID: 18626064]

Marcolini, E.G., Bond, M.C. (2017). Postcardiac Arrest Management.*Emergency Department Resuscitation of the Critically Ill-2017..* Dallas, Texas: American College of Emergency Physicians.

Miraglia, D., Miguel, L.A., Alonso, W. (2020). Esmolol in the management of pre-hospital refractory ventricular fibrillation: A systematic review and meta-analysis. *Am. J. Emerg. Med., 38*(9), 1921-1934.
[http://dx.doi.org/10.1016/j.ajem.2020.05.083] [PMID: 32777667]

National Institue of Health Care Excellence. *Arrhythmias.* https://bnf.nice.org.uk/treatment-summary/arrhythmias.html

Neumar, R.W., Shuster, M., Callaway, C.W., Gent, L.M., Atkins, D.L., Bhanji, F., Brooks, S.C., de Caen, A.R., Donnino, M.W., Ferrer, J.M., Kleinman, M.E., Kronick, S.L., Lavonas, E.J., Link, M.S., Mancini, M.E., Morrison, L.J., O'Connor, R.E., Samson, R.A., Schexnayder, S.M., Singletary, E.M., Sinz, E.H., Travers, A.H., Wyckoff, M.H., Hazinski, M.F. (2015). Part 1: Executive Summary. *Circulation, 132*(18) (Suppl. 2), S315-S367.
[http://dx.doi.org/10.1161/CIR.0000000000000252] [PMID: 26472989]

Nichol, G., Thomas, E., Callaway, C.W., Hedges, J., Powell, J.L., Aufderheide, T.P., Rea, T., Lowe, R., Brown, T., Dreyer, J., Davis, D., Idris, A., Stiell, I. Resuscitation Outcomes Consortium Investigators.. (2008). Regional variation in out-of-hospital cardiac arrest incidence and outcome. *JAMA, 300*(12), 1423-1431.
[http://dx.doi.org/10.1001/jama.300.12.1423] [PMID: 18812533]

Olasveengen, T.M., Sunde, K., Brunborg, C., Thowsen, J., Steen, P.A., Wik, L. (2009). Intravenous drug administration during out-of-hospital cardiac arrest: a randomized trial. *JAMA, 302*(20), 2222-2229.
[http://dx.doi.org/10.1001/jama.2009.1729] [PMID: 19934423]

Olasveengen, T.M., Wik, L., Sunde, K., Steen, P.A. (2012). Outcome when adrenaline (epinephrine) was actually given vs. not given - post hoc analysis of a randomized clinical trial. *Resuscitation, 83*(3), 327-332.
[http://dx.doi.org/10.1016/j.resuscitation.2011.11.011] [PMID: 22115931]

Page, R.L., Joglar, J.A., Caldwell, M.A., Calkins, H., Conti, J.B., Deal, B.J., Estes, N.A., III, Field, M.E., Goldberger, Z.D., Hammill, S.C., Indik, J.H., Lindsay, B.D., Olshansky, B., Russo, A.M., Shen, W.K., Tracy, C.M., Al-Khatib, S.M. Evidence Review Committee Chair‡. (2016). 2015 ACC/AHA/HRS Guideline for the Management of Adult Patients With Supraventricular Tachycardia: A Report of the American College of Cardiology/American Heart Association Task Force on Clinical Practice Guidelines and the Heart Rhythm Society. *Circulation, 133*(14), e506-e574.
[http://dx.doi.org/10.1161/CIR.0000000000000311] [PMID: 26399663]

Panchal, A.R., Berg, K.M., Hirsch, K.G., Kudenchuk, P.J., Del Rios, M., Cabañas, J.G., Link, M.S., Kurz, M.C., Chan, P.S., Morley, P.T., Hazinski, M.F., Donnino, M.W. (2019). 2019 American Heart Association Focused Update on Advanced Cardiovascular Life Support: Use of Advanced Airways, Vasopressors, and Extracorporeal Cardiopulmonary Resuscitation During Cardiac Arrest: An Update to the American Heart Association Guidelines for Cardiopulmonary Resuscitation and Emergency Cardiovascular Care. *Circulation, 140*(24), e881-e894.https://www.ahajournals.org/doi/10.1161/CIR.0000000000000732
[http://dx.doi.org/10.1161/CIR.0000000000000732] [PMID: 31722552]

Perkins, G.D., Ji, C., Deakin, C.D., Quinn, T., Nolan, J.P., Scomparin, C., Regan, S., Long, J., Slowther, A., Pocock, H., Black, J.J.M., Moore, F., Fothergill, R.T., Rees, N., O'Shea, L., Docherty, M., Gunson, I., Han, K., Charlton, K., Finn, J., Petrou, S., Stallard, N., Gates, S., Lall, R. PARAMEDIC2 Collaborators. (2018). A randomized trial of epinephrine in out-of-hospital cardiac arrest. *N. Engl. J. Med., 379*(8), 711-721.
[http://dx.doi.org/10.1056/NEJMoa1806842] [PMID: 30021076]

Reynolds, J.C., Lawner, B.J. (2017). Cardiac arrest updates. In: Winters, M.E., (Ed.), *Emergency Department Resuscitation of the Critically Ill-2017.* Dallas, Texas: American College of Emergency Physicians.

Roden, D. (2006). Antiarrhythmic drugs. In: Brunton, L., Knollman, B., Hilal-Dandan, R., (Eds.), *Goodman and Gilman's The Pharmacological Basis of Therapeutics* (11th ed., pp. 899-932). New York: McGrawHill.

Rosen, M.R., Janse, M.J. (2010). Concept of the vulnerable parameter: the Sicilian Gambit revisited. *J. Cardiovasc. Pharmacol., 55*(5), 428-437.
[http://dx.doi.org/10.1097/FJC.0b013e3181bfaddc] [PMID: 19755918]

Salvage, S.C., Chandrasekharan, K.H., Jeevaratnam, K., Dulhunty, A.F., Thompson, A.J., Jackson, A.P., Huang, C.L. (2018). Multiple targets for flecainide action: implications for cardiac arrhythmogenesis. *Br. J. Pharmacol., 175*(8), 1260-1278.
[http://dx.doi.org/10.1111/bph.13807] [PMID: 28369767]

Sampson, K., Kass, R. (2011). Anti-arrhythmic drugs. In: Brunton, L., Chabner, B., Knollman, B., (Eds.), *Goodman & Gilman's The Pharmaceutical Basis of Therapeutics* (pp. 815-848). New York, NY: McGrawHill.

Sanghavi, P., Jena, A.B., Newhouse, J.P., Zaslavsky, A.M. (2015). Outcomes after out-of-hospital cardiac arrest treated by basic *vs* advanced life support. *JAMA Intern. Med., 175*(2), 196-204.
[http://dx.doi.org/10.1001/jamainternmed.2014.5420] [PMID: 25419698]

Sato, S., Zamami, Y., Imai, T., Tanaka, S., Koyama, T., Niimura, T., Chuma, M., Koga, T., Takechi, K., Kurata, Y., Kondo, Y., Izawa-Ishizawa, Y., Sendo, T., Nakura, H., Ishizawa, K. (2017). Meta-analysis of the efficacies of amiodarone and nifekalant in shock-resistant ventricular fibrillation and pulseless ventricular tachycardia. *Sci. Rep., 7*(1), 12683.
[http://dx.doi.org/10.1038/s41598-017-13073-0] [PMID: 28978927]

Schmitt, N., Grunnet, M., Olesen, S.P. (2014). Cardiac potassium channel subtypes: new roles in repolarization and arrhythmia. *Physiol. Rev., 94*(2), 609-653.
[http://dx.doi.org/10.1152/physrev.00022.2013] [PMID: 24692356]

Stiell, I.G., Hébert, P.C., Wells, G.A., Vandemheen, K.L., Tang, A.S., Higginson, L.A., Dreyer, J.F., Clement, C., Battram, E., Watpool, I., Mason, S., Klassen, T., Weitzman, B.N. (2001). Vasopressin *versus* epinephrine for inhospital cardiac arrest: a randomised controlled trial. *Lancet, 358*(9276), 105-109.
[http://dx.doi.org/10.1016/S0140-6736(01)05328-4] [PMID: 11463411]

Task Force of the Working Group on Arrhythmias of the European Society of Cardiology. (1991). The Sicilian gambit. A new approach to the classification of antiarrhythmic drugs based on their actions on arrhythmogenic mechanisms. *Circulation, 84*(4), 1831-1851.
[http://dx.doi.org/10.1161/01.CIR.84.4.1831] [PMID: 1717173]

van Walraven, C., Stiell, I.G., Wells, G.A., Hébert, P.C., Vandemheen, K. (1998). Do advanced cardiac life support drugs increase resuscitation rates from in-hospital cardiac arrest? The OTAC Study Group. *Ann. Emerg. Med., 32*(5), 544-553.
[http://dx.doi.org/10.1016/S0196-0644(98)70031-9] [PMID: 9795316]

Wang, Y., Tsui, H., Bolton, E.L., Wang, X., Huang, C.L., Solaro, R.J., Ke, Y., Lei, M. (2015). Novel insights into mechanisms for Pak1-mediated regulation of cardiac Ca(2+) homeostasis. *Front. Physiol., 6*, 76.
[http://dx.doi.org/10.3389/fphys.2015.00076] [PMID: 25852566]

Yancy, C.W., Jessup, M., Bozkurt, B., Butler, J., Casey, D.E., Jr, Drazner, M.H., Fonarow, G.C., Geraci, S.A., Horwich, T., Januzzi, J.L., Johnson, M.R., Kasper, E.K., Levy, W.C., Masoudi, F.A., McBride, P.E., McMurray, J.J., Mitchell, J.E., Peterson, P.N., Riegel, B., Sam, F., Stevenson, L.W., Tang, W.H., Tsai, E.J., Wilkoff, B.L. (2013). 2013 ACCF/AHA guideline for the management of heart failure: executive summary: a report of the American College of Cardiology Foundation/American Heart Association Task Force on practice guidelines. *Circulation, 128*(16), 1810-1852.
[http://dx.doi.org/10.1161/CIR.0b013e31829e8807] [PMID: 23741057]

CHAPTER 11

Electrotherapies: Emergency Defibrillation, Cardioversion, and Transcutaneous Pacing

Abstract: Emergency cardioversion and defibrillation are life-saving procedures that exert direct electric current to the heart through the chest wall in order to terminate lethal tachyarrhythmias. Early defibrillation is life-saving in the survival of adult patients who develop sudden cardiac arrest. In the defibrillation process, myocardial cells are depolarized, and VF is terminated by delivering a certain amount of direct current to the heart, passing through the chest wall. Proper timing and accurate performance of these procedures have a vital role in both survival and recovery post-resuscitation neurological functions without sequelae. Return of spontaneous circulation (ROSC) rates in defibrillation performed without losing time (within 20-30 seconds) can be up to 100% following the occurrence of these lethal rhythms. While cardioversion is performed in pulsating contraction rhythms, defibrillation is an electrical stimulation procedure applied in rhythms that do not generate pulses. In the cardioversion, synchronous energy is exerted onto the QRS complex to convert the rhythm into a sinus rhythm.

When there are signs of instability in rhythms with a pulse, emergency cardioversion (ECV) can be preferred over all other treatments if it is known to have acute onset (less than 48 hours) in atrial rhythm disorders, Transcutaneous pacing (TCP) is a recommended practice for temporary stabilization and invasive techniques such as transvenous pacing (TVP) should be attempted for longer pacing requirements. This chapter gives a brief outline on the outstanding features of electrotherapies (*i.e.*, ECV; defibrillation; TCP, TVP) both in case of life-threatening dysrhythmias and also in urgent non-lethal situations.

Keywords: Cardioversion, Defibrillation, Electrotherapies, Transcutaneous pacing, Transvenous pacing.

INTRODUCTION AND DEFINITIONS

Cardioversion and defibrillation can be summarized as passing a direct electric current through the chest wall to terminate tachyarrhythmias. The purpose of the defibrillation process is to provide high electrical current to the thoracic cage from the outside in a very short time to end lethal arrhythmias, namely, ventricular fibrillation (VF) and pulseless ventricular tachycardia (PVT). A certain amount of non-synchronized direct electrical current is exerted in a random moment of the

Ozgur KARCIOGLU

cardiac cycle. With the given current, all the excitable tissue of the heart is depolarized, and in this way, reentry foci are stopped. In brief, the heart is "silenced" totally all of a sudden. The myocardial cells all come in line with the same phase, and the dominant pacemaker (*i.e.*, the sinus node, as a rule) is activated. In this way, we target to line up the heart cells all in the same phase and to precipitate coordinated, organized conduction and contraction. The duration of the direct current applied to the thorax for these procedures lasts for less than one second.

The longer the time between the time the PVT or VF occurs and the defibrillation procedure, the smaller the chance of success in defibrillation. ROSC rates in defibrillation performed without losing time (within 20-30 seconds) can be up to 100% following the occurrence of these lethal rhythms. In real life, healthy discharge rates from the hospital do not exceed 50% in the most advanced systems.

Proper timing and accurate performance of BLS have an important role in both survival and recovery post-resuscitation neurological functions without sequelae.

Early defibrillation is life-saving in the survival of adult patients who develop sudden cardiac arrest (SCA) for the following reasons:

1. The most common initial rhythm is VF in patients with witnessed SCA.

2. The treatment of VF is defibrillation.

3. The probability of success with defibrillation decreases significantly over time.

4. When the VF arrests are not defibrillated, they will degenerate in a few minutes to turn into asystole, which is the arrest rhythm with the worst prognosis.

Each minute increases the mortality rate by 7-10% when BLS cannot be started, and defibrillation is not performed in SCA cases due to the lack of a rescuer at the scene at the moment. Defibrillation performed in the first 4 to 5 minutes by the layperson, bystanders who witnessed the event has the potential to save the lives of many adults without neurological sequelae due to hypoxia in the brain. In cases where the defibrillator cannot be reached immediately, it is very important to continue cardiac compressions until the defibrillator arrives. In this way, with the blood flow provided, the duration of VF can be extended and the impairment of brain functions can be delayed (Fig. **1**).

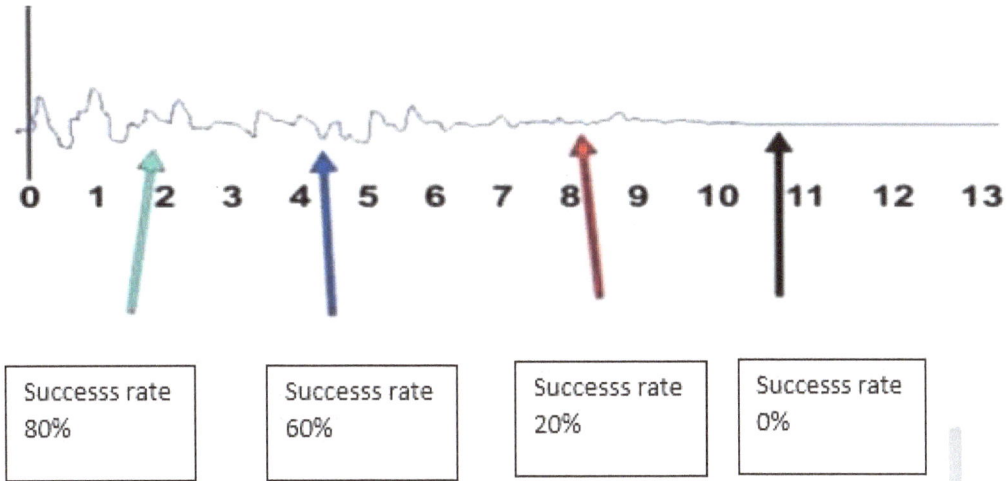

Fig. (1). Delay in defibrillation results in a significant decrease of success rates in time.

The amount of energy to be delivered is adjusted to be the lowest but the most effective energy to terminate VF. The meaning of the success of the defibrillation process is the conversion of VF within 5 seconds following the shock. Although VF may recur after successful defibrillation, these recurrences should not mean that defibrillation has failed. There are many factors that affect the successful outcome of resuscitation, and defibrillation is one of the critical ones. Success in defibrillation procedure and successful resuscitation are separate phenomena. The success of resuscitation includes ROSC, survival and healthy discharge of the patient from the hospital.

Electrical cardioversion (ECV) and defibrillation are different practices. While cardioversion is performed in pulsating contraction rhythms, defibrillation is an electrical stimulation procedure applied in rhythms that do not generate pulses. In the ECV process, synchronous energy is exerted onto the QRS complex to convert the rhythm into a sinus rhythm.

There are only four types of rhythms that are intervened with ECV:

- wide complex tachycardias with a pulse (VT),

- atrial fibrillation,

- atrial flutter and

- paroxysmal supraventricular tachycardias.

Defibrillation is never performed in any patient whose pulse is palpable, and ECV cannot be performed when pulses are not elicited.

AUTOMATED EXTERNAL DEFIBRILLATORS

Every healthcare personnel performing cardiopulmonary resuscitation (CPR) should be able to proceed with defibrillation as an integral part of it. Automatic External Defibrillators (AEDs) have been developed for people with basic training on BLS and ambulance personnel, which they can practically carry out defibrillation within BLS. As a result, defibrillation is now included in both BLS and ACLS procedures. It has been shown that survival and discharge rates from the hospital have boosted significantly with defibrillation that the lay rescuers immediately practice *via* AED after cardiac arrest.

Three main procedures must be undertaken in the first minutes following out of hospital cardiac arrest (OHCA) to increase the chance of survival:

1. 911/112 ambulance systems (EMS) should be activated,
2. BLS including high-quality chest compressions should be commenced immediately,
3. Defibrillation should be performed *via* AED in case of shockable rhythms.

AEDs are easy-to-use smart boxes which can direct trained rescuers *via* audible and visual stimuli to ensure that the person with CA is defibrillated effectively and safely. AEDs with self-adhesive pads have also a system to analyze the rhythm. The sensitivity of this system in recognizing coarse VF is 100%, while it is reduced to 90-92% in fine VF.

Besides ambulances, it is recommended to have AED devices in business centers, schools and airplanes where large numbers of people are passing by in a time unit. AEDs can be used by paramedics, firefighters, police, pilots and hostesses. Physicians and/or paramedic personnel can easily intervene with AEDs in planes, shopping malls, airports, *etc.*

Recently, extracorporeal CPR (ECPR) instruments were combined with AEDs, which were turned into devices that could defibrillate with ongoing CPR.

Many AEDs are sensitive enough to recognize VF in children of all ages and distinguish between shockable and non-shockable rhythms. Some AEDs are equipped with "attenuated dose systems" suitable for children so they can deliver direct current at lower doses. Rescuers should use these attenuated dose systems in children between 1 and 8 years old, when necessary.

AED Usage

AED is applied with two adhesive pads, their cables and the appropriate device connected to them. Once the AED is properly installed, it analyses the rhythm itself and delivers an electric shock when the appropriate button is pressed. On the other hand, fully automated ones announce that it will shock with a warning sound immediately once it identifies the appropriate rhythm and delivers the shock *via* direct current.

Placement of Pads On AED Devices

Many patients do not necessitate any preparation other than removing the clothes on the chest and drying if there is excessive wetness. However, for those with very hairy chest, it may be necessary to clean/shave the hair at the site before the pads are placed, but defibrillation should not be delayed for shaving.

If the patient has an internal "implantable cardiac defibrillator" (ICD) to deliver shock in case of VF, then allow 30 to 60 seconds for the intervention of the ICD and shock *via* AED only if there is nothing done in that time window.

TTS-patches or ointments (such as nitroglycerine, nicotine, analgesic, hormone) adhered to the skin for therapeutic purposes should be removed quickly to allow placement of the pads.

If the victim is in the water, or if the patient's chest is covered with water or excessive sweating, the victim must first be rescued from the water, dried, and then the pads should be placed and defibrillated as appropriate.

DEFIBRILLATION PROCEDURE

In the defibrillation process, myocardial cells are depolarized and VF is terminated by delivering a certain amount of direct current to the heart, passing through the chest wall. The amount of energy to be delivered is predetermined to be the lowest but most effective energy to terminate VF. The meaning of the success of the defibrillation process is the termination of VF within 5 seconds following the shock.

What kind of Defibrillators Can I Use? Depending on the waveform used, defibrillator devices can be divided into monophasic and biphasic waves. Today, almost all AEDs and other defibrillators use biphasic waves as a standard.

Monophasic Wave Defibrillators: Its usage has decreased considerably in the recent decades. The term "monophasic wave" is used to describe the unidirectional flow of electrical current. The current given to the chest wall progresses in only one direction, decreases sharply following exertion and approaches zero. Monophasic waves are classified according to the current decreasing towards zero. If you are using a monophasic defibrillator, the dose of energy for VF is recommended as 360 J for all shocks. If the VF was terminated at the first shock, but then the arrest situation recurred, it is recommended to use the energy level that you delivered in the previous shocks and achieved successful results.

BIPHASIC WAVE DEFIBRILLATORS

Defibrillators producing energy in biphasic wave form were launched in the late 1990s. These devices do not require an increase in the energy level and less energy is delivered to the patient than in monophasic devices.

In biphasic waved defibrillators, the current to the chest wall proceeds in a positive direction for a certain period of time, then rotates to a negative direction. Studies have found that biphasic wave shocks are more effective and reliable in terminating VF when given in the same or lower energy levels than monophasic shocks. This kind of intervention reduces the chances of VF recurrence. However, there are publications stating that monophasic and biphasic defibrillators cause similar clinical results and that there is no significant difference in cases of OHCA, provided that they are administered at an early phase. Although it is not known exactly which energy level is the best, repeated shocks are given initially at doses of 120-200 J. If the practitioner uses a manually adjusted biphasic defibrillator and does not know the effective dose limits to terminate VF, 200 J may be used as the initial dose and the same or higher doses for the second and subsequent shocks.

RESISTANCE IN THE CHEST CAVITY - TRANSTHORACIC IMPEDANCE (TTI)

It is the resistance encountered in the tissues during the procedure until the energy current delivered reaches the heart. It is around 70 to 80 ohms in normal adult (Fig. **2**). When TTI is excessive, the actual energy exerted to the heart is attenuated, which affect defibrillation success. This phenomenon is mostly encountered in patients with COPD, emphysema, and advanced obesity in clinical practice (Table **1**).

To reduce TTI, it is necessary to apply sufficient pressure and use a conductive gel during the procedure. During defibrillation, 10-12.5 nt (kg/cm^2) of force should be applied on the spoons. This would in practice mean that a mid-size adult rescuer would press with all his/her might. If a gel is unavailable, a gauze pad moistened with saline can be used between the skin and the paddles.

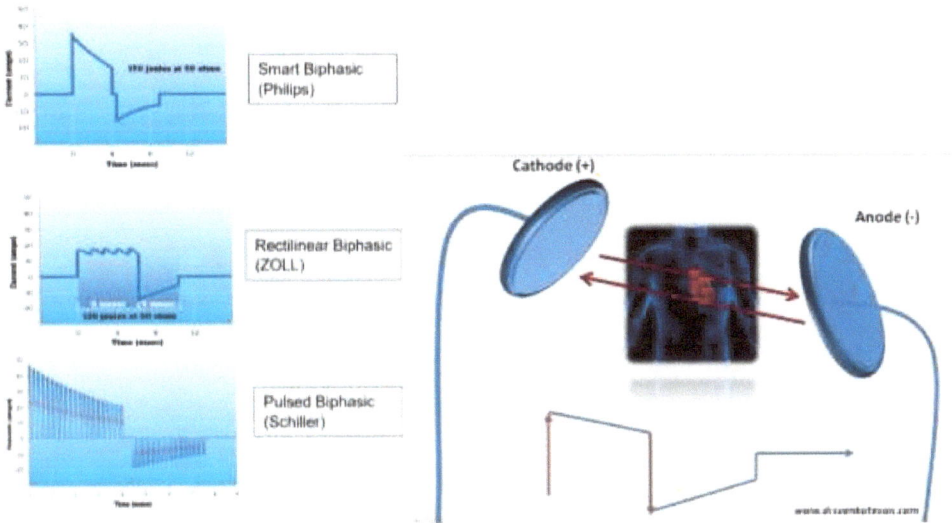

Fig. (2). A. Graphics of electrical energy current delivered by biphasic defibrillators of different brands. **B.** Direction of current and its reflection on the graph in biphasic defibrillators.

Table 1. Factors determining TTI.

• Selected energy level
• The size of the paddles
• Conductive material between the paddles and skin
• Number of shocks previously applied and the time passed after them
• Respiratory phase (TTI increases in diseases that increase dead space in the lungs)
• The distance between the paddles
• Pressure applied to paddles

If defibrillation is going to be done with adhesive electrodes, it is not necessary to apply pressure or apply conductive material. Contact of paddles with ECG and/or monitor cables should be prevented.

WHAT IS IN THE DEFIBRILLATOR?

In general, a defibrillator device has the following buttons, except for two hand-held paddles (Fig. **3**).

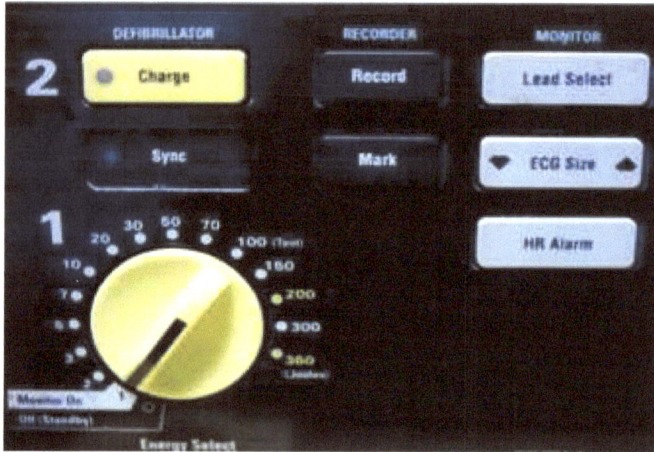

Fig. (3). Buttons on defibrillator devices.

- "On-Off" button.
- The button to select the appropriate energy level "Energy select": has ranges that can vary by brand of the machine.
- Energy charge button "Charge": It is located both on the paddle and the device. It charges at 2 to 5 seconds.
- Synchronization button "SYNC"
- Lead select button "Lead select". Provides "quick-look" when viewed with the paddle as the monitor pads
- Energy discharge-shock buttons "Discharge"
- Paddles: It is indicated with the words STERNUM and APEX.

The equivalents of the buttons are, in general, located on the paddles also for faster access.

Defibrillation Steps are given in Table (**2**).

Table 2. Steps for defibrillation with a standard defibrillator device is summarized below.

• Setting the defibrillator to working position (On)
• Evaluation/analysis of the rhythm from the monitor.
• Energy level selection (360 j for monophasic defibrillators, 200 J. for manual biphasic defibrillators or if unknown)
• Placing the paddles on the chest wall by applying gel (not necessary if pads are placed)
• Pressing the "Charge" button
• Checking that no one is in contact with the patient, giving 3 loud alarms to prevent the patient from touching anybody

(Table 2) cont.....

"I am clear."
"You are clear."
"Everybody clear."
• By applying sufficient force to the paddles, pressing both "discharge" buttons on the paddles at the same time
• The rhythm can be seen on the monitor without removing the paddles after the shock.
• Continuing compressions without wasting time after shock

If the patient is in ambulance, the ambulance must be stopped before defibrillating the patient.

PLACEMENT OF DEFIBRILLATOR PADDLES

In the defibrillator devices, the paddle indicated as "apex" is placed to the lateral side of the left nipple (the region between the midaxillary line and the left 4th to 5th intercostal space). On the other hand, the paddle indicated as "sternum" is placed on the right side of the sternum, just below the right clavicle, 2nd to 3rd intercostal space. The paddle should not be placed directly on the sternum (Fig. **4**).

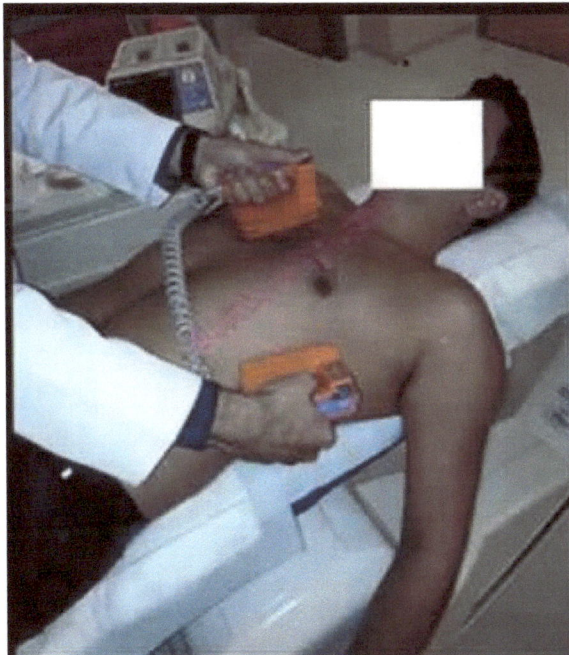

Fig. (4). Placement of defibrillator paddles.

It is important that the paddles are put sufficiently far away from each other and that no electrical arc is allowed to generate between them. Of note, gel should not be smeared on the chest on the clean area between the paddles.

For adults, a diameter of 8 to 12 cm is sufficient for defibrillator paddles and AED pads.

PEDIATRIC ARRESTS, DIFFERENCES IN AED USE AND DEFIBRILLATION

Since coronary artery disease is practically not encountered in children, VF/PVT is very rare. Hypoxemia, hypovolemia, hypoglycemia, acidemia are the triggers in the majority of CA cases. Therefore, PEA, bradycardia and asystole are seen as the final common pathway- the arrest rhythm. On the scene, it was reported that VF was seen in 5-15% of children and adolescents with CA. Only 3% of nontraumatic arrests under the age of 8 are VF arrests. However, hypothermia, some drug effects (such as hydrocarbons) may cause VF. Kawasaki disease, coronary artery aneurysm, vasculitic conditions also affect this risk. AEDs are not used in young children. Standard AED pads are suitable for children over 8 years old.

It is important that there is no gel bridge between them when placing the AED or standard defibrillator pads as the child's chest is quite small (Figs. **5-7**).

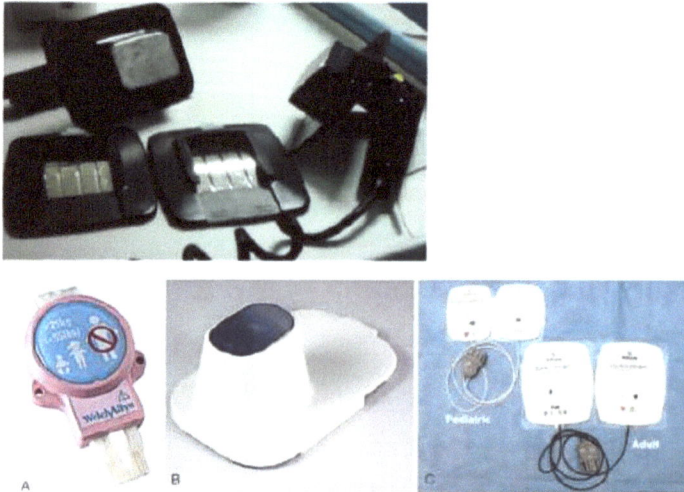

Fig. (5). Pediatric paddles should be easily removable just beneath the adult paddles. AED pads are also provided in some brands differently from adult pads.

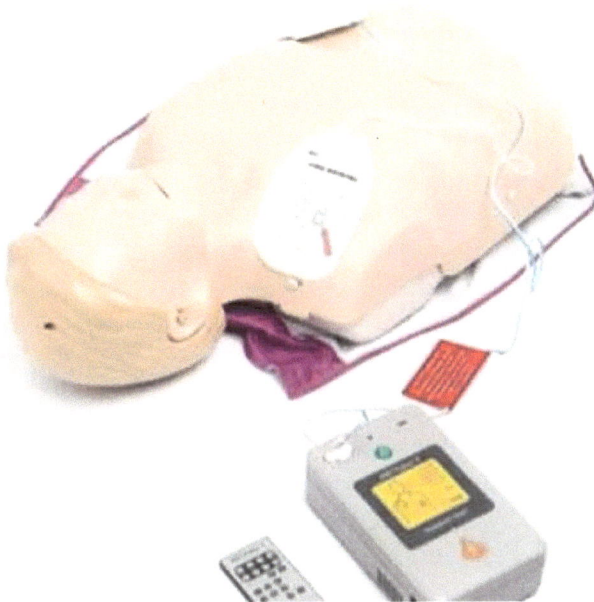

Fig. (6). Automated External Defibrillator device and pads. Rescuers should place the right (sternal) adhesive pad on the right anterior-upper (below the clavicle) part of the patient's chest; the left (apical) pad should be placed on the left-lower side of the patient's chest, lateral to the left nipple. If there is any medical device (*e.g.* permanent pacemaker or ICD) placed beneath the skin in the normal location of the pads, the pad should be put at least 2.5 cm away from the device.

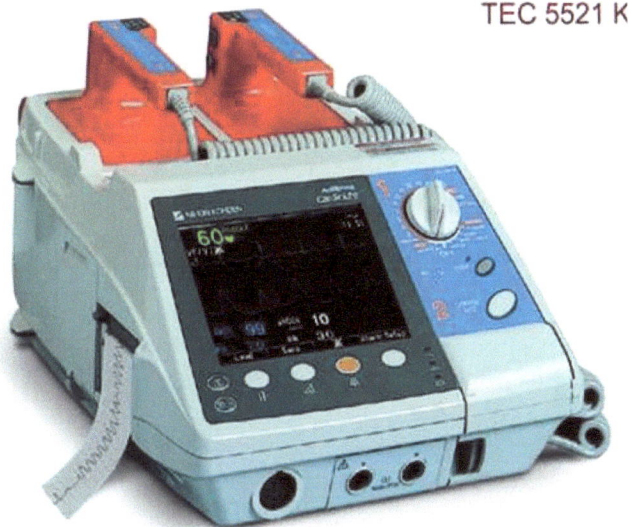

Fig. (7). Standard defibrillator device. It is intended for use by adequately trained healthcare professionals. Each device of different brands can have different properties, thus the machines should be practiced before encountering an emergency patient and all their characteistics should be recognized.

Pediatric paddles are beneath adult paddles which are easily removed in case of a pediatric emergency.

- It is delivered at a dose of 2-4 J/kg.

- Pediatric paddles are used in children up to 10 kg. Its dimensions are around 5 to 8 cm.

DEFIBRILLATION IN PATIENTS WITH PERMANENT PACEMAKERS (PPM)

If patients with PPM will undergo ECV or defibrillation, the paddles should not be placed on or close to these devices. Defibrillation should be performed in an anteroposterior position, at least 10 cm away from the generator or wires. Besides, TCP should be prepared. Paddles are placed on the left lateral chest wall and the right midsternal border if the PPM is in the upper left wall of the chest, and placed on the lower right chest wall or in the upper left wall and if the battery in the upper right chest wall. If the patient has such devices, these should be checked with post-defibrillation studies.

DEFIBRILLATION IN PREGNANT WOMEN

No adverse effects of defibrillation could be found on the fetus. Therefore, it is not contraindicated in pregnant women. However, the left lateral position is recommended if possible.

SYNCHRONOUS ELECTRICAL CARDIOVERSION (ECV)

ECV is the delivery of a shock simultaneously with the QRS complex. All defibrillator devices are switched on in asynchronous (defibrillation) mode when they are first turned on. Synchronization is accomplished by pressing the 'SYNC' button on the defibrillator devices. ECV helps prevent shock delivery during the relative refractory period of the cardiac cycle which could trigger VF. The energy level in synchronized shocks is lower than the shock levels in defibrillation. If these low-dose energies are applied as defibrillation rather than synchronous, they can lead to VF.

In ECV, unlike defibrillation, shock does not occur immediately after pressing the "discharge" buttons on the paddles. Synchronized cardioversion is expected to occur for a few seconds by keeping the paddles in place with the appropriate pressure force.

Emergency ECV is employed in the treatment of atrial fibrillation, atrial flutter and supraventricular tachycardias and in wide complex tachycardias with unstable signs and symptoms thought to be due to tachyarrhythmia. The ECV procedure aims to treat unstable tachyarrhythmias with the QRS complex and to ensure a circulating heart pattern. Signs and symptoms that render the patient diagnosed with unstable tachyarrhythmia include chest pain, shortness of breath, hypotension, confusion, pulmonary edema, shock, CHF, and ACS.

The rhythm identified in the patient determines the energy level to be delivered in the ECV. It has been reported that 200 J in monophasic defibrillators is roughly equivalent to 150 J in biphasic defibrillators. According to the latest data, the recommended initial doses for emergency cardioversion are summarized in Table **2**.

In summary, when there are signs of instability in rhythms with a pulse, emergency ECV is the option to be preferred over all other treatments if it is known to have acute onset (less than 48 hours) in atrial rhythm disorders.

Cardioversion is a painful procedure. Analgesia and sedation should be performed before the procedure, unless the patient's clinical condition is too unstable. Steps to be undertaken for ECV with a standard defibrillator are summarized below:

1. Turn the defibrillator 'on'.
2. Attach the monitor cables to the patient.
3. Synchronize by pressing the 'sync' button.
4. Select the appropriate energy level.
5. Put gel on paddles and placing them on the chest wall.
6. Press the "Charge" button.
7. Check that no one is in contact with the patient, loudly warn on the scene so that no one touches "I am giving shock, I am ready, you are ready, everyone is ready".
8. With enough force applied to the paddles, press both "discharge" buttons at the same time and hold them for a few seconds until the shock process takes place.
9. Monitor the rhythm and increase the energy level according to the guides, if not cardioverted, switch to an alternative plans.
10. Call for a consultation with cardiology and/or intensive care.

Generally, defibrillator devices return to asynchronous mode immediately after ECV is completed and the patient is shocked. For this reason, when the first attempt fails, if the ECV will be tried again with higher energy, the "SYNC" button must be activated again or the operator verifies that the device is in synchronous (SYNC) mode (Fig. **8**).

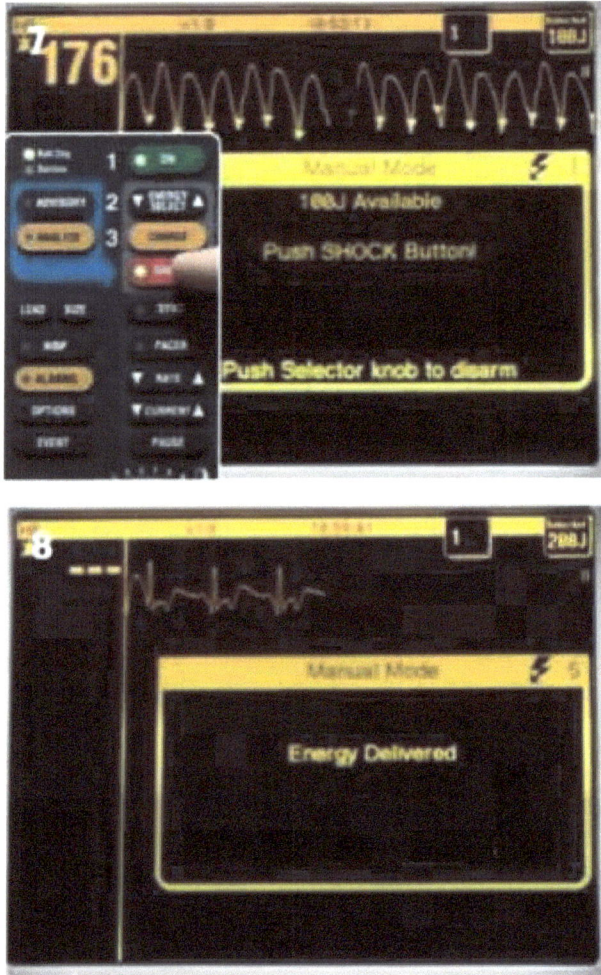

Fig. (8). Patient with VT converted to NSR by synchronized cardioversion. Ischemic appearance emerged following conversion must be confirmed with 12-lead ECG, the patient must be thoroughly examined and differential diagnoses should be reviewed.

SPECIFIC ARRHYTHMIAS AND RECOMMENDATIONS ON CARDIOVERSION DOSES

ECV is performed when there are signs of instability in rhythms with pulses, and is also recommended in patients known to have an acute onset (less than 48 hours) in atrial rhythm disorders. Emergency echocardiography/POCUS is suitable for the exclusion of atrial thrombus (Table **3**).

Table 3. Specific arrhythmias and recommended cardioversion tips.

Arrhythmia	Recommendations on Cardioversion Doses
Wide QRS complex tachycardias (VT with pulse)	In monomorphic VT, it is recommended to start with 100 J with a monophasic wave and gradually increase the energy level (100 J, 200 J, 300 and 360 J) in the stable patients, if the rhythm does not convert. The recommended starting dose when using biphasic wave is 120 to 150 J. If sinus rhythm cannot be achieved with the first shock, the energy level should be increased step by step in subsequent shocks.
Atrial fibrillation	The initial recommended energy level for AF is 100 to 200 J with monophasic wave, while 100 to 150 J with biphasic wave. Energy levels can be titrated up for subsequent shocks.
Atrial flutter and Supraventricular tachycardia	It is recommended to start with 50 J with monophasic wave, 20 to 50 J with biphasic.

COMPLICATIONS OF DEFIBRILLATION AND CARDIOVERSION PROCEDURES

One of the important complications of defibrillation and cardioversion procedures is that the healthcare personnel around the patient can be exposed to electrocution during procedure.

While defibrillation is conducted in narrow places such as ambulances, caution should be exercised not to injure the patient and healthcare personnel.

Other complications are listed below:

1. Direct Myocardial Injury: Although rare, it can be encountered in recurrent high-energy shocks (>325 J).

2. Soft Tissue Injuries: Thermal injuries are commonly encountered in relation with the energy delivered. First-degree burns are the most commonly noted. Usage of conductive gels as necessary would prevent such injuries.

3. Cardiac Dysrhythmias: Ventricular, supraventricular arrhythmias or asystole may occur following defibrillation, The incidence of VF is less than 5% in cardioversion and VF is more likely to occur in patients with digoxin and/or quinidine toxicity, hypokalemia, and acute myocardial infarction. In patients undergoing digoxin therapy, lower energies (50 J and below) may be preferred for cardioversion.

4. Bradycardia: is more common as a complication in patients with an inferior myocardial infarction and multiple defibrillation attempts. Bradycardia is mostly recorded 5 seconds after the shock and is short-lived. It rarely lasts longer than 20 seconds. Likewise, tachycardic rhythms (usually sinus tachycardia) is rare after shock, if any, and usually ends within the first 5 seconds.

5. Ectopic Beats: Atrial, junctional and ventricular ectopic beats are common but benign.

6. ST Segment Changes: Can be observed temporarily and for a short time.

7. Systemic Embolism: It is encountered in 1.2% to 1.5% in patients with chronic atrial fibrillation.

8. Hypotension: It is a rare complication which may last hours. All differential diagnoses (fluid losses, GI hemorrhages, third-space losses, pulmonary embolism, dysrhythmias, drug adverse effects, anaphylaxis *etc.* should be ruled out.

8. Muscle Damage: CK and LDH levels may boost after the procedure. However, more specific cardiac enzymes (CK-MB, troponin) are infrequently affected.

9. Pulmonary Edema: Although rare, it can be seen more frequently in patients with mitral, aortic valve and left ventricular failure.

EMERGENCY APPLICATION OF TRANSCUTANEOUS PACEMAKER

Temporary and emergent placement of transcutaneous pacemaker (TCP) is cardiac electrical stimulation performed until permanent treatment is performed in certain tachyarrhythmias and bradyarrhythmias generating pulses in unstable patients. In 1952, Zoll produced the first practical TCP device.

The purpose of the TCP procedure is to transmit the electrical impulses generated *via* a generator from the electrodes (pads) to the heart and thereby provide myocardial depolarization or stimulation. The electrical stimulation passes through the chest wall and stimulates the myocardium using two pads attached to the chest wall.

Emergency pacing can also be done through central vascular access (transvenous pacing, TVP). However, TCP is preferred in emergency setting because it is easy and fast. TCP devices and pads are often found all in one piece, mounted on defibrillators.

INDICATIONS AND PROCEDURE

TCP can only be placed in patients with palpable pulses. It is recommended in emergency management of bradycardia or tachycardia resulting in instability. In these cases, symptoms indicative of vital organ hypoperfusion such as altered mental status and tachypnea are recorded commonly. Objective monitoring findings such as hypotension and low O2 saturation (SpO2) may or may not accompany clinical findings.

It should be remembered that the technique is only a temporary method and can be used until the TVP is inserted or the underlying cause of the dysrhythmia (such as hyperkalaemia, drug poisoning, acute ischemia) is eliminated.

In clinical practice, the most common conditions which prompt insertionTCP are most frequently reported as high-grade atrioventricular (AV) blocks (such as 2nd degree Mobitz type II AV block and complete-3rd degree AV block). The newly emerged bilateral branch block (right branch and left anterior or left posterior fascicle block) or alternating acute left and right branch block also warrant prophylactic TCP application. The most rational treatment of the left anterior fascicle block accompanying right bundle branch block or a new left bundle branch block is also performed by pacing.

The paramedic personnel who sees the patient with severe symptoms accompanying bradycardia should consult the command control center (CCC) should complete the primary and secondary surveys quickly. If the patient has tight tie and/or collar that may cause bradycardia by triggering carotid sinus compression, they should be loosened.

The procedure starts with the administration of atropine in most cases while preparing the TCP. It should be noted that atropine has no benefit in AMI and high-grade AV blocks. 0.5 mg of atropine can be given initially, and the same dose may be repeated if no response is elicited within a few minutes. Dopamine or adrenaline infusion can also be considered as an option. Preparation of TCP equipments should be commenced immediately following the unstable symptoms and signs are detected, or the patient do not respond to atropine and other agents, or abnormalities in vital signs becomes permanent.

TCP PROCEDURE

Placement of the pads: Correct placement of the pads is important for the best and adequate stimulation of the heart rate. Adhesive pads can be used but are more expensive. If the patient's general status allows, antero-posterior placement can be performed. In this case, the anterior pad (negative electrode) should be placed on the left side of the anterior chest, where the heartbeats are most audible, and the posterior pad should be placed directly above the anterior pad, and to the left of the thoracic vertebrae on the back. Anterior-lateral placement may be preferred if the patient's findings are severe or if there is difficulty in positioning.

In the anterior-lateral placement, the anterior electrode is placed in the same place, and the posterior electrode is placed below the right clavicle, just to the right of the sternum. Also, if defibrillator pads have to be placed, they should be put at least 2-3 cm away from the TCP pads. If CPR is to be performed, it can be applied directly on the pads.

Once the pads are placed, defibrillation and monitoring functions are available, along with TCP. Defibrillation can be done if a complication ensues during the TCP procedure. If pacing stimulus is exerted just on the ventricular repolarization, it can trigger cardiac dysrhythmias (R-on-T phenomenon).

The device has the following modes:

1. Operation mode; Includes asynchronous (fixed) mode and 'demand' mode. Demand mode is more suitable if the patient has palpable beats and blood pressure, albeit inadequate. In this mode, the device detects the patient's own heartbeats and warns if there are no beats. Fixed mode can be selected in patients who are unstable in extremis and do not have a reliable pulse. In this mode, the patient's cardiac activity is disregarded and impulses are exerted with regular intervals.
2. Rate selection: It can be selected between 30 to 200 bpm. However, in practice, values between 50 and 80 are often chosen, more commonly 60 and 70 bpm.
3. Current output: It is usually adjustable between 0-200 mA. It can be titrated upwards or downwards, depending on the severity of the findings and instability.
4. Pulse duration: It ranges from 20 to 40 milliseconds. However, these values cannot be adjusted by the user.

STEPS OF TCP PROCEDURE

The operation sequence in the TCP procedure is as follows:

1. The patient and his family are informed about the intervention. Informed consent is obtained, if possible.
2. The patient's vital signs are recorded.
3. Excessive hair on the skin area of the pads should be shaved/cleaned.
4. Pads are placed as indicated.
5. Pacemaker is turned 'On'.
6. Pace 'demand' mode is selected. It can be entered in fixed mode in unstable or pre-arrest patients.
7. Rate selection is achieved; generally 60 to 70 bpm is suitable.
8. Energy current level (mA) is selected. Starting with 10 to 15 mA, it is gradually

titrated up until it captures pacing beats. The capture of beats is confirmed by the formation of QRS complex and T wave after each pace spike.

The ideal is to achieve the capture state at the minimal current, and it can be maintained at 1.25 times this level (Fig. **9 A,B and C**).

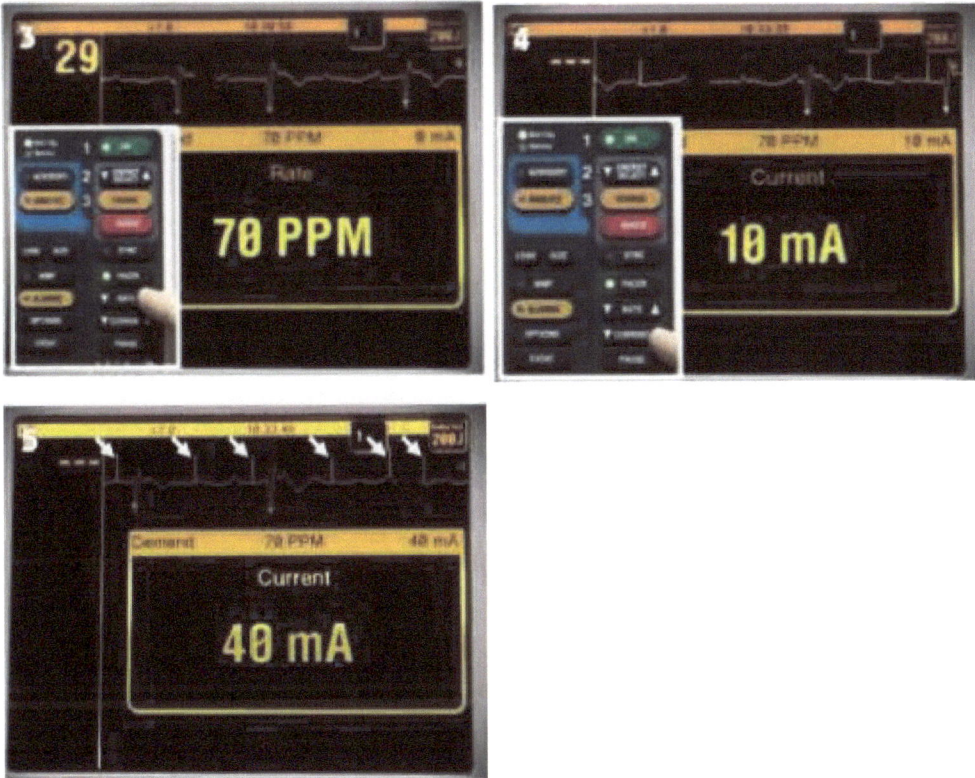

Fig. (9). The target pulse rate is set with the 'rate' button on the defibrillator. 'Current', indicates energy output titrated from the minimal up to the level it captures the beats. It is stated as milliamp (mA).

Overdrive Pacing

Sometimes, TCP can be performed when pharmacological agents do not impact positively in a patient with tachycardia leading to hemodynamic instability (Overdrive pacing). The rationale of this procedure is the suppression of the cardiac rhythm by pacing at a higher rate than the patient's tachyarrhythmia. This technique can sometimes be successful in the treatment of recurrent VT, (*e.g.* torsades de pointes).

TCP Contraindications

Generally, the insertion of TCP is contraindicated in asymptomatic, stable rhythms such as AV rhythm, Mobitz type 1 or a stable escape rhythms (*e.g.*, accelerated idioventricular rhythm). In addition, it may be necessary to perform in Mobitz type 1 patients with wide QRS, for these can turn into complete AV block. TCP should not be conducted in bradycardias associated with hypothermia because they can trigger life-threatening arrhythmias. Likewise, TCP should not be performed in cases of PEA, VF, and arrhythmias that respond to drug treatments. TCP is not applied when an intracardiac conduction block is detected. Again, TCP is not required unless hemodynamic instability ensues in rhythms over 40 bpm.

Complications of TCP

In TCP application, fasciculations and contractions may occur depending on the duration and intensity of the electrical impulse. The major drawback with TCP is that it is not tolerated by some patients. Patients may experience discomfort due to the contraction of the diaphragm and other muscles. Sedative-anxiolytics such as etomidate or midazolam will be required in patients with stable hemodynamics and intact neurological functions.

Although rare, there is a risk of electrical injury, but severe myocardial damage is not expected.

TCP is a recommended practice for temporary stabilization and invasive techniques such as TVP should be attempted for longer pacing requirements.

The most common reasons for failure of electrical capture are the use of improper pads, incorrect placement of pads and poor skin contact with pads.

How can I understand if ACS/AMI develops in a patient treated with TCP?

In TCP, the QRS duration is widened, AMI recognition will warrant to refer to rules in the patient with bundle branch block. "Modified Sgarbossa criteria" are ideally used for this (Table **4**).

Table 4. Properties of Sgarbossa criteria for the diagnosis of AMI in a patient using a ventricular pacemaker.

ECG criteria	Sensitivity (%)	Specificity (%)	p
Discordant ST-elevation >5 mm	53	88	0.025
Concordant ST- elevation >1 mm	18	94	>0.05

(Table 4) cont.....

ECG criteria	Sensitivity (%)	Specificity (%)	p
V1–V3 ST-segment depression >1 mm	2	82	>0.05

CONCLUSIONS

Emergency defibrillation is one of the most important interventions applied in a majority of all cardiac arrest situations, because most of these in the adult population stems from VF and PVT. These situations mostly appear suddenly and unexpectedly, thus only rapid response teams and/or in-hospital teams can imply expedient interventions as necessary. ROSC rates are targeted to be risen to optimal levels, but a more important goal is to discharge the patient from the health institution to normal, productive life in accord with the given patient's basal general health status and life expectancies. Defibrillation should be incorporated mainly into resuscitative protocols of bystander CPR (*i.e. via* AEDs) and advances within EMS as life-saving interventions.

ECV, on the other hand, is applied on the living patient with a palpable pulse, therefore, expectations are at a very high level. The main goals of the procedure are restoration of an adequately perfusing rhythm and maintenance of the stabilized medical status. Caveats such as thromboembolism cannot be underemphasized and specific measures (*i.e.* use of anticoagulants) should be employed as required.

TCP is employed for emergency stabilization for pacing requirements of symptomatic and unstable bradycardias, especially in high-grade AV blocks. TCP should be used as a life-saving bridge which should be replaced by a TVP or other permanent measure to provide prolonged homeostasis. All emergency physicians should be proficient in evaluation and decision making processes, indications and contraindications related to TCP/TVP.

REFERENCES

Antonelli, D., Feldman, A., Freedberg, N.A., Darawsha, A., Rosenfeld, T. (2007). [Biphasic *versus* monophasic shock waveforms for transthoracic cardioversion of atrial flutter in the emergency room]. *Harefuah, 146*(3), 181-183, 247.
[PMID: 17460921]

Bessman, E.S. (2019). Emergency cardiac pacing. In: Roberts, J.R., (Ed.), *Clinical Procedures in Emergency Medicine.* (7th ed., pp. 288-308). Philadelphia: Saunders.

Borgundvaag, B., Ovens, H. (2004). Cardioversion of uncomplicated paroxysmal atrial fibrillation: a survey of practice by Canadian emergency physicians. *CJEM, 6*(3), 155-160.
[http://dx.doi.org/10.1017/S1481803500006849] [PMID: 17433167]

Cummins, R.O. (2003). *Advanced Cardiac Life Support: Principles and Practice (The References Textbook).* American Heart Association.

Deakin, C.D., Nolan, J.P. (2005). European Resuscitation Council guidelines for resuscitation 2005. Section

3. Electrical therapies: automated external defibrillators, defibrillation, cardioversion and pacing. *Resuscitation,* *67*(Suppl. 1), S25-S37.
[http://dx.doi.org/10.1016/j.resuscitation.2005.10.008] [PMID: 16321714]

Electrical Therapies: Automated External Defibrillators, Defibrillation, Cardioversion, and Pacing (Part 5). 2005 American Heart Association (AHA) Guidelines for Cardiopulmonary Resuscitation and Emergency Cardiovascular Care. *Circulation, 112*, IV-35-IV-46.

Faddy, S.C., Jennings, P.A. (2016). Biphasic *versus* monophasic waveforms for transthoracic defibrillation in out-of-hospital cardiac arrest. *Cochrane Database Syst. Rev., 2*, CD006762.
[http://dx.doi.org/10.1002/14651858.CD006762.pub2] [PMID: 26904970]

Higgins, S.L., O'Grady, S.G., Banville, I., Chapman, F.W., Schmitt, P.W., Lank, P., Walker, R.G., Ilina, M. (2004). Efficacy of lower-energy biphasic shocks for transthoracic defibrillation: a follow-up clinical study. *Prehosp. Emerg. Care, 8*(3), 262-267.
[http://dx.doi.org/10.1016/j.prehos.2004.02.002] [PMID: 15295725]

Kudenchuk, P.J., Cobb, L.A., Copass, M.K., Olsufka, M., Maynard, C., Nichol, G. (2006). Transthoracic incremental monophasic *versus* biphasic defibrillation by emergency responders (TIMBER): a randomized comparison of monophasic with biphasic waveform ascending energy defibrillation for the resuscitation of out-of-hospital cardiac arrest due to ventricular fibrillation. *Circulation, 114*(19), 2010-2018.
[http://dx.doi.org/10.1161/CIRCULATIONAHA.106.636506] [PMID: 17060379]

Lim, S.H., Teo, W.S. (2020). Cardiac pacing and implanted defibrillation. In: Tintinalli, J.E., (Ed.), *Emergency Medicine A Comprehensive Study Guide.* (9th ed., pp. 216-223). North Carolina: McGraw-Hill.

Ong, M.E.H., Leong, B.S.H. (2020). Defibrillation and Electrical Cardioversion. *Cardiac Pacing and Implanted Defibrillation.* Tintinalli, JE (2020). Emergency Medicine A Comprehensive Study Guide.(9th ed., pp. 149-153). North Carolina, McGraw-Hill:

Ramzy, M., Hughes, P.G. (2021). Double Defibrillation. *StatPearls*Treasure Island (FL): StatPearls Publishing. PMID: 31334951

CHAPTER 12

Conclusion

"NOTHING WILL BE THE SAME ANYMORE"

The COVID-19 infection, which has been at the forefront of the agenda with the pandemic it has created, harms humanity both by causing death and diseases and by socioeconomic impairments since the end of the year 2019. In this context, public health measures are of vital importance in minimizing losses. The rational use of diagnostic kits, isolation of diagnosed patients, and supportive treatment are indispensable conditions in reducing deaths. Emergency health services, primary care institutions, emergency medicine, internal medicine, infection, and intensive care clinics have to work in cooperation and unison. Algorithms for case management in hospitals should be updated according to contemporary requirements. More importantly, the public should act in cooperation with healthcare professionals and institutions. Both individual and social measures for the prevention and mitigation of the disease can be effective when implemented together with the legislations and regulations of the state. Immediate isolation of the cases with high suspicion or diagnosis and even applying quarantine is key in reducing the famous 'Rt' values below 1.

Combining physical/individual isolation with social solidarity and personal hygiene is vital in order to prevent the production of new cases.

Although the COVID-19 PCR test and antibody tests are important in diagnosis, they are not *sine qua non*, and hospitalization and discharge decisions should be made by keeping the clinical conditions, signs, and symptoms of the patients ahead of the tests. Radiological findings are the most important adjuncts, and sometimes they can be a more important indicator than all other tests.

Our problem with COVID-19 is not limited to diagnostic challenges. New WHO guidelines cite that, there are no specific agents with proven benefit in the treatment of COVID-19. The world, which is far away from creating a truly standardized approach to treatment, has left mankind facing the experience and common sense of local physicians from previous epidemics, and with the knowledge gained from the others to follow on the internet, and the difficulties of the situation itself. Fortunately, some developing countries, including our country, have a long tradition of community medicine, public health, preventive medicine, as well as clinical experience, so this process is being overcome with as little loss as possible.

COVID-19 is not the only item to solve in the agenda of emergency medicine. We are the champion of multi-tasking, especially when faced with problems such as reducing cardiovascular deaths, standardization of education, combating the risks of overcrowding in EDs, and preparing for disasters. However, we have lost many of our colleagues, friends in the pandemic era.

And what about our 'sweet hearts'? Cardiac diseases are still one of the greatest threats to one's health on the planet, despite all technological advances achieved in the last decades. For example, life-threatening cardiac arrhythmias including ventricular fibrillation leads to a loss of cardiac function and sudden cardiac death. Guidelines for contemporary therapeutic interventions and for management of patients with in- or out-of-hospital cardiac arrest and refractory arrhythmias in prehospital and emergency settings are key approaches to increase survival and save lives. Advanced modalities for invasive management, including urgent coronary angiography, extracorporeal membrane oxygenation, and other innovated strategies for managing cardiac emergencies are still in development in most parts of the world. Beyond any doubt, pandemic circumstances represent a real challenge to provide usual care to those in need, both in prevention and management of the deadly cardiac diseases.

In brief, it is clear that we will have long years and new generations to live with masks, sanitizers and hand disinfectants. Therefore, long-term evolution of sociocultural codes should be considered to maintain an everlasting struggle with the disease, while preserving welfare of ourselves as human-being. For this, the education of pre-school and school children and women plays a key role.

In summary, cardiac diseases and pandemic threats will not be defeated only by the heroism of physicians, nurses and healthcare professionals. When social and economic measures adapt to healthcare interventions globally, a sought-after 'peak' of the pandemics will be found in a short time, then the disease will be eradicated safely. Only after this, we will be able to continue our search for a mutual and happily shared future as the peoples of the world and society that had learned lessons and experienced from all of these. Above all, respecting natural habitats will help prevent future pandemics, while healthy foods and exercise opportunities for everyone will alleviate risks of cardiac emergencies.

SUBJECT INDEX

www.ingramcontent.com/pod-product-compliance
Lightning Source LLC
Chambersburg PA
CBHW050816220326
41598CB00006B/226